Selected Papers from the pHealth 2022
Conference, Oslo, Norway,
8–10 November 2022

Selected Papers from the pHealth 2022 Conference, Oslo, Norway, 8–10 November 2022

Editors

Bernd Blobel
Mauro Giacomini
Bian Yang

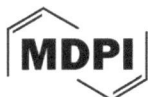

Basel • Beijing • Wuhan • Barcelona • Belgrade • Novi Sad • Cluj • Manchester

Editors

Bernd Blobel
University of Regensburg
Regensburg
Germany

Mauro Giacomini
University of Genoa
Genoa
Italy

Bian Yang
Norwegian University of
Science and Technology
(NTNU)
Gjøvik
Norway

Editorial Office
MDPI AG
Grosspeteranlage 5
4052 Basel, Switzerland

This is a reprint of articles from the Special Issue published online in the open access journal *Journal of Personalized Medicine* (ISSN 2075-4426) (available at: https://www.mdpi.com/journal/jpm/special_issues/36WBUZ3TG0).

For citation purposes, cite each article independently as indicated on the article page online and as indicated below:

Lastname, A.A.; Lastname, B.B. Article Title. *Journal Name* **Year**, *Volume Number*, Page Range.

ISBN 978-3-7258-2341-3 (Hbk)
ISBN 978-3-7258-2342-0 (PDF)
doi.org/10.3390/books978-3-7258-2342-0

© 2024 by the authors. Articles in this book are Open Access and distributed under the Creative Commons Attribution (CC BY) license. The book as a whole is distributed by MDPI under the terms and conditions of the Creative Commons Attribution-NonCommercial-NoDerivs (CC BY-NC-ND) license.

Contents

Preface vii

Bernd Blobel
Selected Papers from the pHealth 2022 Conference, Oslo, Norway, 8–10 November 2022
Reprinted from: *J. Pers. Med.* **2024**, *14*, 947, doi:10.3390/jpm14090947 1

Bernd Blobel, Pekka Ruotsalainen, Frank Oemig, Mauro Giacomini, Pier Angelo Sottile and Frederik Endsleff
Principles and Standards for Designing and Managing Integrable and Interoperable Transformed Health Ecosystems
Reprinted from: *J. Pers. Med.* **2023**, *13*, 1579, doi:10.3390/jpm13111579 4

Flora Nah Asah and Jens Johan Kaasbøll
Challenges and Strategies for Enhancing eHealth Capacity Building Programs in African Nations
Reprinted from: *J. Pers. Med.* **2023**, *13*, 1463, doi:10.3390/jpm13101463 27

Sara Mora, Roberta Gazzarata, Bernd Blobel, Ylenia Murgia and Mauro Giacomini
Transforming Ontology Web Language Elements into Common Terminology Service 2 Terminology Resources
Reprinted from: *J. Pers. Med.* **2024**, *14*, 676, doi:10.3390/jpm14070676 38

Paula Andrea Rosero Perez, Juan Sebastián Realpe Gonzalez, Ricardo Salazar-Cabrera, David Restrepo, Diego M. López and Bernd Blobel
Multidimensional Machine Learning Model to Calculate a COVID-19 Vulnerability Index
Reprinted from: *J. Pers. Med.* **2023**, *13*, 1141, doi:10.3390/jpm13071141 52

Georgy Kopanitsa, Oleg Metsker and Sergey Kovalchuk
Machine Learning Methods for Pregnancy and Childbirth Risk Management
Reprinted from: *J. Pers. Med.* **2023**, *13*, 975, doi:10.3390/jpm13060975 72

Yoram Segal, Ofer Hadar and Lenka Lhotska
Using EfficientNet-B7 (CNN), Variational Auto Encoder (VAE) and Siamese Twins' Networks to Evaluate Human Exercises as Super Objects in a TSSCI Images
Reprinted from: *J. Pers. Med.* **2023**, *13*, 874, doi:10.3390/jpm13050874 84

Olga Irtyuga, Mary Babakekhyan, Anna Kostareva, Vladimir Uspensky, Michail Gordeev, Giuseppe Faggian, et al.
Analysis of Prevalence and Clinical Features of Aortic Stenosis in Patients with and without Bicuspid Aortic Valve Using Machine Learning Methods
Reprinted from: *J. Pers. Med.* **2023**, *13*, 1588, doi:10.3390/jpm13111588 116

Pankaj Khatiwada, Bian Yang, Jia-Chun Lin and Bernd Blobel
Patient-Generated Health Data (PGHD): Understanding, Requirements, Challenges, and Existing Techniques for Data Security and Privacy
Reprinted from: *J. Pers. Med.* **2024**, *14*, 282, doi:10.3390/jpm14030282 130

Pekka Ruotsalainen and Bernd Blobel
Future pHealth Ecosystem-Holistic View on Privacy and Trust
Reprinted from: *J. Pers. Med.* **2023**, *13*, 1048, doi:10.3390/jpm13071048 174

Kerstin Denecke, Richard May, Elia Gabarron and Guillermo H. Lopez-Campos
Assessing the Potential Risks of Digital Therapeutics (DTX): The DTX Risk Assessment Canvas
Reprinted from: *J. Pers. Med.* **2023**, *13*, 1523, doi:10.3390/jpm13101523 192

Subhashis Das and Pamela Hussey
HL7-FHIR-Based ContSys Formal Ontology for Enabling Continuity of Care Data Interoperability
Reprinted from: *J. Pers. Med.* **2023**, *13*, 1024, doi:10.3390/jpm13071024 . . . . **206**

Preface

This reprint presents extended versions of contributions to pHealth 2022, the 19th International Conference on Wearable Micro and Nano Technologies for Personalized Health, held on 8–10 November 2022 in Oslo, Norway, selected for the related Special Issue of *The Journal of Personalized Medicine*. The original papers have been published in the IOS Press Studies in Health Technology and Informatics 2021, volume 299.

The 2022 edition of pHealth focused on the ongoing transformation of health and social care towards personalized, preventive, predictive, participative precision medicine (5PM), considering the individual health status, conditions, genetic, and genomic dispositions in personal social, occupational, environmental, and behavioral contexts, as supported by advanced technologies. Beside mobile technologies and bio-, nano-, and molecular technologies, assistive technologies such as robotics and intelligent autonomous systems must also be deployed. The latter require knowledge representation and management including machine learning and deep learning, natural language processing, and artificial and generic intelligence. The resulting multidisciplinary, highly complex, and dynamic ecosystems offer big chances, but also bear risks to be managed, such as legal, ethical, and humanistic challenges. For designing and managing integration and interoperability, the ecosystems must follow a system-oriented, architecture-centric, ontology-based, and policy-driven approach based on international standards. The volume discusses all those challenges and exemplifies corresponding solutions.

Following the procedure practiced with all former pHealth Special Issues, Bernd Blobel, as the long-term Chair of the pHealth conferences Scientific Program Committee (SPC) as well as the pHealth Steering Committee, has checked and edited every paper invited for publication in the MDPI *JPM* pHealth 2022 Special Issue before giving the green flag for formal submission. That way, we could keep the quality of the volumes extraordinary high. Mauro Giacomini as the SPC Co-Chair has managed the review process performed by at least two independent international experts. Bian Yang was the Chair of the pHealth 2022 Local Organizing Committee, providing the framework for a successful conference.

Bernd Blobel, Mauro Giacomini, and Bian Yang
Editors

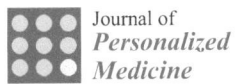

Editorial

Selected Papers from the pHealth 2022 Conference, Oslo, Norway, 8–10 November 2022

Bernd Blobel [1,2,3,4]

1. Medical Faculty, University of Regensburg, 93053 Regensburg, Germany; bernd.blobel@klinik.uni-regensburg.de
2. First Medical Faculty, Charles University Prague, 12800 Prague, Czech Republic
3. Department of Informatics, Bioengineering, Robotics and System Engineering, University of Genoa, 16145 Genoa, Italy
4. Faculty European Campus Rottal-Inn, Deggendorf Institute of Technology, 94469 Deggendorf, Germany

This Special Issue of the Journal of Personalized Medicine presents extended versions of selected contributions to pHealth 2022, the 19th International Conference on Wearable Micro and Nano Technologies for Personalized Health, held on 8–10 November 2022 in Oslo, Norway. The original papers were published in the IOS Press Studies in Health Technology and Informatics 2022, volume 299 (URL https://ebooks.iospress.nl/volume/phealth-2022-proceedings-of-the-19th-international-conference-on-wearable-micro-and-nano-technologies-for-personalized-health-810-november-2022-oslo-norway (accessed on 3 November 2022)).

The 2022 edition of pHealth continues to focus on the advancement of pHealth towards personalized, participative, preventive, predictive, and precision medicine (5P medicine), supported by technologies such as mobile technologies, micro/nano-bio smart systems, artificial intelligence and robotics, big data and analytics, and machine learning and deep learning. The new technologies offer new opportunities and bear new potential risks for security, privacy and safety. Therefore, ethical challenges and solutions for guaranteeing the needed trustworthiness must be addressed. Transformed health and social care ecosystems are highly distributed, complex and dynamic, combining perspectives and knowledge from different disciplines. This requires covering the medical, technological, political, administrative, and social domains, and philosophical or linguistic challenges in designing and managing such ecosystems. Bernd Blobel, the long-term Chair of the pHealth conference Scientific Program Committee as well as the pHealth Steering Committee, checked and edited every paper invited for publication in the MDPI *JPM* pHealth 2022 Special Issue before approving them for formal submission. Mauro Giacomini, as Co-Chair of both committees, managed the review process, which was performed by at least two independent international experts.

The book starts with challenges and solutions for healthcare transformation. In this chapter, a pHealth 2022 Keynote addresses principles and standards for designing and managing intelligent and ethically transformed health ecosystems [1]. After introducing the healthcare transformation towards 5P medicine, the paper explains the formal representation of health ecosystems as systems of systems, representing the different perspectives of the domains involved and all components, their functions and relationships at all granularity levels of interest, but also the viewpoints of the evolutionary or development process the ecosystem is facing. This must be carried out through a system-theoretical, architecture-centric, ontology-based, policy-driven approach, meanwhile standardized as ISO 23903 [2]. Interoperability and Integration Reference Architecture—Model and Framework. The Keynote paper explains the necessary principles and methodologies and references the standards defining them. The second contribution of the introductory chapter is a paper invited to the conference [3]. It observes the obstacles hindering capacity building and innovation promotion for eHealth in low- and medium-income countries exemplified for

Citation: Blobel, B. Selected Papers from the pHealth 2022 Conference, Oslo, Norway, 8–10 November 2022. *J. Pers. Med.* **2024**, *14*, 947. https://doi.org/10.3390/jpm14090947

Received: 14 August 2024
Accepted: 28 August 2024
Published: 6 September 2024

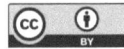

Copyright: © 2024 by the author. Licensee MDPI, Basel, Switzerland. This article is an open access article distributed under the terms and conditions of the Creative Commons Attribution (CC BY) license (https://creativecommons.org/licenses/by/4.0/).

Africa. Here, the lack of financial resources, qualified personnel, but also infrastructure and governance must be mentioned.

The second chapter discusses and exemplifies the role of automation, machine learning and artificial intelligence for advancing pHealth. The first paper discusses the sharing of clinical data between healthcare establishments at a regional level in Italy, thereby guaranteeing the correct understanding of the exchanged data [4]. This requires the representational transformation of data and information shared using the Common Terminology Service Release 2 (CTS2) standard [5]. The second paper presents a methodology for improving the prediction of risks for COVID-19 infections depending on multiple factors such as environmental conditions and mobility of citizens, but also social factors [6]. For assessing the risk factors, a multidimensional analysis using machine learning models has been deployed, which is also applicable for other infectious diseases. As the best-performing model, the Extra Trees Regressor algorithm could be identified. The third paper in the chapter demonstrates the deployment of machine learning methodologies to identify and manage pregnancy and childbirth risks [7]. Thereby, data from clinical and laboratory tests and multiple measurements are deployed. The outcome could advance the decision support in perinatal care provision. The high predictive performance achieved by the models ensures precise support for both individual patient care and overall health organization management. The next paper of this chapter presents a new approach for evaluating human exercises in telehealth services to support remote diagnoses and treatment [8]. Thereby, the movement is defined as a static super object represented by a single two-dimensional image. This allows for analyzing and optimizing movements presented in videos. With proposed and demonstrated methodology, exercises can be simulated and scored. All papers discussed have been invited to the pHealth 2022 conference. The last paper, based on a presentation to pHealth 2021, investigates the improvement in the diagnosis and treatment of aortic stenosis (AS) by earlier detection using echocardiography and machine learning [9]. In this context, prevalence and clinical features of AS in patients with bicuspid aortic valves vs. patients with tricuspid aortic valve were studied. As an outcome, significant features impacting AS patients such as age, hypertension, aortic regurgitation, ascending aortic dilatation, and bicuspid aortic valves could be identified.

The third chapter is dedicated to security, privacy and safety as important prerequisites for the usability and acceptability of pHealth and dHealth solutions. The chapter starts with two papers invited to the pHealth 2022 conference. The first paper addresses one 5P medicine aspect, the individualization of the system according to the personal social, environmental, occupational and behavioral context of the subject of care, putting people at the center of the business system [10]. This is especially supported by Patient-Generated Health Data (PGHD). For understanding and correctly assessing opportunities and risks for the security, privacy and accuracy of PGHD, the actors involved, the technologies used, the specific types of data, their source and way of generation, etc., must be analyzed. Thereby, the Preferred Reporting Items for Systematic Reviews and Meta-Analyses (PRISMA) methodology was followed. The second paper presents a holistic view on privacy and trust, considering that pHealth ecosystems are multi-domain, highly distributed and dynamic, increasingly autonomous ecosystems deploying advanced technologies such as mobile and implantable sensors and actuators, big data and analytics as well as artificial intelligence [11]. Such systems enable the monitoring of the person's physical and social life and behavior, making privacy and trust an illusion. Therefore, it is necessary to start the development of next-generation pHealth ecosystems according to ISO 23903 to formally and correctly present and manage intentions and objectives of the ecosystem actors as well as related consequences in each business use case. Thereby, personal health information (PHI) must be considered as personal property, and trust as a fiduciary duty, for the service provider and other stakeholders processing PHI in the ecosystem. The ecosystem's behavior must be controlled by legally binding smart contracts stored in a blockchain-based repository. The last paper in this chapter deals with the assessment of potential risks of digital therapeutics (DTX) including health and wellness apps for patient safety, and possible adverse events [12]. By carrying this out, the authors developed a risk assessment canvas as a tool to calculate the risks bound to DTX. For defining relevant aspects, they used ISO/TS 82304-2 [13]. and performed a literature review.

The book concludes with a short eHealth solutions chapter, consisting of one paper on systems interoperability [14]. It demonstrates a practical solution for enabling the continuity of care. The challenges of continuity of care are the communication and cooperation between experts from different domains. For enabling this interoperability, a system of concepts to support continuity of care (ContSys) is inevitable. To formally represent ContSys, a ContSys ontology is necessary. For developing an IT solution, the business viewpoint components represented by the aforementioned ontology must be transformed into implementable artifacts. Here, HL7 Fast Health Interoperability Resources (FHIRs) are used.

The editors thank all authors and reviewers for their important contribution to the success of this volume. Furthermore, they are deeply indebted to the MDPI *Journal of Personalized Medicine* and its Editorial Office, especially to Penny Su, but also to Joanna Krefft, Marilyn Zhang, Calla Zhu and Jane Jin, for their continuous support. Without such efforts, this volume would not have been possible.

Conflicts of Interest: The author declares no conflicts of interest.

References

1. Blobel, B.; Ruotsalainen, P.; Oemig, F.; Giacomini, M.; Sottile, P.A.; Endsleff, F. Principles and Standards for Designing and Managing Integrable and Interoperable Transformed Health Ecosystems. *J. Pers. Med.* **2023**, *13*, 1579. [CrossRef]
2. *ISO 23903:2021*; Health Informatics—Interoperability and Integration Reference Architecture – Model and Framework. ISO: Geneva, Switzerland, 2021.
3. Asah, F.N.; Kaasbøll, J.J. Challenges and Strategies for Enhancing eHealth Capacity Building Programs in African Nations. *J. Pers. Med.* **2023**, *13*, 1463. [CrossRef]
4. Mora, S.; Gazzarata, R.; Blobel, B.; Murgia, Y.; Giacomini, M. Transforming Ontology Web Language Elements into Common Terminology Service 2 Terminology Resources. *J. Pers. Med.* **2024**, *14*, 676. [CrossRef] [PubMed]
5. Object Management Group. *Common Terminology Services 2*; OMG: Needham, MA, USA, 2015.
6. Rosero Perez, P.A.; Realpe Gonzalez, J.S.; Salazar-Cabrera, R.; Restrepo, D.; López, D.M.; Blobel, B. Multidimensional Machine Learning Model to Calculate a COVID-19 Vulnerability Index. *J. Pers. Med.* **2023**, *13*, 1141. [CrossRef]
7. Kopanitsa, G.; Metsker, O.; Kovalchuk, S. Machine Learning Methods for Pregnancy and Childbirth Risk Management. *J. Pers. Med.* **2023**, *13*, 975. [CrossRef] [PubMed]
8. Segal, Y.; Hadar, O.; Lhotska, L. Using EfficientNet-B7 (CNN), Variational Auto Encoder (VAE) and Siamese Twins' Networks to Evaluate Human Exercises as Super Objects in a TSSCI Images. *J. Pers. Med.* **2023**, *13*, 874. [CrossRef] [PubMed]
9. Irtyuga, O.; Babakekhyan, M.; Kostareva, A.; Uspensky, V.; Gordeev, M.; Faggian, G.; Malashicheva, A.; Metsker, O.; Shlyakhto, E.; Kopanitsa, G. Analysis of Prevalence and Clinical Features of Aortic Stenosis in Patients with and without Bicuspid Aortic Valve Using Machine Learning Methods. *J. Pers. Med.* **2023**, *13*, 1588. [CrossRef] [PubMed]
10. Khatiwada, P.; Jang, B.; Lin, J.-C.; Blobel, B. Patient-Generated Health Data (PGHD): Understanding, Requirements, Challenges, and Existing Techniques for Data Security and Privacy. *J. Pers. Med.* **2024**, *14*, 282. [CrossRef]
11. Ruotsalainen, P.; Blobel, B. Future pHealth Ecosystem-Holistic View on Privacy and Trust. *J. Pers. Med.* **2023**, *13*, 1048. [CrossRef]
12. Denecke, K.; May, R.; Gabarron, E.; Lopez-Campos, G.H. Assessing the Potential Risks of Digital Therapeutics (DTX): The DTX Risk Assessment Canvas. *J. Pers. Med.* **2023**, *13*, 1523. [CrossRef]
13. *TS 82304-2:2021*; Health Software—Part 2: Health and Wellness Apps—Quality and Reliability. ISO: Geneva, Switzerland, 2021.
14. Das, S.; Hussey, P. HL7-FHIR-Based ContSys Formal Ontology for Enabling Continuity of Care Data Interoperability. *J. Pers. Med.* **2023**, *13*, 1024. [CrossRef]

Disclaimer/Publisher's Note: The statements, opinions and data contained in all publications are solely those of the individual author(s) and contributor(s) and not of MDPI and/or the editor(s). MDPI and/or the editor(s) disclaim responsibility for any injury to people or property resulting from any ideas, methods, instructions or products referred to in the content.

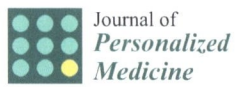

Article

Principles and Standards for Designing and Managing Integrable and Interoperable Transformed Health Ecosystems

Bernd Blobel [1,2,3,*], Pekka Ruotsalainen [4], Frank Oemig [5], Mauro Giacomini [6], Pier Angelo Sottile [7] and Frederik Endsleff [8]

[1] Medical Faculty, University of Regensburg, 93053 Regensburg, Germany
[2] Faculty European Campus Rottal-Inn, Deggendorf Institute of Technology, 94469 Deggendorf, Germany
[3] First Medical Faculty, Charles University Prague, 11000 Staré Město, Czech Republic
[4] Faculty of Information Technology and Communication Sciences, Tampere University, 33100 Tampere, Finland; pekka.ruotsalainen@tuni.fi
[5] IT-Consulting in Healthcare, 45472 Mülheim, Germany; frank@oemig.de
[6] Department of Informatics, Bioengineering, Robotics and System Engineering, University of Genoa, 16145 Genoa, Italy; mauro.giacomini@dibris.unige.it
[7] BI Health Srl, 00185 Rome, Italy; p.sottile@bihealth.it
[8] IT Architecture, Centre for IT and Medical Technology (CIMT), The Capital Region of Denmark, 2100 Copenhagen, Denmark; frederik.endsleff@regionh.dk
* Correspondence: bernd.blobel@klinik.uni-regensburg.de

Citation: Blobel, B.; Ruotsalainen, P.; Oemig, F.; Giacomini, M.; Sottile, P.A.; Endsleff, F. Principles and Standards for Designing and Managing Integrable and Interoperable Transformed Health Ecosystems. *J. Pers. Med.* **2023**, *13*, 1579. https://doi.org/10.3390/jpm13111579

Academic Editor: Marcelo Saito Nogueira

Received: 8 September 2023
Revised: 25 October 2023
Accepted: 31 October 2023
Published: 4 November 2023

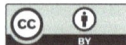

Copyright: © 2023 by the authors. Licensee MDPI, Basel, Switzerland. This article is an open access article distributed under the terms and conditions of the Creative Commons Attribution (CC BY) license (https://creativecommons.org/licenses/by/4.0/).

Abstract: The advancement of sciences and technologies, economic challenges, increasing expectations, and consumerism result in a radical transformation of health and social care around the globe, characterized by foundational organizational, methodological, and technological paradigm changes. The transformation of the health and social care ecosystems aims at ubiquitously providing personalized, preventive, predictive, participative precision (5P) medicine, considering and understanding the individual's health status in a comprehensive context from the elementary particle up to society. For designing and implementing such advanced ecosystems, an understanding and correct representation of the structure, function, and relations of their components is inevitable, thereby including the perspectives, principles, and methodologies of all included disciplines. To guarantee consistent and conformant processes and outcomes, the specifications and principles must be based on international standards. A core standard for representing transformed health ecosystems and managing the integration and interoperability of systems, components, specifications, and artifacts is ISO 23903:2021, therefore playing a central role in this publication. Consequently, ISO/TC 215 and CEN/TC 251, both representing the international standardization on health informatics, declared the deployment of ISO 23903:2021 mandatory for all their projects and standards addressing more than one domain. The paper summarizes and concludes the first author's leading engagement in the evolution of pHealth in Europe and beyond over the last 15 years, discussing the concepts, principles, and standards for designing, implementing, and managing 5P medicine ecosystems. It not only introduces the theoretical foundations of the approach but also exemplifies its deployment in practical projects and solutions regarding interoperability and integration in multi-domain ecosystems. The presented approach enables comprehensive and consistent integration of and interoperability between domains, systems, related actors, specifications, standards, and solutions. That way, it should help overcome the problems and limitations of data-centric approaches, which still dominate projects and products nowadays, and replace them with knowledge-centric, comprehensive, and consistent ones.

Keywords: 5P medicine; ecosystem; system architecture; knowledge representation; knowledge management; modeling; integration; interoperability

1. Introduction

The paper at hand is a revised and extended version of the pHealth 2022 Keynote paper, published in [1]. It addresses the globally ongoing transformation of health and social care systems and provides a model and framework for representing and managing them. To realize sustainable and compatible health ecosystems, their design, implementation, and management must follow internationally accepted principles and standards. The authors introduce a theoretical approach, common principles, standards, and practical solutions for designing and managing integrable and interoperable health ecosystems that are proven through some practical demonstrations. The described solution has also been successfully applied to and integrated into the standards from ISO, CEN, IEEE, and other standardization organizations. The paper explains those principles and how to navigate the related standards jungle.

An ecosystem is a system or network of living and nonliving interconnecting and interacting elements to meet specific objectives [2]. The transformation aims at mastering challenges such as the ongoing demographic changes towards aging, multi-diseased societies, the related development of human resources, health and social services consumerism, medical and biomedical progress, and exploding costs for health-related R&D as well as health services delivery [3]. An overview of requirements and solutions for managing healthcare transformation towards 5P medicine can be found in [4] or [5]. A detailed description of the architectural approach is available in [6]. The transformation is bound to fundamental organizational, methodological, and technological paradigm changes [7]. Thereby, the care type advances from empirical or phenomenological medicine through evidence-based medicine, person-centered medicine, personalized medicine, 5P medicine, and ubiquitous personal health. Organizationally, the systems turn from organization-centered local services through cross-organizational local services and distributed local and remote services to ubiquitous care. Regulated professionals manage the first three organizational settings, while for the other three regulated and non-regulated professionals, non-professionals such as the subject of care and his/her relations and technical systems play the role of actors. In the phenomenological medicine care type, domain-specific general services are provided to humanity as one solution fits all. In evidence-based medicine, domain-specific services are provided to disease-specifically defined groups. In person-centered medicine, individuals are served with multiple domains' disease-specifically interrelated services, including telemedicine. Personalized medicine provides multiple domains' services to the individual's personal disposition. Systems medicine—also called 5P medicine, i.e., personalized, preventive, predictive, participative precision medicine—provides integrated cross-domain services to the individual in personal, environmental, social, occupational, and behavioral contexts, thereby deploying life sciences, social sciences, and engineering sciences, as well as specialties such as the bunch of omics disciplines and others. Ubiquitous personal health serves the individual under comprehensive focus with integrated services. From a methodological perspective, empirical medicine practices are based more or less on objectivized observations, justified with pattern recognition or experiences. Evidence-based medicine advances observations through objective evaluations, statistically justified with group-specific treatment outcomes stored in records, registries, etc. Person-centered medicine is realized as managed care, leading the subject of care through the care process and justifying the process through process management and best medical practice guidelines. A big advancement is provided through personalized medicine based on the pathology of the individual disease, clinically justified with the individual's status and context. Systems medicine understands the detailed pathology based on multiple domains, scientifically justified through individual status and context. Ubiquitous personal health provides services dynamically tailored for the subject of care, anywhere and anytime. The methodological paradigm changes are accompanied by transformations regarding the representation style of the practice outcome. Phenomenological medicine represents the observations as data stored in local data repositories. As evidence-based medicine contains data from multiple sources stored in central data repositories, the meaning of the data must be justified and verified against the source's intent, leading to information. For representing the outcome of person-centered medicine, agreed-upon terminologies deployed in the Disease Management Program (DMP) Best Practice Guidelines are used, representing a cross-organizational business process. Personalized medicine requires the representation of disciplinary concepts in the situational context in the sense of knowledge representation and management. Systems medicine is represented through multi-disciplinary concepts in a comprehensive context, requiring knowledge space management. The different care types and related representation styles require different standards to manage them. Those standards range from data standards through information modeling standards, terminology, and process standards up to domain ontology standards, and for systems medicine, finally, top-level ontology standards guiding the management of multiple ontologies.

Interoperability advances thereby from signal sharing through data sharing, information sharing, knowledge sharing at the IT concept level, knowledge sharing at the business concept level, knowledge sharing at the domain level (cross-domain cooperation), up to skills-based knowledge sharing (moderated end-user collaboration). Such transformation must be supported using appropriate technologies from mobile devices through wearable and implantable sensors and actuators, pervasive sensors, actuators, and network connectivity, up to the micro, molecular, and quantum levels. By combining the advancements in societies, sciences, including data sciences, and technologies, health and social care systems are transformed into 5P medicine ecosystems. The outcome of the process enables early identification, proactive intervention, and a full understanding of the course of disease, i.e., its pathology and its effective treatment. It allows for health service provision everywhere, anytime, thereby individualizing the system according to the status, context, needs, expectations, wishes, etc., of the subject of health and social care. More details can be found at [1]. Table 1 summarizes the organizational, methodological, technological, and standardization paradigm changes in transformed health and social care ecosystems.

Table 1 clarifies that the advancement in health and social care paradigms must be accompanied by related advancements in the standard world. Healthcare transformation must be supported through appropriate technologies. The "Standards" column just addresses minimal needs for the representation and specification of real-world business systems and documents the increasing requirements. The design and implementation of information and communication technology (ICT) solutions require, of course, other standards and specifications, which are also discussed in this paper.

Table 1. Organizational, methodological, technological, and standardization paradigm changes in transformed health and social care ecosystems.

Care Type	Organization, Service Provision	Actors	Services	Target	Way of Practicing	Justification	Representation Style	Electronic Comm./Co-op.	Standard
Phenomenological medicine	Organization-centered, local services	Regulated professionals	Domain-specific general services	Humanity	Observation	Pattern recognition	Data	Local data repository; inside the unit	Data standards
Evidence-based medicine	Organization-centered, local services	Regulated professionals	Domain-specific, group-specific services	Disease-specific defined group	Observation with objective evaluation	Statistical justification, group-specific treatment outcome	Information	Central data repositories	Information standards
Person-centered medicine	Cross-organizational local services	Regulated professionals	Multiple domains' services	Individual	Managed care	Process mgmt., best medical practice guidelines	Agreed terminology, DMP Best Practice Guidelines	Cross-organizational business process	Terminology standards; process standards

Table 1. Cont.

Care Type	Organization, Service Provision	Actors	Services	Target	Way of Practicing	Justification	Representation Style	Electronic Comm./Co-op.	Standard
Personalized medicine	Distributed local and remote services	Regulated and non-regulated professionals, laymen, technical systems	Multiple domains' services—telemedicine	Individual's personal disposition	Considering the pathology of disease	Clinically justified individual status and context	Disciplinary concepts in situational context	Knowledge management	Domain ontology standards
5P medicine	Distributed cross-domain services, smart healthcare	Regulated and non-regulated professionals, laymen, technical systems	Cross-domain services—consumerism, telemedicine	Individual in personal, environmental, social, occupational, and behavioral contexts	Understanding the pathology of disease	Scientifically justified individual status and context	Multidisciplinary concepts in comprehensive context	Knowledge space management	Multiple ontologies guided via top-level ontology standards
Ubiquitous personal health and social care	Ubiquitous services	Regulated and non-regulated professionals, laymen, technical systems	Integrated services—consumerism, ubiquitous medicine	Individual under comprehensive focus		Dynamically and scientifically justified individual status			

Table 2 presents the objectives of 5P medicine, the requirements (characteristics) for enabling those objectives, as well as the methodologies and technologies to realize them [8,9].

Table 2. 5P medicine objectives, characteristics, and methodologies/technologies to meet objectives (after [8], changed).

Objective	Characteristics	Methodologies/Technologies
Provision of health services everywhere, anytime	• Openness • Distribution • Mobility • Pervasiveness • Ubiquity	• Wearable and implantable sensors and actuators • Pervasive sensor, actuator, and network connectivity • Embedded intelligence • Context awareness
Individualization of the system according to status, context, needs, expectations, wishes, environments, etc., of the subject of care	• Flexibility • Scalability • Cognition • Affect and behavior • Autonomy • Adaptability • Self-organization • Subject of care involvement • Subject of care centration	• Personal and environmental data integration and analytics • Service integration • Context awareness • Knowledge integration • Process and decision intelligence • Presentation layer for all actors
Integration of different actors from different disciplines/domains (incl. the participation/empowerment of the subject of care), using their own languages, methodologies, terminologies, ontologies, thereby meeting any behavioral aspects, rules, and regulations	• Architectural framework • End-user interoperability • Management and harmonization of multiple domains including policy domains	• Advanced systems architecture • Terminology and ontology management and harmonization • Knowledge harmonization • Language transformation/translation

Table 2. *Cont.*

Objective	Characteristics	Methodologies/Technologies
Usability and acceptability of 5P Medicine solutions	• Preparedness of the individual subject of care—security, privacy, trust, and ethics framework • Consumerization • Subject of care empowerment • Subject of care as manager • Information-based assessment and selection of services, service quality, and safety as well as trustworthiness • Lifestyle improvement and Ambient Assisted Living (AAL) services	• Tool-based ontology management • Individual terminologies • Individual ontologies • Tool-based enhancement of individual knowledge and skills • Human-centered design of solutions • User experience evaluation • Individual, context-sensitive privacy agreements • Trust calculation services

In the following, we will provide a comprehensive and scientifically sound representation of 5P medicine ecosystems as well as the standards for defining, modeling, and implementing the related system components.

2. Representation of 5P Medicine Ecosystems

To represent any system, we can deploy systems theory. The simplest way is the black-box methodology, which characterizes any living or non-living system's coarse behavior and functionality through an input-output analysis. However, we cannot understand the functionality without considering the structure and functionality of the system components according to the white-box approach. Figure 1 represents an architectural system model by considering three aspects or dimensions:

- The system's architectural perspective, representing the system's composition/decomposition or specialization/generalization;
- The system's domain perspective, representing the involved domains and their actors;
- The system's evolutionary or development perspective.

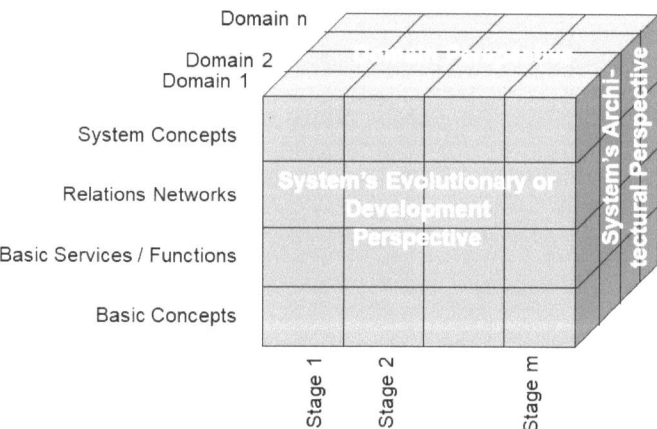

Figure 1. Generic model to represent ecosystems (after [10], changed).

Therefore, 5P medicine ecosystems must be structurally and functionally represented in a comprehensive way. For describing such ecosystems, universal type theory and universal logics, formally represented using the Barendregt Cube [11], can be deployed.

Thereby, all domains involved, specific objectives and contexts, the system elements, their composition and decomposition, including internal and external relationships, and all steps in the development process represented as system views must be considered, thereby strictly following the good modeling best practices [12].

P5 medicine requires the communication and cooperation of actors from multiple disciplines with specific perspectives, contexts, and objectives, using their special methodologies, languages, knowledge, and skills to name and define the business use case concepts and relations for correctly deriving the system requirements. The challenge of P5 medicine ecosystems is the proper representation, mapping, and matching of their domain-specific knowledge at any representation level. The knowledge spaces for the different viewpoints range from the business view through the enterprise view, the information view, and the computational view up to the technology view, as defined in ISO/IEC 10746 Open Distributed Processing [13]. The business view addresses the real-world business system. The enterprise view of the ICT system considers the management of the business process. The information view and the computational view deal with the semantic interpretation of data as information, while the engineering and technology views' concerns are the implementable solution and its maintenance based on data. The business view is represented by domain ontologies, while the last five views are defined using corresponding ICT ontologies. For representing the different viewpoints, different presentation language types with increasing expressivity and increasing constraints according to the Chomsky grammar level are used. However, a highly expressive knowledge representation is less likely to properly consider context and implicit knowledge as being complete and decidable. Therefore, the limitations on data spaces and data interoperability are insufficient for correctly and consistently representing ecosystems. Consequently, for correctly defining relations for integration or interoperability in a more constraint view, we have always had to start representing the business system at the view with the highest generative power and transform thereafter the models up to the view to be managed. The language types start with domain-specific or natural languages to represent the business system, by domain experts. At the next level, business process modeling languages like BPML and BPML+ are used, followed by information representation languages such as vocabularies, thesauri, taxonomies, glossaries, data dictionaries, or information models, and finally data representation languages such as data/meta-data definitions, database management system (DBMS) schemes, or programming languages (see Table 3). In their data modeling hierarchy, Hoberman et al. [14] call the aforementioned representation levels as very high level, high level, logical level, and physical level, respectively. The corresponding representation of a multi-domain, ontology-based, policy-driven P5 ecosystem using the model and framework of the ISO 23903 Interoperability and Integration Reference Architecture [15], discussed in the next section, is shown in Figure 2.

Table 3. Representation tools for the different ISO 10746 viewpoints [9].

Viewpoint	Language/Grammar	Representation Level
Business View	Domain-specific and/or natural languages	
Enterprise View	Business Process Modeling Language (BPML)	Very high
Information View	Unified Modeling Language (UML)	High level
Computational View	Object Constraint Language (OCL)	Logical level
Engineering View	Programming languages with different levels of grammar	Physical level
Technology View		

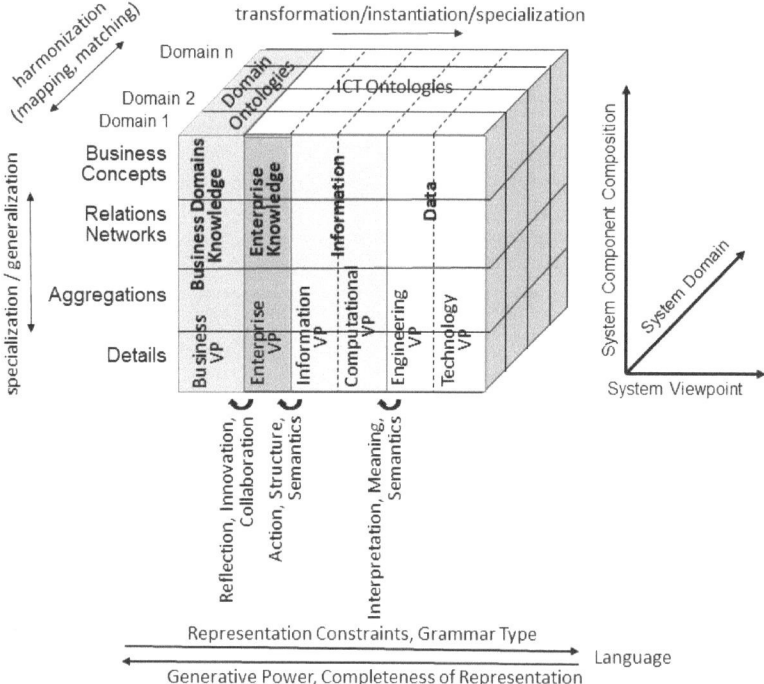

Figure 2. Model and framework for representing multi-domain, knowledge-based, ontology-based, policy-driven ecosystems [1].

The mapping between elements from different domains or different viewpoints can only be performed at the horizontal level, i.e., at the same level of granularity. To get there, components must be specialized or generalized, respectively.

For designing, developing, and implementing P5 medicine ecosystems, we must generically model the system architecture and the unified process around it. Thereafter, we have to formally represent the domains involved in the use case of the business system considered. Then, we have to represent the different views in the contexts and from the perspectives of the domain experts participating in the business use case. A domain controlling the business system behavior and therefore being relevant across all specific use cases is, e.g., the policy domain, covering procedural, legal, administrative, security, privacy, and trustworthiness, as well as ethical aspects.

For managing organizations to meet their objectives, interests, and needs, strategic, operational, and tactical aspects must be considered. In that context, related standards and procedures have to be established alongside policies to create a strong governance structure. Security and privacy policies address operational needs [16].

Consequently, we need architecture standards, knowledge representation, and management standards, including ontology standards and terminology standards, for all domains involved in the ecosystem. Furthermore, policy standards, business process modeling standards, information standards, and data standards to model and implement the 5P medicine ecosystem in a compliant and conformant way are necessary. In that context, we cannot ignore quality criteria standards to enable quality assessment (self-assessment and/or assessment by certified assessors) of pHealth digital tools such as IEC 82304-2:2021 Health Software-Part 2: Health and wellness apps-Quality and reliability [17]. Each standard family will be discussed and exemplified in some detail in the next sections.

3. Standards for Modeling 5P Medicine Ecosystems

The solution for designing, managing, and implementing the intended ecosystem is a system-theoretical white box, architecture-centric, ontology-based, and policy-controlled approach, meanwhile standardized as ISO 23903 Interoperability and Integration Reference Architecture–Model and Framework and re-used by many international Standards Developing Organizations (SDOs) such as ISO, CEN, IEC, IEEE, OMG, and HL7. Besides the definition of the modeling and system development process, ISO 23903 also covers challenges such as domain-specific knowledge representation and management at the epistemological level, as well as its harmonization. In that context, it supports not only the ontology development and harmonization but also the implementation of good modeling best practices. ISO 23903 enables integration of and interoperability between any systems and their components, any domains and their actors, any specifications or products, and any IT-specific view of ISO/IEC 10764. Without following the ISO 23903 model and framework, the integration of and interoperability between specifications and standards are usually not feasible.

3.1. Architecture Standards

Regarding the architectural approach, ISO 23903 builds on ISO/IEC/IEEE 42010:2011 Systems and Software Engineering–Architecture Description (ISO/IEC/IEEE 42010 is originally based on ANSI/IEEE 1471-2000 Recommended Practice for Architectural Description of Software-Intensive Systems) [18] and ISO/IEC/IEEE 42020:2019 Software, Systems and Enterprise–Architecture Processes [19]. On that basis, ISO/IEC 10746 Open Distributed Processing [13] has been widely introduced, which is a family of international standards for describing and developing distributed systems and applications. Regarding the system development process, ISO 23903 refers to ISO/IEC 10746 and the Rational Unified Process (RUP) [20]. Another architectural approach, reusing the Reference Model of Open Distributing Processing (RM-ODP), is the HL7 Version 3 Development Framework (HDF), advancing the messaging approach HL7 started with. In the context of HL7, ISO/IEC 7498-1:1994 Information technology-Open Systems Interconnection-Basic Reference Model: The Basic Model, providing the basics for HL7, should be mentioned here as well [21].

Almost all architecture standards focus on the ICT perspective and ignore the importance of real-world communication and cooperation between the domain experts, which is, however, crucial for all ecosystems and especially for the 5P medicine ecosystems. ISO 23903 extended the aforementioned standards like, ISO/IEC 10746, from the business perspective represented by domain experts. Contrary to those standards, ISO 23903 introduced a three-dimensional model with the additional domain perspective dimension to represent multiple domains involved in the ecosystem's specific use cases and with the additional component composition dimension, thereby reusing the OMG Model Driven Architecture (MDA) hierarchy [22]. The latter starts with the computation-independent model (CIM) or requirement model defining the system in its environment. CIM is transformed into the platform-independent model (PIM), or analysis and design model, defining the system's architecture. PIM is then transformed into the platform-specific model (PSM) or realization model, defining how the system is built using specific technologies and programming languages. At the end, the code of the system and configuration artifacts are generated [23]. An overview of architecture standards and approaches, including their relation to ISO 23903, is provided in [24]. Table 4 compares the aforementioned data model levels as well as the dimensions of modeling with the model and framework of ISO 23903 and ISO/IEC 10746.

Table 4. Comparing data model levels and dimensions of modeling with ISO 23903 and ISO 10746 (after [25], changed).

Data Model Level	Modeling Actors	Model Scope	Dimension of Modeling	Interop. Reference Architecture	Examples		
Very-high-level data model	Business domain stake-holders	Scope, requirements, and related basic concepts of business case	Knowledge space	Business View	OMG CIM		ISO 23903 Interoperability and Integration Reference Architecture
High-level data model	Business domain stake-holders	Relevant information and representation and relationships of basic concepts	Knowledge	Enterprise View	OMG PIM, HL7 DCM, CSO		
Logical data model	Data modelers and analysts	Layout and types of data and object relationships	Information	Information View	OMG PSM, HL7 V3 (CMETs), HL7 CIMI, openEHR Archetypes, FHIM	ISO 10746 ODP-RM	
				Computational View			
Physical data model	Data modelers and developers	Implementation-related and platform-specific aspects	Data	Engineering View	HL7 FHIR		

All architecture standards presented so far are business-domain-independent. However, there are also domain-specific architecture standards such as ISO 12967 Health informatics–Service architecture [26].

3.2. Knowledge Representation and Knowledge Management Standards

Regarding the business system representation from the perspective and context of the domain experts involved by formally representing their knowledge, we deploy the related domain ontologies. An ontology provides an explicit specification of a conceptualization [27]. It is a collection of terms, relational expressions and associated natural-language definitions in combination with formal theories [28] to represent that knowledge.

Medical/clinical domain terminologies and ontologies for 5P medicine ecosystems are, e.g.,: the Unified Medical Language System (UMLS) [29]; the SNOMED International products Systematized Nomenclature of Medicine–Clinical Terms (SNOMED CT) and Systematized Nomenclature of Medicine Clinical Term Ontology (SCTO) [30]; ISO 25,720 Genomic Sequence Variation Markup Language [31]; Human Phenotype Ontology (HPO) [32]; Infectious Diseases Ontology (IDO) [33]; Epilepsy and Seizures Ontology (EPSO) [34]; Alzheimer's Disease Ontology (ADO) [35]; the Gene Ontology (GO) [36], and many more. A specific representation of care systems is provided by ISO 13940 Health informatics–System of concepts to support Continuity of care [37]. Its representation style is placed below formal ontologies but above IT systems representation in the enterprise view because of the definition of clinical concepts. An overarching medical ontology, not limited to a specific medical domain but covering the entire health business, has been recently published in [38].

For mapping and matching different ontologies to enable cross-domain communication and collaboration, the ontologies have to be represented or re-engineered, respectively, as formal entities, including their contexts, constraints, and relationships, by using attributes and relations according to ISO/IEC 21838:2021 Information Technology–Top Level Ontologies (TLO) [28] (Figure 3). In case no ontologies are available for representing a specific domain or subdomain, a preliminary ontology can be derived from the TLO base classes.

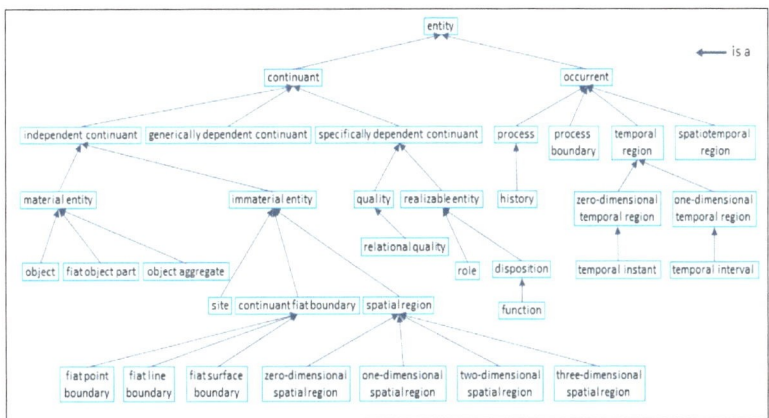

Figure 3. Basic Formal Ontology (BFO) is a hierarchy (after ISO/IEC 21838:2020) [28].

3.3. The Policy Domain

A policy defines a set of legal, regulatory, procedural, ethical, and contextual requirements and obligations for communication and cooperation, including privacy and trustworthiness. That way, controlling the intended behavior of business systems, a policy domain representing policy knowledge, concepts, and relations, is crucial for defining, designing, and running any type of ecosystem. Using the ISO 23903 model and framework, Figure 4 demonstrates the specialization of the policy domain into the sub-policy domains relevant for P5 medicine ecosystems. The user policy domain—sometimes also called personal policy domain or individual's policy domains—represents the intentions, expectations, wishes, etc., of the individual engaged in the business case, such as a patient.

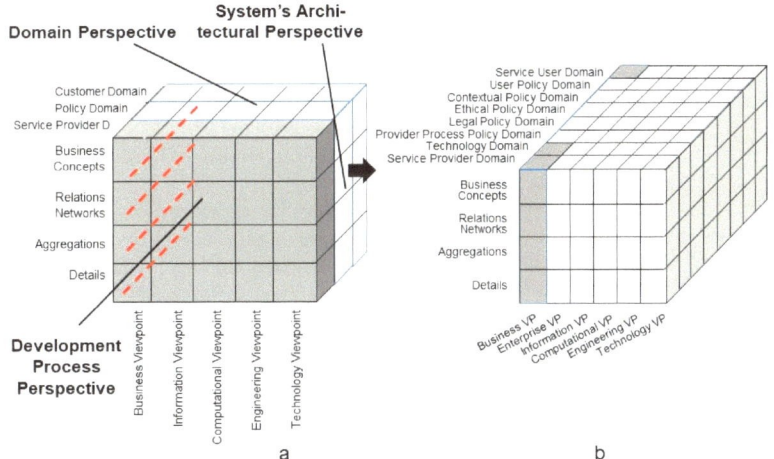

Figure 4. Specialization of the policy domain into sub-policy domains relevant for P5 medicine ecosystems (after [39], changed).

Examples for a provider process policy domain instance are best practice clinical guidelines. All sub-policy domains must be represented using related ontologies.

Based on the Ponder Language specification [40], a policy ontology to formalize the rules and constraints controlling the behavior of a business system has been provided by ISO 22600 [41], instantiated for the security and privacy domain (Figure 5).

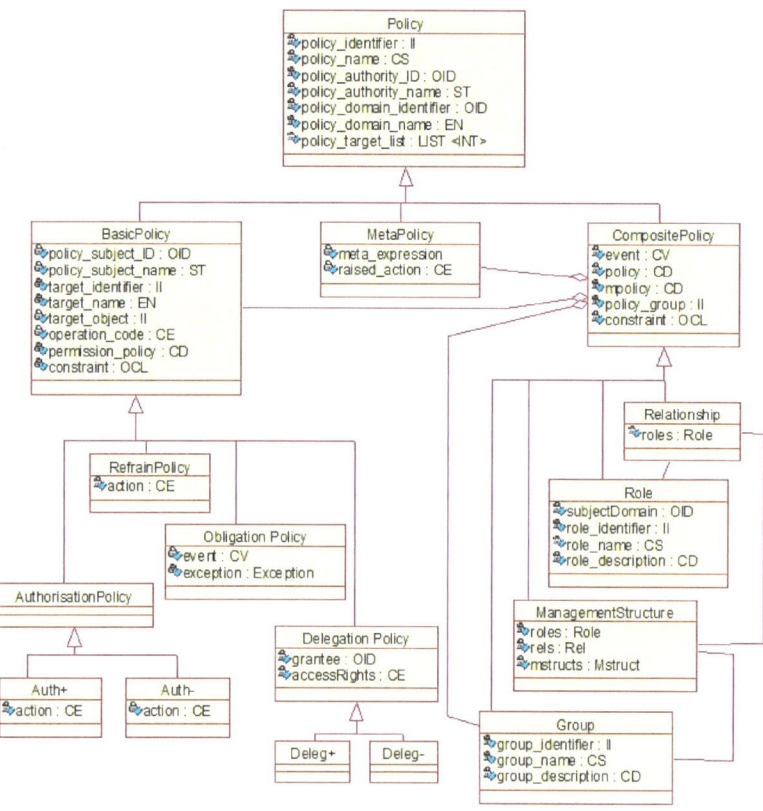

Figure 5. Policy domain components according to ISO 22600-2 [41].

The integration of that policy ontology in an ecosystem for managing security and privacy, using ISO 23903, has been performed in the HL7 Privacy and Security Logical Data Model, Release 1, June 2021 [42] (Figure 6). There are also more ontology-based approaches available [43,44].

For managing ethical and trust aspects of autonomous and intelligent 5P medicine ecosystems, IEEE defined the IEEE 7000 Standard Model Process for Addressing Ethical Concerns during System Design [45] as a framework for specifying ethical issues in IT systems. On that basis, a series of standards with the involvement of the first author have been developed at IEEE. A foundational specification for designing and managing transformed 5PM ecosystems according to the ISO 23903 model and framework is the first global ontological standard for ethically driven robotics and automation systems (ERAS) [46]. More information can be found in [3].

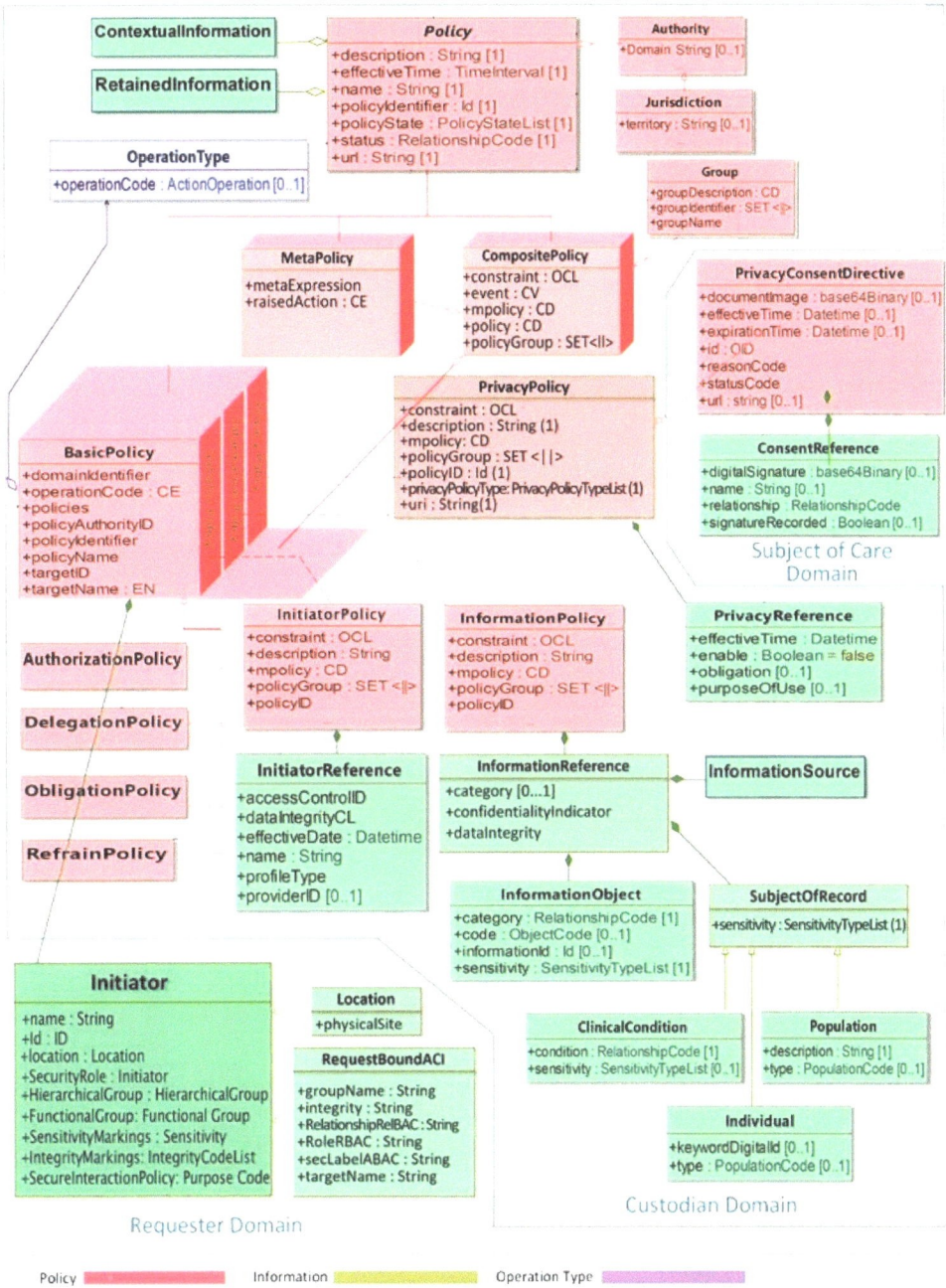

Figure 6. HL7 Privacy and Security Logical Data Model, Release 1, June 2021 [42].

4. A Short Overview on Standard Classes and Related Specifications

Table 5, presents for the classes architecture standards; modeling standards; terminology and ontology standards; communication standards; policy, security, and privacy standards; safety standards; and identifier and identification standards some international specifications relevant in the context of P5 medicine ecosystems. Of course, the presented standard types and examples list is not intended to be complete.

Table 5. Standard classifications and related international standard examples.

Standards Classification	Examples
Architecture standards	HL7 Version 2.x/3, OMG CORBA, OMG MDA, ISO 12967 Health informatics–Service architecture (HISA), ISO 7498-2:1989, Information processing systems—Open Systems Interconnection—Basic Reference Model—Part 2: Security Architecture, ISO 13407:1999 Human-centred design processes for interactive systems
Modelling standards	OMG Unified Modeling Language (UML), ISO/IEC 19505-2:2012 Unified Modeling Language (UML), CEN 15300 CEN Report: Framework for formal modelling of healthcare security policies
Terminology and ontology standards	UMLS, Systematized Nomenclature of Medicine Clinical Terms (SNOMED CT), Systematized Nomenclature of Medicine Clinical Term Ontology (SCTO), ISO 25720 Genomic sequence variation markup language, ISO/IEC 2382-8:1998 Information technology—Vocabulary—Part 8: Security, CEN-ENV 13608-1:2000 Health informatics—Security for healthcare communication—Part 1: Concepts and terminology, ISO 13940:2015 Health informatics—System of concepts to support continuity of care, Logical Observation Identifiers Names and Codes (LOINC), Unified Code for Units of Measure (UCUM)
Communication standards	ISO/IEC 7498-1:1994 Information technology—Open Systems Interconnection—Basic Reference Model: The Basic Model, HL7 V2.x/3, HL7 FHIR (Fast Healthcare Interoperability Resource), X12 EDI, UN EDIFACT, H.PRIM, xDT, Odette FTP, CEN 13606 Electronic healthcare record communication, ISO/IEEE 11073 Health informatics—Point-of-care medical device communication, ISO 17113 Health informatics–Exchange of information between healthcare information systems–Development of messages, CDISC and DICOM specifications, Classification Markup Language (ClaML), EN ISO 27269:2022 Health informatics-International patient summary (ISO 27269:2021)
Policy, security, and privacy standards	ISO/IEC 2700 Information security management, ISO 22600:2014 Health informatics–Privilege management and access control, ISO 17090 Public key infrastructure, ETSI TS 101733 Electronic Signature Formats, ASTM E1987-98 Standard guide for individual rights regarding health information, CEN 13608 Security for healthcare communication, CEN 13729 Secure user identification-Strong authentication using microprocessor cards, ISO 25237:2017 Health informatics—Pseudonymization, ISO/IEC PDTS Pseudonymisation Practices for the Protection of Personal Health Information and Health Related Services, ISO/IEC 27018:2019 Information technology—Security techniques—Code of practice for protection of personally identifiable information (PII) in public clouds acting as PII processors, ISO/IEC 29151:2017 Information technology—Security techniques—Code of practice for personally identifiable information protection, ISO 21298:2017 Health informatics—Functional and structural roles, ISO/IEC 9594-8:2008, Information technology—Open Systems Interconnection—The Directory: Public-key and attribute certificate frameworks, ISO/IEC 9798-3:1998, Information technology—Security techniques—Entity authentication—Part 3: Mechanisms using digital signature techniques, ISO/IEC 10181-1:1996, Information technology—Open Systems Interconnection—Security frameworks for open systems: Overview, ISO/TS 17090-1:2013 Health informatics—Public key infrastructure—Part 1: Overview of digital certificate services, ENV 13729:1999, Health informatics—Secure user identification for healthcare strong authentication using microprocessor cards, ISO 21091:2013 Health informatics—Directory services for healthcare providers, subjects of care and other entities, ISO/IEC 15408-1:2009 Information technology—Security techniques—Evaluation criteria for IT security—Part 1: Introduction and general model
Safety standards	CEN 13694 CEN Report: Safety and security related software quality standards for healthcare, ISO/DTS 25238 Classification of Safety Risks, IEC 82304-1 Health Software–Part 1: General requirements for product safety. IEC 82304-2 Health Software–Part 2: Health and wellness apps–Quality and reliability
Identifier and identification standards	LOINC, ASTM E1714-00 Standard guide for properties of a Universal Healthcare Identifier
Document standards	HL7 V3/CDA (Clinical Document Architecture), DICOM SR (Structured Reporting), HL7 FHIR Bundle+Composition

Table 5. *Cont.*

Standards Classification	Examples
Data representation (visualization) standards	HTML, PDF, PDF/A, MS Word, ClaML
Encoding standards	XML, JSON, ASN.1, ER7, xDT
Character representation standards	ASCII, EBCDIC, Unicode

5. Managing the Modeling and Development Process of 5P Medicine Ecosystems

5.1. Representation of 5P Medicine Ecosystems through Standards

When modeling and developing 5PM ecosystems or managing the integration and interoperability challenge, we are inevitably bound to the good modeling best practices [12] realized by ISO 23903 model and framework [15] by strictly performing a top-down approach. In other words, we cannot jump to a specific viewpoint to correctly interrelate models and artifacts. Instead, we must first solve the mapping between the involved domains represented by domain ontologies to correctly and formally represent the considered multi-disciplinary business system use case. Thereafter, we have to perform the transformation into the ICT-specific views from the enterprise viewpoint through the information view, the computational view down to the engineering viewpoint representing the implementable artifacts. Thereby, we must deploy the related ICT ontologies, from business process modeling through information modeling up to data modeling. While this process, including the representation styles, is clearly specified for the ICT domain perspective by using ISO/IEC 10746 Open Distributed Processing [13] and related specifications, the ontologies and representation styles in health informatics may be healthcare-specific and changing over time. Healthcare-specific standards for representing domain-specific business views are, e.g., the HL7 Domain Analysis Models (DAM) or the ISO or CEN Health Informatics Functional Models (FM) or Services Functional Models (SFM). An example for the first group is the HL7 Composite Security and Privacy Domain Analysis Model (CSP-DAM), meanwhile replaced by the aforementioned HL7 Privacy and Security Logical Data Model, R1 [42]. Examples for the latter group are the HL7 EHR-System Functional Model, R2 (HL7 EHR-S FM), the HL7 PHR-System Functional Model, R2 (HL7 PHR-S FM), or the HL7 Service Functional Models like the HL7 Common Terminology Services 2 Functional Model or the HL7 Version 3 Standard Identification Service R1. Also, the ISO 13940 System of Concepts to Support Continuity of Care [37] must be mentioned here. A newer example for representing health enterprise view components are clinical information models according to ISO 139722 Clinical Information Models [47] or the openEHR [48] and ISO 13606 Electronic Health Record Communication [49,50] archetypes. Thereby, some aspects of the business view as well as the informational representation (information view) are covered. Standards for healthcare-specific information view representations have been established in the HL7 Clinical Document Architecture (HL7 CDA) series [51]. Computational view representation examples are HL7 Implementable Technology Specifications (ITS) but also the globally pushed HL7 Fast Healthcare Interoperability Resources (HL7 FHIR) [52]. Figures 7 and 8 represent the different standards and representation styles in the ISO 23903 Interoperability and Integration Reference Architecture model and framework. Regarding FHIR, starting as an implementable resource as expressed in Figure 8, five levels are meanwhile supported. The highest Level 5 covers knowledge-related aspects such as clinical reasoning, Level 4 covers process-related aspects, Level 3 covers semantic interpretations, Level 2 covers service implementations, and Level 1 covers technical representations.

5.2. Integrating Existing Standards in 5P Medicine Ecosystems

After discussing some detail in the modeling and development of 5P medicine ecosystems, we will now address the challenge of mapping/matching or integrating existing specifications and artifacts using the model and framework of the ISO 23903 Interoperability and Integration Reference Architecture. To meet this challenge, we must understand the perspectives, objectives, concepts, contexts, etc., that the designer and developer of the component had in mind. Without that knowledge, which is normally not provided with the specification, any integration, mapping, or matching is not decidable. Therefore, we must re-engineer that missing knowledge. As the aforementioned conditions might change from use case to use case, the provided interoperability and integration outcome are specific to the considered use case or related classes of use cases, and the procedure has to be performed again for any new settings and contexts.

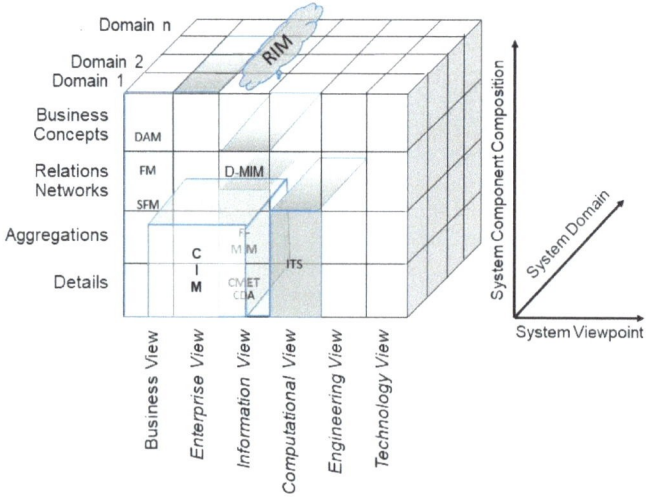

Figure 7. Healthcare-specific specifications representing different ISO 23903 views.

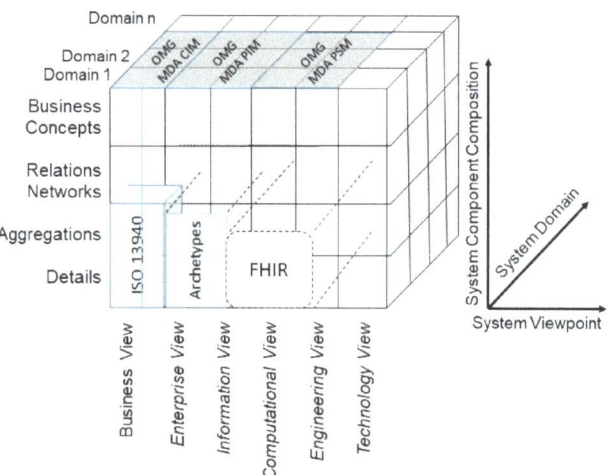

Figure 8. Healthcare-specific specifications representing different ISO 23903 views.

In the first step, the components in question must be correctly placed into the ISO 23903 model regarding the domain, the granularity level, and the represented development process viewpoint. Thereafter, the concepts represented by the considered components must be formally modeled in the business view using the corresponding domain ontologies as well as top-level ontologies for interrelating them. The concepts must be completed to correctly and operationally represent the real-world business system and business processes for the use case to be enabled or supported. The resulting business system representation must then be transformed into views according to the development process up to the considered components' view. This includes a re-engineering of the components and relationships, i.e., classes, attributes, operations, and relations needed to represent the full business use case must be added or modified. Figure 9 represents the described procedure.

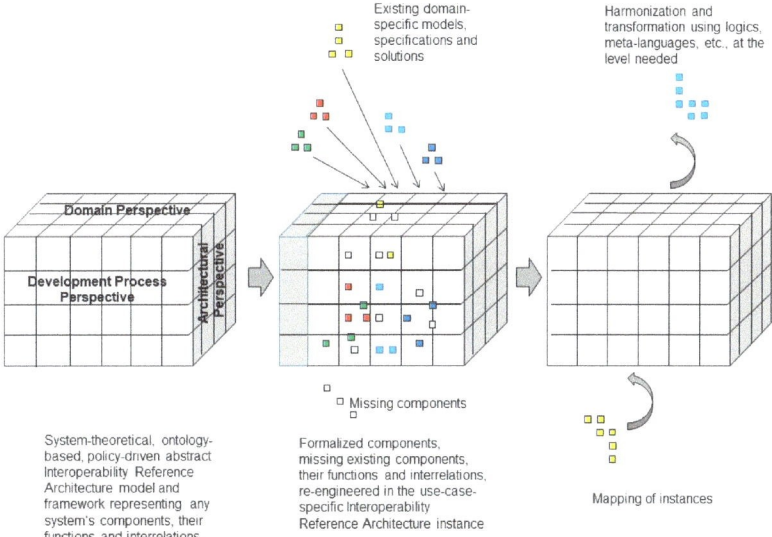

Figure 9. Integration of standards and specifications using the ISO 23903 Reference Architecture model and framework.

Following, we will exemplify the procedure of integrating and mapping specifications for enabling comprehensive interoperability as presented in ISO 23903:2021. First, we demonstrate the integration of security and privacy aspects specified in different standards, such as ISO 13606-1:2019 Health informatics-Electronic health record communication-Part 1: Reference model [49] (Figure 10a) and the HL7® Composite Security and Privacy Domain Analysis Model [53] (Figure 10b). Reengineering and mapping both standards by using the ISO 23903 model and framework is demonstrated in Figure 10c. That way, the more advanced security and privacy specifications provided by HL7 can be integrated into EHR solutions based on ISO 13606.

Another example deals with mapping HL7 V2 and HL7 V3 models and specifications. While HL7 V3 is based on the standardized HL7 Development Framework (HDF) related to ISO/IEC 10746 [13] or the Rational Unified Process (RUP) [20], respectively, HL7 V2 does not have a formal development framework or foundation but has been specified "on the fly" by borrowing from another ASTM standard and simply adjusting it to healthcare needs. Therefore, the HL7 V2 process must first be formally analyzed and represented (re-engineered), following the ISO 23903 principles. Furthermore, it must be ontologically represented using the Communication Standards Ontology (CSO) developed by Frank Oemig in the context of his PhD work [54] (Figure 11). The CSO elements integrated into the aforementioned BFO [28] are presented in bold [55].

The outcome of re-engineering HL7 V2 and V3 according to ISO 23903 and representing them using the Communication Standards Ontology for mapping the specifications is shown in Figure 12.

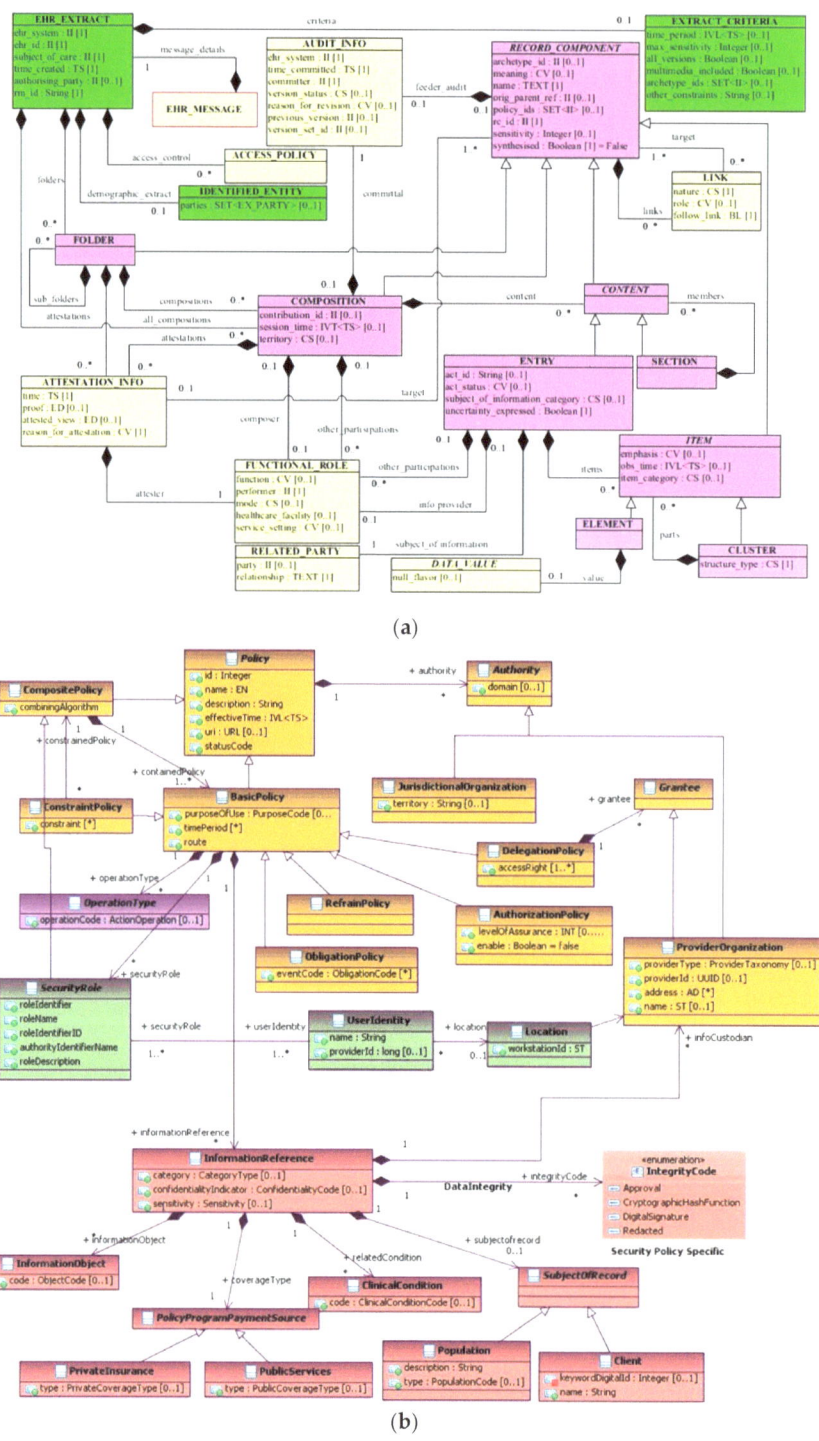

Figure 10. Cont.

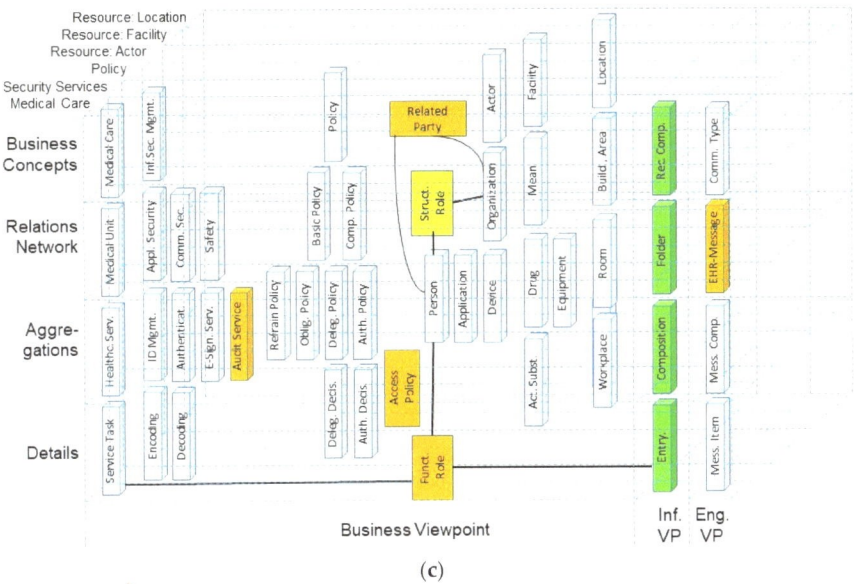

(c)

Figure 10. (**a**) ISO 13606-1 Reference Model [49]. (**b**) HL7 V3 Composite Security and Privacy DAM [53]. (**c**) Integrating ISO 13606-1 Reference Model and the HL7 V3 Composite Security and Privacy DAM regarding security and privacy aspects using ISO 23903.

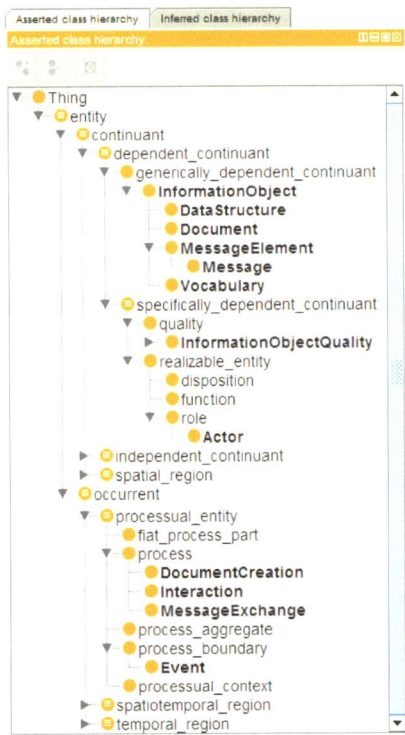

Figure 11. The Communication Standards Ontology presented in Protégé [55].

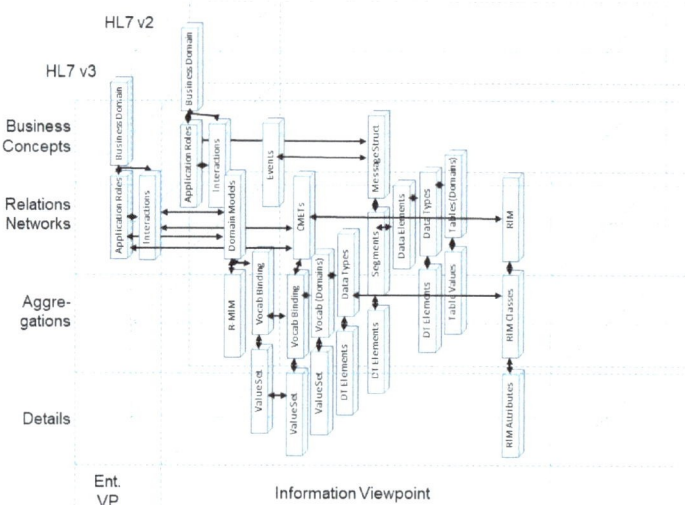

Figure 12. Re-engineering the development process model of HL7 v2® and HL7v3® for integrating the two communication standards [15].

Another integration example is provided in Figure 13, demonstrating the re-engineering and mapping of the higher-level specifications ISO 12967 Health Informatics Service Architecture [26] and ISO 13940:2015 System of concepts to support continuity of care [37].

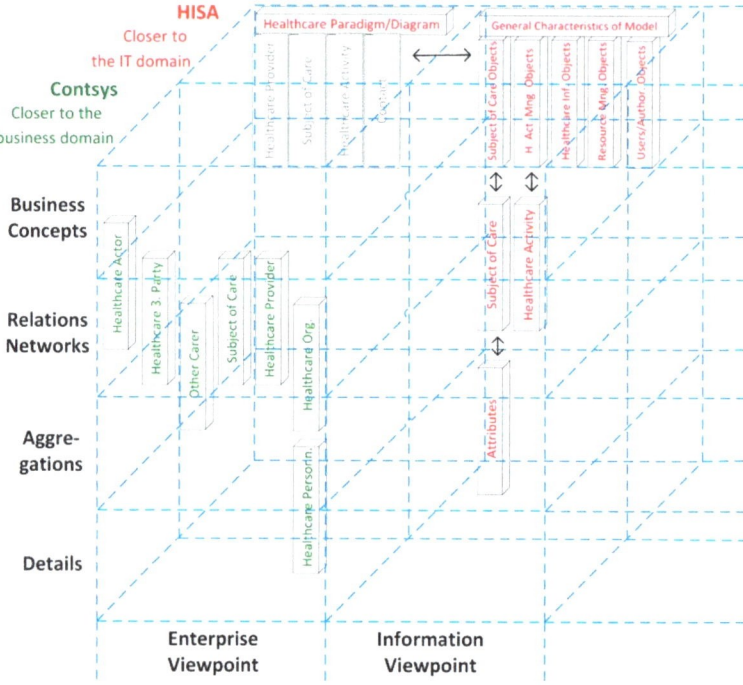

Figure 13. Re-engineering example of selected parts of ISO 12967 (all parts) and ISO 13940.

6. Summary and Conclusions

For designing, implementing, and managing transformed health ecosystems, we cannot simply integrate system components (specifications, standards, and artifacts) from a specific IT system viewpoint perspective, i.e., enterprise concepts representing enterprise knowledge, terms representing information, or data. When this has been completed, e.g., by combining special FHIR resources or mapping specifications from different standards just based on representational characteristics in one viewpoint, such as terminologies, naming conventions, etc., performed in some ISO/TC 215 projects, the outcome is incompatible, inconsistent, and therefore unsuitable. Instead, we must understand and formally represent the ecosystem using a system-oriented, architecture-centric, ontology-based, and policy-controlled approach, acknowledging the limitations of the data focus for specifying ecosystems.

Building on many years of work in health care with responsibilities for designing, implementing, and using related information systems, including necessary infrastructure services for interoperability, security, privacy, etc., but also for advancing health with telemedicine, pHealth, and eHealth, the first author developed the cross-domain and technology-independent interoperability and integration reference model and framework, domain-specifically supported by some of the co-authors. The basis for the approach, the Generic Component Model (GCM), dates from the early nineties of the last century and has successfully evolved over time. Meanwhile, the Health Informatics TCs of ISO and CEN, as well as other SDOs, mandated the use of ISO 23903 for any project covering multiple aspects or domains, as well as for realizing integration and interoperability between system components, including specifications and artifacts. The described limitations of constraint representation language result in the need to advance from data sharing interoperability to knowledge sharing interoperability in dynamic and complex intercultural, interdisciplinary, and inter-jurisdictional environments. Additionally, this was the driving factor for replacing the EU Data Protection Directive [56] by the EU General Data Protection Regulation (GDPR) [57], i.e., advancing from a privacy-related data classification towards the detailed consideration of processes and contexts of creating, collecting, using, and sharing personally identifiable information (PII) [58]. Projects such as the European Health Data Space [59] are therefore more than questionable (see, e.g., [9]). The nature of 5P medicine requires a concept- and context-based approach, including accompanying privacy and ethical aspects.

The presented approach enables comprehensive and consistent integration of and interoperability between domains, systems, related actors, specifications, standards, and solutions without limiting the used languages and methodologies. Thereby, it advances interoperability beyond the still dominant syntactic and semantic level towards knowledge sharing at the business concept level (agreed cooperation), knowledge sharing at the domain level (cross-domain cooperation), and even knowledge sharing in the individual context of education, experiences, and skills (moderated end-user collaboration).

Author Contributions: B.B. drafted this paper. B.B., P.R., F.O., M.G., P.A.S. and F.E. reviewed and edited the article. F.O. provided meaningful amendments to the HL7 standards world. P.A.S. added aspects from CEN/TC 251 and ISO/TC 215 perspectives. Furthermore, the authors have been involved in the development of most of the standards mentioned. All authors have read and agreed to the published version of the manuscript.

Funding: This research received no external funding.

Institutional Review Board Statement: Not applicable.

Informed Consent Statement: Not applicable.

Data Availability Statement: The original contributions presented in the study are included in the article. Further inquiries can be directed to the corresponding author.

Acknowledgments: The authors are indebted to their colleagues from IEEE, HL7 International, ISO TC 215, and CEN TC 251 for their kind and constructive support and co-operation.

Conflicts of Interest: The authors declare no conflict of interest.

References

1. Blobel, B.; Ruotsalainen, P.; Giacomini, M. Standards and Principles to Enable Interoperability and Integration of 5P Medicine Ecosystems. *Stud. Health Technol. Inform.* **2022**, *299*, 3–19. [PubMed]
2. Byju's. Structure, Functions, Units and Types of Ecosystem. Available online: https://byjus.com/biology (accessed on 28 June 2023).
3. Blobel, B.; Ruotsalainen, P.; Brochhausen, M.; Prestes, E.; Houghtaling, M.A. Designing and Managing Advanced, Intelligent and Ethical Health and Social Care Ecosystems. *J. Pers. Med.* **2023**, *13*, 1209. [CrossRef] [PubMed]
4. Blobel, B.; Kalra, D. Managing Healthcare Transformation Towards 5P Medicine. Lausanne: Frontiers Media SA. Available online: https://www.frontiersin.org/research-topics/21049/managing-healthcare-transformation-towards-p5-medicine (accessed on 11 October 2023).
5. Blobel, B. Challenges and Solutions for Designing and Managing pHealth Ecosystems. *Front. Med.* **2019**, *6*, 83. [CrossRef] [PubMed]
6. Blobel, B.; Oemig, F.; Ruotsalainen, P.; Lopez, D.M. Transformation of Health and Social Care Systems—An Interdisciplinary Approach Toward a Foundational Architecture. *Front. Med.* **2022**, *9*, 802487. [CrossRef] [PubMed]
7. Blobel, B.; Giacomini, M. Interoperability is more than just technology—Editorial. *Eur. J. Biomed. Inform.* **2016**, *12*, en1–en2. [CrossRef]
8. Blobel, B.; Ruotsalainen, P.; Lopez, D.M.; Oemig, F. Requirements and Solutions for Personalized Health Systems. *Stud. Health Technol. Inform.* **2017**, *237*, 3–21. [PubMed]
9. Blobel, B.; Ruotsalainen, P.; Oemig, F. Why Interoperability at Data Level Is Not Sufficient for Enabling pHealth? *Stud. Health Technol. Inform.* **2020**, *273*, 3–19. [PubMed]
10. Blobel, B. Architectural approach to eHealth for enabling paradigm changes in health. *Methods Inf. Med.* **2010**, *49*, 123–134. [CrossRef] [PubMed]
11. Kamareddine, F.; Laan, T.; Nederpelt, R. *A Modern Perspective on Type Theory*; Kluwer Academic Publishers: New York, NY, USA, 2004.
12. Rebstock, M.; Fengel, J.; Paulheim, H. *Ontologies-Based Business Integration*; Springer: Berlin/Heidelberg, Germany, 2008.
13. *ISO/IEC 10746*; Information Technology—Open Distributed Processing—Reference Model. International Organization for Standardization: Geneva, Switzerland, 2009.
14. Hoberman, S.; Burbank, D.; Bradley, C. *Data Modeling for the Business: A Handbook for Aligning the Business with IT Using High-Level Data Models*; Technics Publications, LLC.: Bradley Beach, NJ, USA, 2009.
15. *ISO 23903:2021*; Health Informatics—Interoperability and Integration Reference Architecture—Model and Framework. International Organization for Standardization (ISO): Geneva, Switzerland, 2021.
16. ComplianceForge. Introduction-Guide to Information-Security-Policy-Cybersecurity-Program-Documentation, Version 2022.3; ComplianceForge LLC: 2022. Available online: https://www.complianceforge.com (accessed on 28 June 2023).
17. *IEC 82304-2:2021*; Health Software-Part 2: Health and wellness apps-Quality and reliability. International Electrotechnical Commission (IEC): Geneva, Switzerland, 2021.
18. *ISO/IEC/IEEE 42010:2011*; Systems and Software Engineering—Architecture Description. International Organization for Standardization (ISO): Geneva, Switzerland, 2011.
19. *ISO/IEC/IEEE 42020:2019*; Software, Systems and Enterprise—Architecture Processes. International Organization for Standardization (ISO): Geneva, Switzerland, 2019.
20. Péraire, C.; Edwards, M.; Fernandes, A.; Mancin, E.; Carroll, K. *The IBM Rational Unified Process for System Z*; IBM International Technical Support Organization: Armonk, NY, USA, 2007.
21. *ISO/IEC 7498-1:1994*; Information technology—Open Systems Interconnection—Basic Reference Model: The Basic Model. International Organization for Standardization (ISO): Geneva, Switzerland, 2000.
22. Object Management Group. *Model Driven Architecture (MDA). MDA Guide rev. 2.0. Milford*; Object Management Group: Needham, MA, USA, 2014.
23. Roubi, S.; Erramdani, M.; Mbarki, S. A Model Driven Approach for generating Graphical User Interface for MVC Rich Internet Application. *Comput. Inf. Sci.* **2016**, *9*, 91–98.
24. Blobel, B.; Oemig, F. The Importance of Architectures for Interoperability. *Stud. Health Technol. Inform.* **2015**, *211*, 18–56. [PubMed]
25. Blobel, B.; Oemig, F. Solving the Modeling Dilemma as a Foundation for Interoperability. *Eur. J. Biomed. Inform.* **2018**, *14*, 3–12. [CrossRef]
26. *ISO 12967*; Health Informatics—Service Architecture (HISA). International Organization for Standardization (ISO): Geneva, Switzerland, 2021.
27. Gruber, T.R. Toward principles for the design of ontologies used for knowledge sharing? *Int. J. Hum. Comput. Stud.* **1995**, *43*, 907–928. [CrossRef]
28. *ISO/IEC 21838:2021*; Information Technology—Top-Level Ontologies (TLO). International Organization for Standardization (ISO): Geneva, Switzerland, 2021.

29. Bodenreider, O. The Unified Medical Language System (UMLS): Integrating Biomedical Terminology. *Nucleic Acids Res.* **2004**, *32*, D267–D270. [CrossRef] [PubMed]
30. SNOMED International. Available online: https://www.snomed.org (accessed on 28 June 2023).
31. *ISO 25720:2009*; Health informatics—Genomic Sequence Variation Markup Language (GSVML). International Organization for Standardization (ISO): Geneva, Switzerland, 2018.
32. Robinson, P.N.; Mundlos, S. The human phenotype ontology. *Clin. Genet.* **2010**, *77*, 525–534. [CrossRef] [PubMed]
33. Cowell, L.G.; Smith, B. Infectious disease ontology. In *Infectious Disease Informatics*; Springer: Berlin/Heidelberg, Germany, 2010; pp. 373–395.
34. Sahoo, S.S.; Lhatoo, S.D.; Gupta, D.K.; Cui, L.; Zhao, M.; Jayapandian, C.; Bozorgi, A.; Zhang, G.-Q. Epilepsy and seizure ontology: Towards an epilepsy informatics infrastructure for clinical research and patient care. *J. Am. Med. Inform. Assoc.* **2014**, *21*, 82–89. [CrossRef] [PubMed]
35. Malhotra, A.; Younesi, E.; Gundel, M.; Muller, B.; Heneka, M.T.; Hofmann-Apitius, M. ADO: A disease ontology representing the domain knowledge specific to Alzheimer's disease. *Alzheimers Dement.* **2014**, *10*, 238–246. [CrossRef] [PubMed]
36. Gene Ontology Consortium. The Gene Ontology; Geneontology: 2022. Available online: http://geneontology.org (accessed on 28 June 2023).
37. *ISO 13940:2015*; Health Informatics—System of Concepts to Support Continuity of Care. International Organization for Standardization (ISO): Geneva, Switzerland, 2015.
38. Benis, A.; Dornauer, V.; Grosjean, J.; Crisan-Vida, M. Medical Informatics and Digital Health Multilingual Ontology (MIMO): A tool to improve international collaborations. *Int. J. Med. Inform.* **2022**, *167*, 104860. [CrossRef] [PubMed]
39. Blobel, B.; Ruotsalainen, P.; Brochhausen, M. Autonomous systems and artificial intelligence—Hype or prerequisite for P5 medicine? *Stud. Health Technol. Inform.* **2021**, *285*, 3–14. [PubMed]
40. Damianou, N.; Dulay, N.; Lupu, E.; Sloman, M. Ponder: A Language for Specifying Security and Management Policies for Distributed Systems; The Language Specification, Version 2.3. Imperial College Research Report DoC 2000/1. 2000. Available online: https://www.researchgate.net/publication/243241194_Ponder_A_Language_for_Specifying_Security_and_Management_Policies_for_Distributed_Systems(accessed on 7 September 2023).
41. *ISO 22600:2014*; Health Informatics—Privilege Management and Access Control. International Organization for Standardization (ISO): Geneva, Switzerland, 2014.
42. Health Level 7 International Inc. HL7 Privacy and Security Logical Data Model, Release 1, June 2021. Ann Arbor: HL7 International. 2021. Available online: https://www.hl7.org (accessed on 28 June 2023).
43. Tsoumas, B.; Gritzalis, D. Towards an Ontology-based Security Management. In Proceedings of the 20th International Conference on Advanced Information Networking and Applications—Volume 1 (AINA'06), Vienna, Austria, 18–20 April 2006. [CrossRef]
44. Palmirani, M.; Martoni, M.; Rossi, A.; Bartolini, C.; Robaldo, L. PrOnto: Privacy Ontology for Legal Reasoning. In *Electronic Government and the Information Systems Perspective: 7th International Conference, EGOVIS 2018, Regensburg, Germany, 3–5 September 2018*; Kő, A., Francesconi, E., Eds.; Proceedings 7; Springer International Publishing: Berlin/Heidelberg, Germany, 2018; pp. 139–152.
45. *IEEE 7000:2021*; IEEE Standard Model Process for Addressing Ethical Concerns during System Design. IEEE: Piscataway, NJ, USA, 2021.
46. *IEEE 7007:2021*; IEEE Ontological Standard for Ethically Driven Robotics and Automation Systems. IEEE: Piscataway, NJ, USA, 2021.
47. *ISO 13972:2022*; Health Informatics—Clinical Information Models—Characteristics, Structures and Requirements. International Organization for Standardization (ISO): Geneva, Switzerland, 2022.
48. openEHR International. Available online: https://openehr.org (accessed on 28 June 2023).
49. *ISO 13606-1:2019*; Health Informatics—Electronic Health Record Communication—Part 1: Reference Model. International Organization for Standardization (ISO): Geneva, Switzerland, 2019.
50. *ISO 13606-3:2019*; Health Informatics—Electronic Health Record Communication—Part 3: Reference Archetypes and Term Lists. International Organization for Standardization (ISO): Geneva, Switzerland, 2019.
51. Health Level 7 International Inc. *HL7 V3 Standard: Clinical Document Architecture, Release 2*; HL7 International: Ann Arbor, MI, USA, 2021; Available online: https://www.hl7.org (accessed on 28 June 2023).
52. Health Level 7 International Inc. *HL7 Fast Healthcare Interoperability Resources Release 4B*; HL7 International: Ann Arbor, MI, USA, 2021; Available online: https://hl7.org/FHIR/ (accessed on 28 June 2023).
53. Health Level 7 International Inc. *HL7 Version 3 Domain Analysis Model: Composite Security and Privacy, Release 1*; HL7 International: Ann Arbor, MI, USA, 2020; Available online: https://www.hl7.org (accessed on 28 June 2023).
54. Oemig, F. Development of an Ontology-Based Architecture for Ensuring Semantic Interoperability between Communication Standards in Healthcare. Ph.D. Thesis, Medical Faculty, University of Regensburg, Regensburg, Germany, 2011. (In German). Available online: http://epub.uni-regensburg.de/20076/1/Dissertation_v39_final.pdf (accessed on 28 June 2023).
55. Oemig, F.; Blobel, B. A Communication Standards Ontology Using Basic Formal Ontologies. *Stud. Health Technol. Inform.* **2010**, *156*, 105–113. [PubMed]
56. European Parliament and Council. *Directive (EU) 95/46/EC Data Protection Directive*; EC: Brussels, Belgium, 1995.
57. European Parliament and Council. *Regulation (EU) 2016/679 General Data Protection Regulation*; EC: Brussels, Belgium, 2016.

58. Blobel, B.; Ruotsalainen, P. How Does GDPR Support Healthcare Transformation to 5P Medicine? *Stud. Health Technol. Inform.* **2019**, *264*, 1135–1339. [PubMed]
59. European Parliament and Council. *Proposal for a Regulation on the European Health Data Space*; EC: Strasbourg, France, 2022.

Disclaimer/Publisher's Note: The statements, opinions and data contained in all publications are solely those of the individual author(s) and contributor(s) and not of MDPI and/or the editor(s). MDPI and/or the editor(s) disclaim responsibility for any injury to people or property resulting from any ideas, methods, instructions or products referred to in the content.

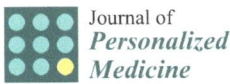

Brief Report

Challenges and Strategies for Enhancing eHealth Capacity Building Programs in African Nations

Flora Nah Asah * and Jens Johan Kaasbøll

HISP Centre, Department of Informatics, University of Oslo, Gaustadallen 30, 0373 Oslo, Norway; jens@ifi.uio.no
* Correspondence: asahflora@outlook.com

Abstract: eHealth applications play a crucial role in achieving Universal Health Coverage. (1) Background: To ensure successful integration and use, particularly in developing and low/middle-income countries (LMIC), it is vital to have skilled healthcare personnel. The purpose of this study was to describe challenges that hinder capacity-building initiatives among healthcare personnel in developing and LMIC and suggest interventions to mitigate them. (2) Methods: Adopted a descriptive research design and gathered empirical data through an online survey from 37 organizations. (3) Results: The study found that in developing and LMIC, policymakers and eHealth specialists face numerous obstacles integrating and using eHealth including limited training opportunities. These obstacles include insufficient funds, inadequate infrastructure, poor leadership, and governance, which are specific to each context. The study suggests implementing continuous in-service training, computer-based systems, and academic modules to address these challenges. Additionally, the importance of having solid and appropriate eHealth policies and committed leaders were emphasized. (4) Conclusions: These findings are consistent with previous research and highlight the need for practical interventions to enhance eHealth capacity-building in LMICs. However, it should be noted that the data was collected only from BETTEReHEALTH partners. Therefore, the results only represent their respective organizations and cannot be generalized to the larger population.

Keywords: eHealth; ICTs; Capacity building activities; BETTEReHEALTH

Citation: Asah, F.N.; Kaasbøll, J.J. Challenges and Strategies for Enhancing eHealth Capacity Building Programs in African Nations. *J. Pers. Med.* **2023**, *13*, 1463. https://doi.org/10.3390/jpm13101463

Academic Editors: Bernd Blobel, Mauro Giacomini and Bian Yang

Received: 11 July 2023
Revised: 28 September 2023
Accepted: 28 September 2023
Published: 5 October 2023

Copyright: © 2023 by the authors. Licensee MDPI, Basel, Switzerland. This article is an open access article distributed under the terms and conditions of the Creative Commons Attribution (CC BY) license (https://creativecommons.org/licenses/by/4.0/).

1. Introduction

According to a recent United Nations (UN) report, almost half of the global population lacks access to essential healthcare services [1]. This is primarily due to over 800 million individuals allocating less than 10% of their household budget toward health expenses. As a result, millions worldwide are facing significant challenges and cannot afford necessary healthcare services [2]. The World Health Organization (WHO) Director-General urged leaders and policymakers, particularly those from developing countries, to embrace eHealth to improve healthcare. By integrating digital health services, access to and quality of health service delivery can be enhanced, ultimately contributing to achieving the United Nations Sustainable Development Goals [3,4]. This manuscript is an adapted version of a paper originally published in the IOS SHTI pHealth 2022 Proceedings [5].

eHealth refers to the provision of health services and information through the Internet, utilizing digital technologies such as information communication technologies (ICTs) and data to offer healthcare services [6,7]. These services may include physical and psychological diagnosis and treatment, telepathology, vital signs monitoring, electronic prescribing, and teleconsultation [8]. The literature has extensively documented the benefits of integrating eHealth in healthcare, such as improving healthcare delivery, efficacy, and quality of care [9]. eHealth applications are considered a potential "game changer" that could improve access to affordable and effective healthcare services [10,11]. Additionally, eHealth services can enhance patients' health-related knowledge and behavior, facilitate information exchange between healthcare providers and patients, and improve coordination and continuity of care while reducing the cost of healthcare delivery. In the long term, eHealth has the potential to transform the workflow of healthcare and support the achievement of Universal Health Coverage (UHC) [11–13].

Factors Influencing the Integration and Use of eHealth

Ensuring access to quality healthcare without financial barriers is essential to achieving Universal Health Coverage (UHC) [3]. eHealth technologies have been identified as key enablers of UHC. However, their integration and widespread use are limited, particularly in developing countries where they are most needed [14]. This is due to several factors, including the high cost of IT infrastructure and a need for more skilled personnel to adopt eHealth [15]. A study on integrating eHealth in Tanzania found that inadequate ICT skills, high cost of ICT, under-developed IT infrastructure, and a need for more information about appropriate ICT solutions were major hindrances [16]. While eHealth services can improve healthcare quality, factors such as insufficient budget for ICT infrastructure, security, privacy, and confidentiality concerns can hinder their integration [17]. A qualitative study on implementing a standardized information system in Cameroon found that centralized structures deter the allocation of finance to ICT equipment, particularly at lower health system levels [18]. According to Mars & Scott [19], LMIC governments need more financial resources, resulting in cautious spending on health activities. Adebesin et al. [20] also pointed out that the lack of interoperability of Health Information systems (HIS) hinders eHealth integration. A survey on eHealth adoption obstacles in Africa revealed limited participation in eHealth standards development beyond the International Organization for Standardization's requirements. Stiawan [21] further explained that the inability of information systems to exchange and share data and information among government agencies is a significant obstacle to eHealth integration. Similarly, Sluijs et al. [22] noted that the need for standards prevents government institutions, such as hospitals, from achieving their targets. The data and information needed by health personnel, such as population data, health insurance data, and patients' medical records, are often stored on different systems and managed by various government departments, making interoperability crucial. S. Masud et al. [23] emphasized standardizing data and information formats to achieve interoperability.

Issues with eHealth policies [24] and leadership [25] within the public sector have been identified as areas of concern in LMICs. Poor coordination among government departments and inadequate policies are challenges in integrating eHealth initiatives, according to Luna et al. [26]. In a study assessing eHealth policies in four African countries, authors noted that strategic goals were vague and lacked consolidated plans [27]. Weak leadership within the government can also hinder the coordination of eHealth projects at the national level, as noted by Mburu et al. [28]. Additionally, developing long-term strategies can be challenging in unstable political environments. However, the political will to embrace eHealth is growing in Sub-Saharan Africa, with the African Union and WHO working with LMIC governments to harmonize eHealth activities on the continent, according to Mars [19].

Various challenges impede the successful integration and use of eHealth services in the healthcare sector. These include the lack of computer equipment, poor internet connectivity, and inconsistent electricity supply [10,29]. Studies have revealed that healthcare workers' reluctance to embrace technology significantly limits their participation in eHealth activities. This is often due to their need for sufficient knowledge and skills to operate eHealth services, which results in denial and resistance towards information technologies [30–32]. Furthermore, the low usage of the internet among doctors in Pakistan is attributed to their insufficient IT skills. In low- and middle-income countries, inadequate human resources pose a significant threat to the successful integration and use of eHealth [33]. The current capacity-building activities for IT professionals need improvement, as studies have shown that the need for qualified health professionals is a persistent problem. Sufficient knowledge and skills are crucial for healthcare providers to use eHealth services effectively and keep up with technical advancements in an ever-changing eHealth environment [34–37].

Research conducted in LMICs suggests that enhancing the ICT skills of health personnel through education and training is crucial [9,38]. Prior studies have primarily focused on the availability of human resources and ease of use rather than the competencies and skills of health personnel in eHealth in Africa and LMICs. While these studies are informative, they challenge policymakers in comprehending, evaluating, and addressing obstacles. Our review unveiled a scarcity of articles on capacity-building endeavors among health personnel, underscoring the importance of this study.

2. Objectives

This study delves into the challenges that hinder capacity-building initiatives among healthcare personnel in developing and LMIC and suggests interventions to mitigate them. The data from this study was extracted from a large study conducted within the BETTEReHEALTH project identifying challenges of integrating digital health policies and gaps in developing digital health capacity among healthcare professionals within the BETTEReHEALTH project. However, in this article, we focused on identifying gaps in eHealth capacity-building activities and suggested approaches to mitigate them. The study gathered empirical data from an online survey on capacity-building activities in Africa. The significance of building the capacity of healthcare personnel in eHealth cannot be overstated, as a well-trained workforce in this field will strengthen health systems and enhance access to and quality of healthcare delivery [39]. The results of this study will guide the provision of health-related information and resources to BETTEReHEALTH partners and others and serve as a roadmap to measure and alleviate the barriers.

BETTEReHEALTH is a European Union project and funded by European Union Horizon 2020. The project aims to strive to increase the level of international cooperation in eHealth, inform and strengthen end-user communities and policy makers in making the right decisions for the successful implementation of e-Health. The project's purpose is to increase opportunities for stakeholders in Africa and Europe with the overall aim of better health outcomes through better healthcare accessibility and higher quality. BETTEReHEALTH provides a platform for stakeholders to network, disseminate and communicate, and provide information on best practices, lessons learnt and policy guidance on eHealth. The project has four hubs: Ghana (Western region), Malawi (Southern region), Ethiopia (Central and Eastern regions), and Tunisia serving the Northern region.

3. Methods

In the research on which this article is based, a descriptive design was adopted, and data was gathered through an online survey created with Google Forms. A links to the following files (i) information form explaining the purpose of the study, (ii) informed consent form, (iii) survey, were sent to project leaders of four BETTEReHEALTH hubs i.e., Ghana, Malawi, Ethiopia, and Tunisia. They then forwarded the survey to eHealth organizations/institutions in their respective countries. The online survey had four sections and five questions per section. The four sections were:

1. eHealth capacity building activities.
2. Factors hindering eHealth capacity building among health professionals.
3. Health workers IT literacy.
4. Proposed suggestions to build IT skills among health professionals.

The project leader, who was the second author, developed the questionnaire, and the BETTEReHEALTH project managers in the hubs were asked to review it. To ensure the accuracy of the questionnaire, it was pre-tested among master students from the Department of Informatics at the University of Oslo. This helped to assess if the questions were unambiguous and easily understood by the respondents and provided direct evidence of questionnaire data validity. Based on feedback from the pre-test, some questions were modified and clarified to improve their quality.

The survey questions were written in English and were open to participation for two months. The questions were closed-ended and were scored on a five-point Likert type scale ranging from strongly agree to strongly disagree. Managers in decision-making positions responded to the questionnaire. Three follow-up participation requests were sent out every two weeks. Ethical clearance for this study was granted as part of a larger BETTEReHEALTH project. In addition, all participants were informed about the study; a consent form and information sheet were attached to the questionnaire. A total of 37 organizations/institutions responded from 13 countries, with one excluded from analysis due to not indicating the name of the country. In addition, four managers were selected at random and interviewed informally to gain insight into eHealth capacity-building activities within their organizations.

Quantitative and Qualitative Data Analyses

The responses to the survey questions were collected and exported to an Excel spreadsheet. To ensure the anonymity of respondents, all metadata was removed from the file. The data gathered was processed with SPSS statistical software. To help us in analyses, the data were arranged in the following sections including general characteristics of the respondents, capacity-building activities and gaps in capacity-building programs, factors hindering eHealth capacity-building activities, health workers IT literacy, and suggestions to building IT skills of health personnel. Thereafter, the institutions were grouped by countries and then by regional hubs. Since there were only 37 respondents, descriptive analyses were employed to summarize the results.

The interviews were analyzed using content analysis, which involves identifying and categorizing themes within text data. Comments from the online survey were also analyzed using this method. The results were supported by quotes from the interviews. However, it should be noted that the survey results only represent their respective organizations and cannot be generalized to the larger population.

4. Results

4.1. General Characteristics of Respondents i.e., Organizations

Thirty-seven organizations from 13 countries responded to the survey. The BETTEReHEALTH project has four hubs namely Ghana (Western), Malawi (Southern), Tunisia (Northern), and Ethiopia (Central and Eastern) serving four geographical regions. We divided the responses (37) per regional hub to ascertain the number of responses per hub. Most responses came from the Southern region and the least number of responses came from the Northern and Western regions. See Table 1.

Table 1. Description of Respondents.

Names of Country	No. of Responses	Regions
Malawi	6	Southern
Tanzania	2	Southern
South Africa	2	Southern
Mozambique	4	Southern
Ethiopia	5	Central & Eastern
Kenya	3	Central & Eastern
Uganda	1	Central & Eastern
Ghana	4	Western
Togo	3	Western
Tunisia	3	Northern
Mauritania	2	Northern
Morocco	1	Northern
Algeria	1	Northern

After analyzing the responses, they were sorted based on the types of organizations. The findings reveal that 36% (13) were institutes of higher education, 34% (12) were government agencies, and 11% (4) were NGOs. Refer to Figure 1 for a visual representation of the respondents/organizations that participated in the study.

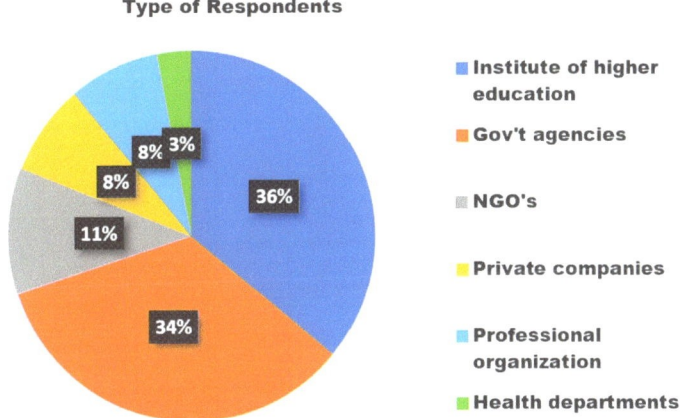

Figure 1. Type of Respondents who participated.

4.2. Capacity Building Activities

We evaluated capacity-building activities and discovered that organizations engage in various types of such activities. These include pre-education, in-service training, and support from external specialists, among others. Although pre-education and in-service training were the most prevalent activities, we observed that "support from specialists outside the organization" was the least employed activity, as shown in Figure 2. We asked the participants why this activity was not widely used, and one manager explained that it involves hiring a specialist, which has financial implications that most organizations cannot afford.

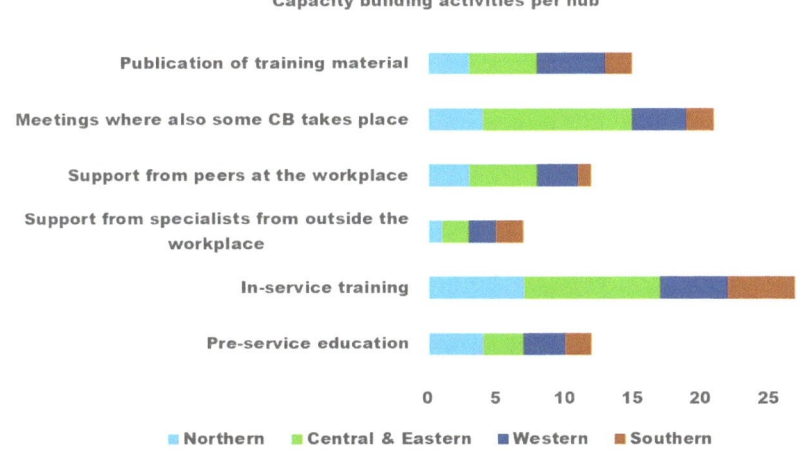

Figure 2. eHealth capacity building activities by hubs.

Gaps in Capacity Building Activities

Though the organizations surveyed had different capacity-building activities, our survey observed some gaps. For instance, the current capacity-building programs do not cater to IT professionals, manager/administrative health personnel, eHealth specialists, and policymakers as shown in Figure 3.

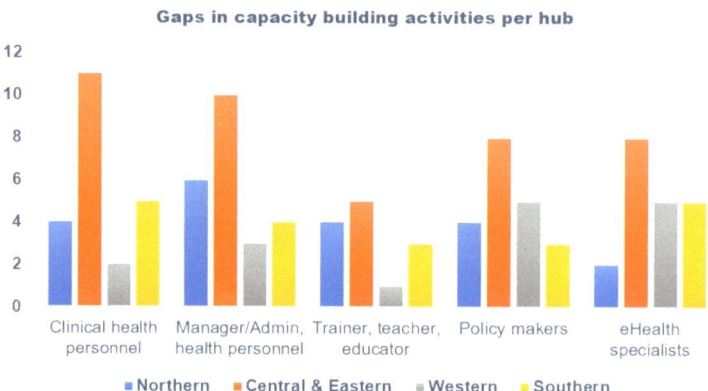

Figure 3. Professional groups targeted for capacity-building activities per hub.

4.3. Factors Hindering eHealth Capacity-Building Activities

The importance of having digital skills is widely recognized, but our survey revealed that there are several challenges that hinder eHealth capacity-building efforts. In this section, the data was further analyzed according to the four geographical regions. The findings revealed that in the Northern hub, infrastructural constraint and lack of motivation were factors hindering eHealth capacity building. While lack of financial support and infrastructural constraint were the most frequent factors that hinder eHealth capacity building in the Southern, Central and Eastern hubs, as illustrated in Figure 4.

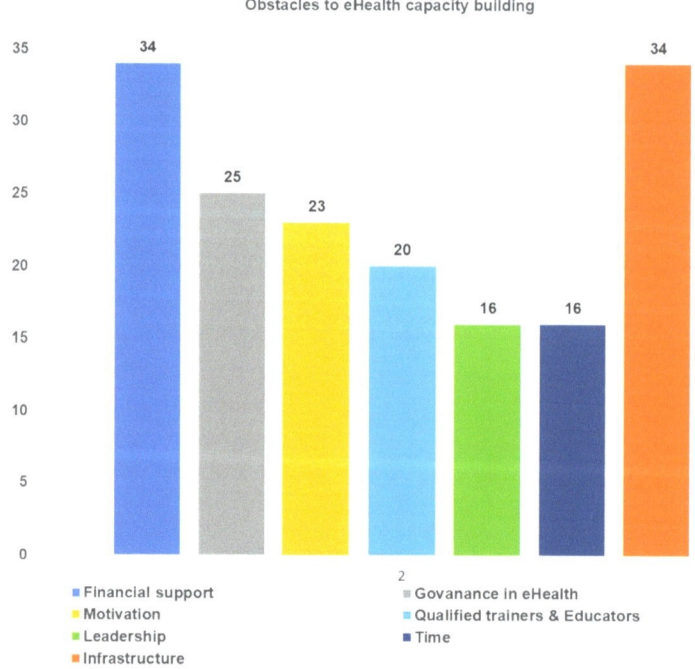

Figure 4. Obstacles to capacity building activities.

4.4. Health Workers' IT Literacy

Regardless of their profession or level of digital expertise, it is widely agreed that possessing eHealth skills will greatly impact an individual's career. IT skills were found to be the most valuable in our study. The data was also analyzed based on income levels of countries, we observed that more individuals in low- and middle-income countries have access to and use smartphones over computers. As a result, more people are becoming proficient in using smartphones, as depicted in Figure 5.

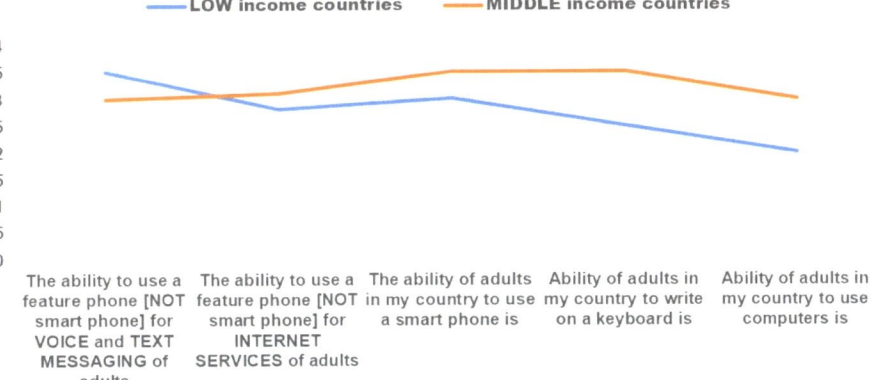

Figure 5. ICT level of the General Public. 1 = very low, 6 = very high.

4.5. Proposed Suggestions to Build ICT Skills of Health Personnel

During the analysis of the interviews, the most frequent recommendations made were to offer ICT in-service training, introduce computer-based systems, and enhance Internet accessibility. Additionally, one respondent highlighted the importance of providing health workers with visual presentation skills, while another emphasized the need for more pre-and in-service training activities. For further suggestions, refer to Figure 6.

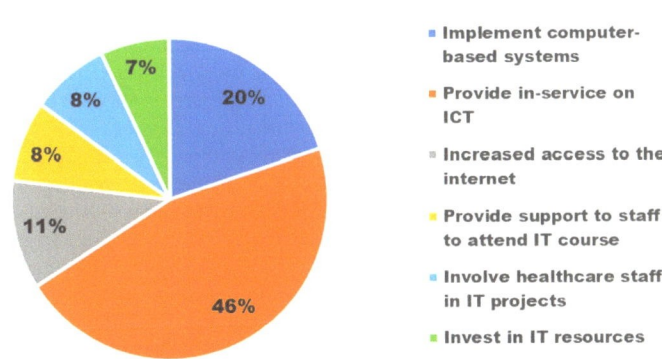

Figure 6. Suggestion to build IT skills of health workers.

5. Discussion

Our research aimed to uncover the challenges faced by healthcare professionals when developing eHealth capacity-building initiatives within the BETTEReHEALTH community. Our findings revealed several factors that hinder the progress of such programs, with the lack of comprehensive eHealth capacity-building policies being a significant obstacle [20].

These policies are essential in creating a shared understanding of eHealth objectives and prioritizing associated efforts [28]. Our study also found that in low- and middle-income countries (LMICs), eHealth policies are often too broad and require more specific delineation of the roles and responsibilities of various stakeholders. For instance, inadequate eHealth policies in Ethiopia and Ghana have resulted in disparities in how the government and research communities implement mHealth activities [40]. For example, mHealth activities are uncoordinated and do not align with national health priorities. As Khoja et al. [41] highlighted, policymakers must take a proactive approach in developing policies that enable seamless and reliable planning of eHealth programs.

Our survey revealed that eHealth training options are diverse, but limited for policymakers, IT professionals, and managers. This supports the findings of a previous study by [35], which highlighted the importance of continuous and practical capacity building for IT specialists and professionals. Our recent online survey also uncovered various obstacles that hinder capacity-building activities, ranging from systemic issues like insufficient infrastructure, low budgets, weak government policies, and poor governance at the national level, to individual barriers such as lack of time, skills, and motivation. Our findings are in line with other researchers who have emphasized the critical role of national eHealth policies in bridging gaps in eHealth activities [19,20,33,42,43]. It's worth noting that while adequate financing is crucial for infrastructure development, technological tools, training workshops, and qualified personnel, it can only be utilized effectively and efficiently with strong policies, political commitment, and good leadership [36].

Our survey has clearly indicated that individuals living in rural areas who have access to smartphones and other technologies tend to develop more IT skills in comparison to those who use computers and keyboards. Our findings support previous studies that highlight the importance of high mobile service penetration in aiding healthcare efforts in areas with limited resources [44]. We emphasize that the skills and knowledge of health personnel are vital, as eHealth tools cannot be effectively utilized without them.

The American Medical Informatics Association advocates for a system-wide approach that integrates digital skills training early in students' education as a compulsory aspect of existing school programs to address skill gaps. As a result, we established a partnership with five universities—Eduardo Mondlane in Mozambique, University of the Western Cape in South Africa, University of Dar Es Salaam in Tanzania, University of Malawi, and University of Gondar in Ethiopia—for the DEDICATED project (BETTEReHEALTH project). We have designed ten eHealth modules that will be taught to undergraduate and postgraduate students at these universities, with the aim of building the capacity of future eHealth professionals [45]. The DEDICATED initiative is in its infancy, but the concept is used at other institutions. The European Health Parliament, for instance, has recommended establishing mandatory customized training programs on digital skills for health professionals. This training should start from the early education phase and extend to professional development programs [45]. Similarly, RAFT uses the same approach to train medical doctors in 15 francophone central and West African countries [19] and capacity building through professional bodies and societies—for example, edX for business. edX is a learning management system (LMS) offering learning solutions that align with the growth objectives of every staff member within an organization. LMS platform offers a simple and efficient set-up process with advanced real-time learning opportunities. Our research has shown that local capacity-building initiatives are effective strategies to develop skilled healthcare staff [9]. In addition, we strongly recommend that educational curricula for health personnel should also include eHealth skills training. While training is essential, it can only succeed with solid eHealth policies and committed leaders.

6. Conclusions

The healthcare industry is characterized by constant evolution, necessitating professionals who can adapt to its changing demands. Nonetheless, for eHealth education and training services to be fully effective, it is crucial to have adequate funding, infrastructure, leadership, governance, and qualified human resources at all levels of the health system. Despite the potential advantages of integrating eHealth services, many low- and middle-income countries (LMICs) face numerous obstacles. Our research underscores the importance of providing healthcare professionals with eHealth skills that are context-specific and tailored to diverse groups. By addressing the challenges facing eHealth capacity building, we can improve health service delivery and contribute to realizing universal health coverage (UHC). Our study offers valuable insights into eHealth capacity building and innovation promotion initiatives for public health and healthcare professionals, adding to the ongoing conversation on promoting innovation and building eHealth capacity. While the data is based on a relatively small sample of 37 respondents from 15 African countries, the findings raise broader issues relevant to implementing eHealth in resource-constrained settings. It is important to note that the study had some limitations, but we took steps to enhance its validity. We ensured that the data collection method was appropriate, and that the questionnaire was clear, concise, and reviewed by project managers. Additionally, we pilot-tested the questionnaire to avoid ambiguity. The survey respondents were managers, and their in-depth knowledge of the subject lends weight to our results. Furthermore, we collected the data systematically and rigorously, enhancing the study's validity and reliability. It is worth noting that the results only reflect the perspective of the organizations and cannot be applied to the larger population. While future studies with a larger sample size would yield more comprehensive results, our findings are consistent with previous research.

Author Contributions: J.J.K. developed the survey and collected the data; F.N.A. analyzed the data, writing–original draft preparation; J.J.K. and F.N.A. writing–review and editing. All authors have read and agreed to the published version of the manuscript.

Funding: The project was funded by the European Union's Horizon 2020 program under grant agreement No. 101017450 (https://betterehealth.eu/, accessed on 27 September 2023).

Institutional Review Board Statement: The study was performed in accordance with the Declaration of Helsinki. Informed consent was obtained from all participating subjects.

Informed Consent Statement: Informed consent from the participants was obtained by BETTEReHEALTH regional hub managers from the various hubs as part of the project.

Data Availability Statement: The datasets used and analyzed during the current study are available from the corresponding authors on reasonable request.

Acknowledgments: We are grateful to the BETTEReHEALTH Consortium members and partners who participated in the online survey.

Conflicts of Interest: The authors declare no conflict of interest.

References

1. Labrique, A.B.; Wadhwani, C.; Williams, K.A.; Lamptey, P.; Hesp, C.; Luk, R.; Aerts, A. Best practices in scaling digital health in low and middle income countries. *Glob. Health* **2018**, *14*, 103. [CrossRef] [PubMed]
2. World Health Organization. *Fifty-Eighth World Health Assembly, Geneva, 16–25 May 2005: Resolutions and Decisions, Annex [Internet]*; WHO: Geneva, Switzerland, 2005; Available online: https://apps.who.int/iris/handle/10665/20398 (accessed on 20 July 2022).
3. WHO. *Global Strategy on Digital Health 2020–2025*; WHO: Geneva, Switzerland, 2021.
4. Manyazewal, T.; Woldeamanuel, Y.; Blumberg, H.M.; Fekadu, A.; Marconi, V.C. The potential use of digital health technologies in the African context: A systematic review of evidence from Ethiopia. *NPJ Digit. Med.* **2021**, *4*, 125. [CrossRef] [PubMed]
5. Asah, F.N.; Kaasbøll, J.J.; Anthun, K.S. Obstacles of eHealth Capacity Building and Innovation Promotion Initiative in African Countries. *Stud. Health Technol. Inform.* **2022**, *299*, 33–43. [PubMed]
6. Eysenbach, G. What is e-health? *J. Med. Internet Res.* **2001**, *3*, e833. [CrossRef]
7. World Health Organization. *Global Action Plan on Physical Activity 2018–2030: More Active People for a Healthier World*; World Health Organization: Geneva, Switzerland, 2019.
8. Kluge, E.-H.W. (Ed.) Chapter 5—Framework considerations. In *Electron Health Rec [Internet]*; Academic Press: Cambridge, MA, USA, 2020; pp. 105–133. Available online: https://www.sciencedirect.com/science/article/pii/B9780128220450000058 (accessed on 3 January 2023).

9. Koivu, A.; Mavengere, N.; Ruohonen, M.J.; Hederman, L.; Grimson, J. Exploring the Information and ICT Skills of Health Professionals in Low- and Middle-Income Countries. In Proceedings of the IFIP TC 3 International Conference on Stakeholders and Information Technology in Education: SaITE 2016, Guimarães, Portugal, 5–8 July 2016; Revised Selected Papers 1. Brinda, T., Mavengere, N., Haukijärvi, I., Lewin, C., Passey, D., Eds.; Springer International Publishing: Cham, Switzerland, 2016; pp. 152–162.
10. Vishwanath, A.; Scamurra, S.D. Barriers to the adoption of electronic health records: Using concept mapping to develop a comprehensive empirical model. *Health Inform. J.* **2007**, *13*, 119–134. [CrossRef]
11. Mehl, G.L.; Tamrat, T.; Bhardwaj, S.; Blaschke, S.; Labrique, A. Digital health vision: Could MomConnect provide a pragmatic starting point for achieving universal health coverage in South Africa and elsewhere? *BMJ Glob. Health* **2018**, *3*, e000626. [CrossRef]
12. Al-Shorbaji, N. Improving Healthcare Access through Digital Health: The Use of Information and Communication Technologies [Internet]. *Healthc. Access. IntechOpen* **2021**. Available online: https://www.intechopen.com/chapters/undefined/state.item.id (accessed on 14 July 2022).
13. Kraus, S.; Schiavone, F.; Pluzhnikova, A.; Invernizzi, A.C. Digital transformation in healthcare: Analyzing the current state-of-research. *J. Bus. Res.* **2021**, *123*, 557–567. [CrossRef]
14. World Health Organization. *Seventh Meeting of the European Health Information Initiative Steering Group: Copenhagen, Denmark, 21–22 March 2017*; World Health Organization, Regional Office for Europe: Geneva, Switzerland, 2017.
15. van Gemert-Pijnen, J.E.; Wynchank, S.; Covvey, H.D.; Ossebaard, H.C. Improving the credibility of electronic health technologies. *Bull. World Health Organ.* **2012**, *1*, 323–323A. [CrossRef]
16. Hamad, W.B. CURRENT Position and Challenges of E-health in Tanzania: A review of literature. *Glob. Sci. J.* **2019**, *7*, 14.
17. Anderson, J.G. Social, ethical and legal barriers to e-health. *Int. J. Med. Inf.* **2007**, *76*, 480–483.
18. Asah, F.N. *Challenges and Approaches of Implementing Standard Health Indicators in Hierarchical Organizations: A Multisited Study*; The University of Oslo: Oslo, Norway, 2021.
19. Mars, M. Building the capacity to build capacity in e-health in sub-Saharan Africa: The KwaZulu-Natal experience. *Telemed. E-Health* **2012**, *18*, 32–37. [CrossRef] [PubMed]
20. Mars, M.; Scott, R.E. Global e-health policy: A work in progress. *Health Aff.* **2010**, *29*, 237–243. [CrossRef] [PubMed]
21. Adebesin, F.; Kotzé, P.; Van Greunen, D.; Foster, R. Barriers & Challenges to the Adoption of E-Health Standards in Africa. In Proceedings of the Health Informatics South Africa Conference (HISA), Port Elizabeth, South Africa, 3–5 July 2013.
22. Stiawan, D. Interoperability framework for integrated e-health services. *Bull. Electr. Eng. Inform.* **2020**, *9*, 354–361.
23. Sluijs, M.; Veeken, H.; Overbeke, A. Deficient information in developing countries: Internet alone is no solution. *Ned. Tijdschr. Geneeskd.* **2006**, *150*, 1351–1354.
24. Masud, M.; Hossain, S.; Alamri, A. Data Interoperability and Multimedia Content Management in e-Health Systems. *IEEE Trans. Inf. Technol. Biomed.* **2012**, *16*, 1015–1023. [CrossRef]
25. Ahern, D.K.; Kreslake, J.M.; Phalen, J.M. What is eHealth (6): Perspectives on the evolution of eHealth research. *J. Med. Internet Res.* **2006**, *8*, e490. [CrossRef]
26. Mburu, S.; Kamau, O. Framework for Development and Implementation of Digital Health Policies to Accelerate the Attainment of Sustainable Development Goals: Case of Kenya eHealth Policy (2016–2030). *J. Health Inform. Afr.* **2018**, *5*, 32–38. [CrossRef]
27. Luna, D.; Almerares, A.; Mayan, J.C.; de Quirós, F.G.B.; Otero, C. Health informatics in developing countries: Going beyond pilot practices to sustainable implementations: A review of the current challenges. *Healthc. Inform. Res.* **2014**, *20*, 3–10. [CrossRef]
28. Larbi, D.; Anthun, K.S.; Asah, F.N.; Debrah, O.; Antypas, K. Assessing Strategic Priority Factors in eHealth Policies of Four African Countries. In Proceedings of the 2022 IST-Africa Conference (IST-Africa), Virtual, 16–20 May 2022; pp. 1–9.
29. Jamil, S. From digital divide to digital inclusion: Challenges for wide-ranging digitalization in Pakistan. *Telecommun. Policy* **2021**, *45*, 102206. [CrossRef]
30. Staton, R.; Bautista, A.; Harwell, J.; Jensen, L.; Minister, A.; Roller, S. Computerized provider order entry awareness for nursing: Unintended consequences and remediation plan. *CIN Comput. Inform. Nurs.* **2013**, *31*, 401–405. [CrossRef] [PubMed]
31. Alshahrani, A.; Stewart, D.; MacLure, K. A systematic review of the adoption and acceptance of eHealth in Saudi Arabia: Views of multiple stakeholders. *Int. J. Med. Inf.* **2019**, *128*, 7–17. [CrossRef] [PubMed]
32. Asangansi Macleod, B.; Meremikwu, M. Improving the routine HMIS in Nigeria through mobile technology for community data collection. *J. Health Inform. Dev. Ctries.* **2013**, *7*, 76–87.
33. Qureshi, Q.A.; Shah, B.; Najeebullah; Kundi, G.M.; Nawaz, A.; Miankhel, A.K.; Chishti, K.A.; Qureshi, N.A. Infrastructural barriers to e-health implementation in developing countries. *Eur. J. Sustain. Dev.* **2013**, *2*, 163.
34. Cardellino, P.; Finch, E. Evidence of systematic approaches to innovation in facilities management. *J. Facil. Manag.* **2006**, *4*, 150–166. [CrossRef]
35. Steen, L.; Mao, X. Digital Skills for Health Professionals. 2016, pp. 37–47. Available online: https://www.researchgate.net/publication/311271370_Digital_skills_for_health_professionals#fullTextFileContent (accessed on 10 July 2023).
36. Detmer, D.E. Capacity Building in E-Health and Health Informatics: A Review of the Global Vision and Informatics Educational Initiatives of the American Medical Informatics Association. 2010. Available online: https://www.thieme-connect.com/products/ejournals/pdf/10.1055/s-0038-1638698.pdf (accessed on 10 July 2023).
37. Shegaw, A.M. Analysing the Challenges of IS implementation in public health institutions of a developing country: The need for flexible strategies. *J. Health Inform. Dev. Ctries.* **2010**, *4*, 1–17.

38. Tchao, E.T.; Acquah, I.; Kotey, S.D.; Aggor, C.S.; Kponyo, J.J. On Telemedicine Implementations in Ghana. *Int. J. Adv. Comput. Sci. Appl.* **2019**, *10*, 193–201. [CrossRef]
39. Curioso, W.H. Building Capacity and Training for Digital Health: Challenges and Opportunities in Latin America. *J. Med. Internet Res.* **2019**, *21*, e16513. [CrossRef]
40. Mengiste, S.A.; Antypas, K.; Johannessen, M.R.; Klein, J.; Kazemi, G.; Kassbøll, J. Research Landscape and Research Priorities in eHealth in four African Countries-A survey. *EGOV-CeDEM-EPart* **2022**, *2022*, 130.
41. Khoja, S.; Durrani, H.; Nayani, P.; Fahim, A. Scope of policy issues in eHealth: Results from a structured literature review. *J. Med. Internet Res.* **2012**, *14*, e1633. [CrossRef]
42. Omary, Z.; Lupiana, D.; Mtenzi, F.; Wu, B. Analysis of the challenges affecting e-healthcare adoption in developing countries: A case of Tanzania. *Int. J. Inf. Stud.* **2010**, *2*, 38–50.
43. Vatsalan, D.; Arunatileka, S.; Chapman, K.; Senaviratne, G.; Sudahar, S.; Wijetileka, D.; Wickramasinghe, Y. Mobile technologies for enhancing eHealth solutions in developing countries. In Proceedings of the 2010 Second International Conference on eHealth, Telemedicine, and Social Medicine, Saint Maarten, Netherlands Antilles, 10–16 February 2010; pp. 84–89.
44. DEDICATED Project 2020. Available online: https://www.mn.uio/hisp/english. (accessed on 9 July 2022).
45. European Health Parliament. Digital Skills for Health Professionals. 2016. Available online: https://www.healthparliament.eu/wp-content/uploads/2017/09/Digital-skills-for-health-professionals.pdf (accessed on 9 September 2023).

Disclaimer/Publisher's Note: The statements, opinions and data contained in all publications are solely those of the individual author(s) and contributor(s) and not of MDPI and/or the editor(s). MDPI and/or the editor(s) disclaim responsibility for any injury to people or property resulting from any ideas, methods, instructions or products referred to in the content.

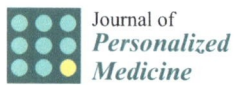

Article

Transforming Ontology Web Language Elements into Common Terminology Service 2 Terminology Resources

Sara Mora [1,†], Roberta Gazzarata [2,†], Bernd Blobel [3], Ylenia Murgia [4] and Mauro Giacomini [4,*]

1. UO Information and Communication Technologies, Istituto di Ricovero e Cura a Carattere Scientifico Ospedale Policlinico San Martino, 16132 Genoa, Italy; sara.mora@hsanmartino.it
2. Healthropy Società a Responsabilità Limitata (S.R.L.), 17100 Savona, Italy; roberta.gazzarata@healthropy.it
3. Medical Faculty, University of Regensburg, 93053 Regensburg, Germany; bernd.blobel@klinik.uni-regensburg.de
4. Department of Informatics, Bioengineering, Robotics and System Engineering (DIBRIS), University of Genoa, 16145 Genova, Italy; ylenia.murgia@edu.unige.it
* Correspondence: mauro.giacomini@unige.it; Tel.: +39-010-353-6546
† These authors contributed equally to this work.

Abstract: Communication and cooperation are fundamental for the correct deployment of P5 medicine, and this can be achieved only by correct comprehension of semantics so that it can aspire to medical knowledge sharing. There is a hierarchy in the operations that need to be performed to achieve this goal that brings to the forefront the complete understanding of the real-world business system by domain experts using Domain Ontologies, and only in the last instance acknowledges the specific transformation at the pure information and communication technology level. A specific feature that should be maintained during such types of transformations is versioning that aims to record the evolution of meanings in time as well as the management of their historical evolution. The main tool used to represent ontology in computing environments is the Ontology Web Language (OWL), but it was not created for managing the evolution of meanings in time. Therefore, we tried, in this paper, to find a way to use the specific features of Common Terminology Service—Release 2 (CTS2) to perform consistent and validated transformations of ontologies written in OWL. The specific use case managed in the paper is the Alzheimer's Disease Ontology (ADO). We were able to consider all of the elements of ADO and map them with CTS2 terminological resources, except for a subset of elements such as the equivalent class derived from restrictions on other classes.

Keywords: ontology; CTS2; semantic interoperability; terminology resources; biomedical field

Citation: Mora, S.; Gazzarata, R.; Blobel, B.; Murgia, Y.; Giacomini, M. Transforming Ontology Web Language Elements into Common Terminology Service 2 Terminology Resources. *J. Pers. Med.* **2024**, *14*, 676. https://doi.org/10.3390/jpm14070676

Academic Editor: Salvatore Scacco

Received: 26 March 2024
Revised: 17 June 2024
Accepted: 21 June 2024
Published: 24 June 2024

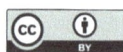

Copyright: © 2024 by the authors. Licensee MDPI, Basel, Switzerland. This article is an open access article distributed under the terms and conditions of the Creative Commons Attribution (CC BY) license (https://creativecommons.org/licenses/by/4.0/).

1. Introduction

The paper at hand presents an extended version of the invited paper provided to the pHealth 2022 conference [1].

Healthcare systems are currently undergoing a transformation towards integrated, interoperable, knowledge-based, policy-driven, highly dynamic, and fully distributed ecosystems according to the personalized, preventive, predictive, participative precision (P5) medicine paradigm [2]. This requires communication and cooperation of actors from multiple disciplines with specific perspectives, contexts, objectives, using their special methodologies, languages, knowledge, and skills. The challenge of P5 medicine ecosystems is the proper representation, mapping, and matching of their domain-specific knowledge. This knowledge representation, mapping, and matching must be performed at any representation level from the real-world business system through the related IT system viewpoints, the information to represent them, and, finally, the data used, deploying more and more constrained languages from natural languages up to computational ones. Thereby, mapping between the system's components from the perspective of different domains or different viewpoints can only be performed at a horizontal level, i.e., at the same level of granularity. To get there, components must be specialized or generalized, respectively. The corresponding representation of system-theoretical, architecture-centric, ontology-based, policy-driven multi-domain P5 ecosystems, standardized in ISO 23903 [3], is shown in Figure 1. Thereby, the Information and Communication Technology (ICT) system development process according to the ISO/IEC 10746 Reference Model Open Distributed Processing [4], just representing the five viewpoints, Enterprise Viewpoint (VP), Information VP, Computational VP, Engineering VP, and Technology VP, must be extended by the Business VP. The Business VP is an inevitable starting point for representing the real-world system and defining the requirements and objectives of the ICT system to be developed from the perspective of the involved domains experts.

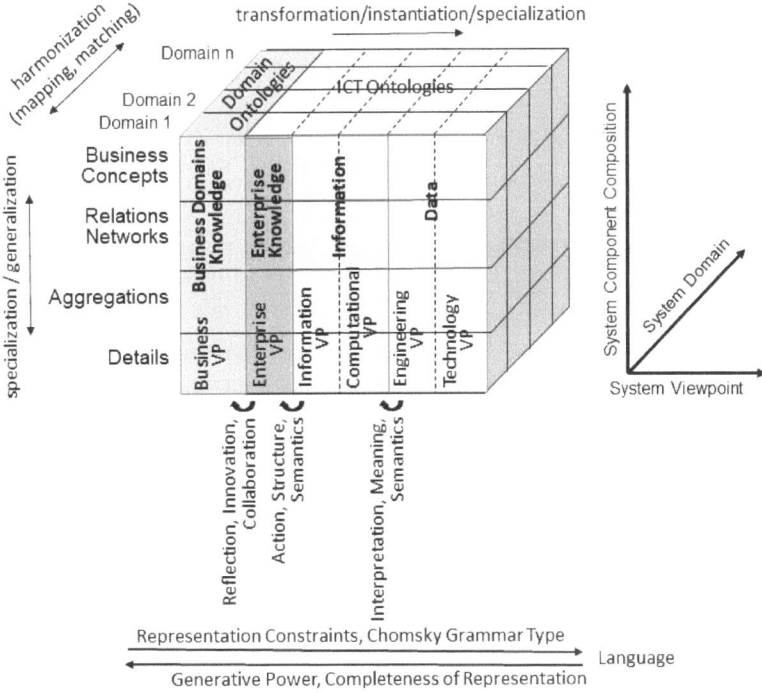

Figure 1. Model and framework for representing multi-domain, knowledge-based, ontology-based, and policy-driven ecosystems.

While, from an ICT system development-process perspective, the transformation into the viewpoint-specific representation style is clearly defined in the aforementioned standard ISO/IEC 10746 [4]. The correct and consistent concept transformation in knowledge-driven transformed health systems is a challenge to be addressed in this paper. Thereby, we have to solve the mapping between domains represented by domain ontologies and the representational transformation of the corresponding concepts between different viewpoints. Examples for the data view representation are database management system schemas or coding systems regarding the semantical representation, terminologies, thesauri, taxonomies, glossaries, data dictionaries, or vocabularies used. The aforementioned semantical resources are collections of terms (entities) that are linked to a specific domain. They aim at creating a complete documentation that supports the correct usage of such terms.

While the domain ontologies representing the concepts of the Business VP usually deploy natural languages, the ICT VPs must be represented by more expressive, computational logic-based languages to be exploited in computing environments. The W3C Web Ontology Language OWL [5] is such a computational logic-based language that can be used to express knowledge and verify the consistency of that knowledge or to make implicit knowledge explicit [6].

Although there are many examples of transforming ontology resources (such as OWL) into other types of languages [7–9], the authors are not aware of any tools for organizing OWL resources using the methodology suggested by Common Terminology Service Release 2 (CTS2). This choice was made by the authors in order, on the one hand, to be able to use all of the features of ontologies encoded rigorously in OWL and, on the other hand, to be able to manage their temporal evolution through the standardized tools provided by CTS2. The need to follow the temporal evolution of said ontologies is obvious when considering ontologies defined in medical fields for which updating is rather frequent [10–12].

The Common Terminology Standard Version 2 (CTS2) is a HL7/OMG specification providing a generic class model and necessary interfaces for managing and sharing terminologies and ontologies by using web services. It is based on a conceptual model representing data by class models and a functional model specifying the terminology server services. The standard is distributed through the HL7 Service Functional Model (SFM) and the Object Management Group (OMG) Service Technical Model (STM), which provide both service interface specification at a functional level and technical requirements of the service. In the present paper, we use the OMG model [13].

Finally, we aimed at developing a web-based user interface that allows for the visualization and management of the terminological content of an ontology. This has been achieved using, in a standard way, functions defined using CTS2.

2. Materials and Methods

The purpose of this paper is to present in detail all of the choices we made to transform an ontology into CTS2 terminology resources. Therefore, a deep analysis of the key aspects, similarities, and differences of the two representations was performed.

2.1. Ontology Elements and Relations

An ontology is a formal explicit specification of a shared conceptualization of a domain of interest [14,15]. One widely used tool to represent ontologies within the computer science environment is the Web Ontology Language (OWL) defined by W3C [16] that is an extension of Resource Description Framework (RDF) [17] to support the definition of the semantic web. RDF is formed by two parts, as follows: the RDF model and syntax, which represents the model structure and describes the syntax, and the RDF Schema (RDFS), which describes the syntax to define the schema and vocabularies for the metadata. RDF and RDFS are used by the Simple Knowledge Organization System (SKOS) language family, created to represent glossaries, classifications, or structured vocabularies for publication purposes.

Some examples of relevant medical ontologies representing different domains are as follows: Human Phenotype Ontology (HPO) [18], Infectious Diseases Ontology (IDO) [19], and Epilepsy and Seizures Ontology (EPSO) [20]. For mapping different domain ontologies, the ISO/IEC 21838 Top-level ontologies (TLO) standard should be used [21]. In cases where a domain ontology is not available, the domain can be preliminary presented using that TLO. Within an ontology, the various objects are defined and interact with each other according to logical properties, reciprocal restrictions between and on objects, and groups and semantic sets. An ontology is characterized by three main components, as listed below.

- **Class:** Every single object belonging to the domain.
- **Annotation Properties:** Further information purely attributable to the Class itself, independent of the others. Examples of annotation properties are synonym, comment, and label.
- **Object Properties:** A restriction, which places a limit on the values of a certain Class that respects a certain Property. In most cases, the considered Property is defined within the ontology, and so its logical value scope only within it.

The interactions between the classes are defined by specific constructs called class axioms. For example, the rdfs: subClassOf construct, defined within the RDF schema and inherited by OWL, allows us to define the hierarchical relations as follows: if a Class C1 is defined as a subClassOf of another Class C2, then the set of elements that make up C1 they must at least be a subset of those that make up C2. A Class is therefore, by definition, a subClass of itself, as the subset can also be the whole set.

Another class axioms is the owl:equivalentClass construct, which indicates that the set of elements of Class C1 are equivalent to those of Class C2. Therefore, the two sets must have exactly the same number and the same elements.

2.2. CTS2 Terminology Resources and Profiles

The main CTS2 terminology resources involved in this process are as follows: CodeSystem, CodeSystemVersion, EntityDescription, Map, MapVersion, and MapEntry (Figure 2).

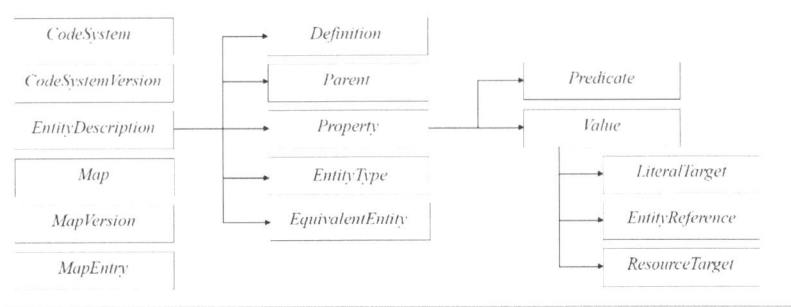

Figure 2. The CTS2 terminology resources and the detail of the EntityDescription elements considered in this paper.

A **CodeSystem** can be a classification system, a code system, an ontology, or a thesaurus, etc. Together with some identifying information such as the name, it includes information about the publisher, release cycles, purpose, etc. However, as this kind of terminological resources may evolve over time, it is necessary to manage the versioning option. Therefore, to each CodeSystem may correspond one or more **CodeSystemVersions** containing information about release date, release format, contact information, etc. Then, each CodeSystemVersion contains one or more **EntityDescriptions** describing a class, a role, or an individual from the specific CodeSystemVersion.

The EntityDescription is the most complex but also the most interesting item to investigate. During the translation process, to maintain the characteristics of the specific element of the ontology, it was necessary to include different metadata. Among others, we considered the following (Figure 2):

- **Definition:** An explanation of the intended meaning of a concept. An EntityDescription may have multiple definitions, each derived from a different source, represented in a different language or having a different purpose.
- **Parent:** The set of direct "parents" defined in the same CodeSystemVersion. It is the responsibility of the service to determine what predicate(s) represent "parent/child" relationships.
- **Property:** Additional "non-semantic" (annotation) assertions about the entity being described that do not fit into the other categories.
- **EntityType:** The set of type(s) a resource can take, and it should include owl:Class, owl:Individual, rdf:Property, or skos:Concept, although it may carry many other types as well.
- **EquivalentEntity:** An entity that has been determined to be equivalent to the about entity in the context.

The element we mainly focused on is **Property** and its two main components are as follows:

- **Predicate:** The name or URI of the property predicate. It can be literal or an EntityDescription itself, namely, an Annotation Property or an Object Property.
- **Value:** The target(s) of the property. Note that this can only represent the literal format of the property. The details about the original property will be found in the *CorrespondingStatement* if the CTS2 implementation supports the statement profile. So, the attribute value of a property is of Class *StatementTarget*, and it can be from three of the following types:
    ○ Literal Target: When the statement type is LITERAL. It can be used for properties like the entity "label" or "comment".
    ○ Entity Reference Target: The URI and optional namespace/name when the target type is ENTITY. It can be used when a property refers to another entity.
    ○ Resource Target: When the statement type is RESOURCE.

An entity may have more than one value for the same predicate, so it is necessary to create a list of *StatementTargets* containing all the items and then assign the list to *Property.Value*, while *Property.Predicate* remains unchanged.

Finally, it could be necessary to link resources across CodeSystems and CodeSystemVersions. To this aim, the CTS2 standard provides the following three terminology resources: Map, MapVersion, and MapEntry. A **Map** is a collection of rules necessary to transform entities of a CodeSystem into others represented in a second one. It also includes information about creators, intended use, CodeSystem involved, etc. As mentioned previously, it is necessary to deal with changes over time in the terminological resource. Therefore, it is possible to identify a specific version of the Map, called **MapVersion**. Then, to each MapVersion, correspond one or more MapEntries, i.e., the definition of a set of rules identifying how a single Entity that belongs to the original CodeSystemVersion maps onto null, one, or more target Entities that belong to the destination CodeSystemVersion.

The CTS2 standard defines, for each terminology, resources (also known as structural profiles) and different functional profiles. The most important ones for this paper are the following: Read, Query, Update, and Maintenance (which has the capability to create resources). The CTS2 specification defines the implementation of a specific server for each couple of structural profile/functional profile (for example, CodeSystem Catalog Maintenance).

2.3. Translation Process Pipeline

The ontology that we considered testing our mapping system on was the Alzheimer's Disease Ontology (ADO) [22], a knowledge-based ontology which encompasses concepts related to Alzheimer'S Disease. In order to show how an ontology can be mapped with another terminology using CTS2, the Analitica Avanzata su Dati Complessi (ADA Lab), a more general ontology, was used to model relations in a complex and interdisciplinary environment [23].

The pipeline of the translation process is composed by the following main steps.

Create CodeSystem (I) using the CodeSystem Catalog Maintenance Service functional profile. Within this phase, we provided the following input parameters: *Uniform Resource Identifier* (URI), i.e., an external link of the resource; and *Name*, i.e., the identifier of the catalog that we want to create, to use locally (Enterprise VP).

Create CodeSystemVersion (II) using the CodeSystemVersion Catalog Maintenance Service. Equally to the CodeSystem, one of the input parameters is *Name*, which uniquely identifies the specific version in the CodeSystem. The other input parameter that we considered is *VersionOf*, which contains the name or URI of the CodeSystem that the version belongs to (Information VP).

Create EntityDescription (III) using the Entity Description Maintenance Service. For each entity, we set two important input parameters, as follows: *EntityID*, i.e., the entity code and/or namespace identifier; and DescribingCodeSystemVersion, which contains the URI or local identifier of the CodeSystemVersion this entity belongs to (Computational VP).

Update EntityDescription (IV) using the Entity Description Maintenance Service. We completed each entity with all of the information linked to the single ontology class or property.

In general, the components of an ontology resource can be distinguished in the following:
(i) the components directly mappable into an element of the CTS2 EntityDescription, as
displayed in Table 1; (ii) the components that could not fit into any predefined item, but
which can be mapped into properties, as displayed in Table 2; and (iii) the components that
could not fit into any predefined item, but which can be mapped into a CTS2 terminology
resource, i.e., the properties devoted to Map elements among ontologies and/or other
coding systems (Engineering VP).

Table 1. Correspondence between elements of an ontology class that can be directly mapped to the
CTS2 EntityDescription components.

Ontology Concept Metadata	CTS2 Resource Metadata	Data Type
Example	.Example	List (0...N)
IsDefinedBy	.Definition	List (0...N)
SubClassOf	.Parent	Class (1...N)
EquivalentClass	.EquivalentEntity	Class (0...N)

Table 2. Four cases to which all of the elements of an ontology class/property not contained in Table 1
can belong to, as follows: (a) the predicate is a text and the value is a text, (b) the predicate is a text
and the value is an entity, (c) the predicate is an entity and the value is a text, and (d) the predicate is
an entity and the value is an entity.

	Value Is a Text	Value Is an Entity
Predicate is a text	The **predicate** contains the name and namespace of the statement predicate (*type: EntityNameOrURI*). The **value** element is a statement target of type LITERAL (*type: Opaque-Data*).	The **predicate** contains the name and namespace of the statement predicate (*type: EntityName-OrURI*). The **value** element is a statement target of type ENTITY (*type: EntityNameOrURI*).
Predicate is an Entity	The **predicate** contains the URI of the entity of type Annotation Property (*type: EntityNameOrURI*). The **value** element is a statement target of type LITERAL (*type: Opaque-Data*).	The **predicate** contains the URI of the entity of type Object Property (*type: EntityNameOrURI*). The **value** element is a statement target of type ENTITY (*type: Entity-NameOrURI*).

Create MapCatalogEntry (V) using the Map Catalog Maintenance Service. We provided
the following input parameters: *MapName*, i.e., the name the new entry will be known as
within a local context; *FromCodeSystem*, i.e., the name or URI of the CodeSystem that the
"from" entities belong to; and *ToCodeSystem*, i.e., the name or URI of the CodeSystem that
the "to" entities belong to.

Create MapVersion (VI) using the Map Version Maintenance Service. The considered
input parameters are as follows: *MapVersionURI*, i.e., the state of the resource version which
can be "OPEN" or "FINAL", and once the MapVersion is finalized it becomes immutable;
MapVersioneName, i.e., an identifier to uniquely identify the MapVersion in a local context;
FromCodeSystemVersion, i.e., the identifier (name or URI) of the specific CodeSystemVersion
that the "from" entities belong to; and *ToCodeSystemVersion*, i.e., the identifier (name or
URI) of the specific CodeSystemVersion that the "to" entities belong to.

Create MapEntry (VII) using the Map Entry Maintenance Service. This is a set of mappings
having the same entity identifier as *MapFrom*.

Update MapEntry (VIII) using the Map Entry Maintenance Service. After we defined the
entity of the "FROM" side, it is necessary to define one or more entities on the "TO" side,
e.g., ones belonging to other CodeSystems. To perform that, the following two operations
need to be executed.

Add MapSet (VIII.i). Specifically, each MapEntry may contain one or more MapSets, defining rules and characteristics of the Map. Considering each Mapset, it is necessary to perform the function below.

Add MapTarget (VIII.ii). In detail, the item MapTarget identifies the entity to include it in the Map on the "TO" side.

3. Results

The architecture that we used to develop the transformation of a semantical resource from an OWL standard format to a CTS2 standard resource allows the user to visualize and manage the terminological content of an ontology, and is formed by the following three components: a CTS2-compliant service, a ASP.NET Console Application (.NET Framework), and a ASP.NET Web Application (.NET Framework).

The CTS2-compliant service is represented by HQuantum© Technology Service (HTS) powered by Healthropy s.r.l. [24,25]. In this way, HTS provides a standard interface to access to read, query, and manage terminological content into the database where the ontology has been stored. The ASP.NET Console Application (.NET Framework) is a client of HTS and was implemented to allow for the first import of an OWL ontology into the HTS, as was made for the Alzheimer's Disease Ontology (ADO). In fact, this application was used to create the CodeSystem "ADO" (by calling CTS2 operation Code System Catalog Maintenance Service/CreateCodeSystem) and its first version "ADPV1" (by calling CTS2 operation Code System Version Catalog Maintenance Service/CreateCodeSystemVersion) and each EntityDescription. In detail, the application opens the XML, which contains the ontology, and, for each OWL class, converts it to the corresponding CTS2 EntityDescription, creates it in HTS (by calling CTS2 operation Entity Description Catalog Maintenance Service/CreateEntityDescription), and updates it by indicating all of the needed EntityDescription elements, as described in Section 2 (by calling CTS2 operation Entity Description Catalog Maintenance Service/UpdateEntityDescription). In Figure 3 is represented an example of the OWL class "Behavioral_therapies", defined in the ADO. Following the same process, also, the "AdaLab" CodeSystam, its first version "AdaLab1", and some EntityDescriptions were uploaded in HTS.

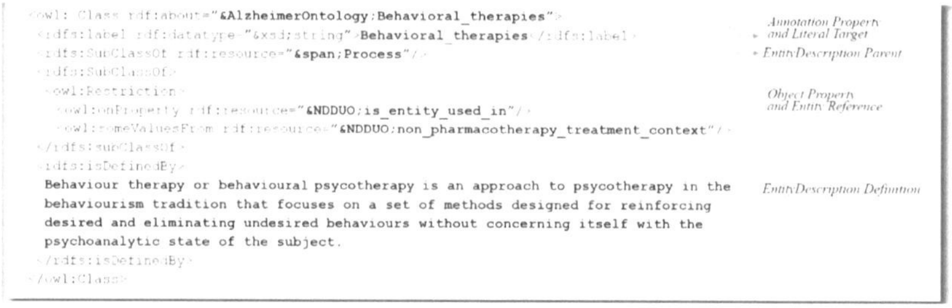

Figure 3. An example of an OWL class defined in ADO, with an indication of the corresponding CTS2 EntityDescription element in which every OWL element can be mapped.

The Console Application was adopted to store, in HTS, some examples of maps between the entities of "ADOV1" and "AdaLab1" available in an Excel spreadsheet which contains two rows: one for the EndityDesctiption source (i.e., the entity defined in ADOV1), and another one for the EndityDesctiption target (i.e., the entity defined in AdaLab1). In fact, this application was used to create the MapCatalogEntry "FromADOToAdaLab" (by calling CTS2 operation Map Catalog Maintenance Service/createMapCatalogEntry) and its first version "FromADOV1ToAdaLab1" (by calling CTS2 operation Map Version Maintenance Service/CreatemapVersion) and each MapEntry. In detail, the application opens the Excel spreadsheet, which contains the maps, and for each row, converts it to the corresponding MapEntry, creates it in HTS by indicating the entity source (by calling

CTS2 operation Map Entry Maintenance Service/CreateMapEntry), and updates it by indicating the entity target, as indicated in Section 2 (by calling CTS2 operations Map Entry Maintenance Service/addMapSet and AddMapTarget).

Once an ontology is created in HTS, it is available to the user through the ASP.NET Web Application (.NET Framework), which, after login, can access four main sections for each CodeSystem: Read, Query, Maintenance, and Map.

The Read section of the web application allows the user to browse all of the entities stored within the HTS, both classes and properties, through a tree-view visualization or a term search. The tree view presents the concepts following the hierarchical organization in the ontology through the CTS2 EntityDescription elements Parent or Children. To fill the elements of this web object, the application interacts with HTS by calling the CTS2 operations provided by the Entity Description Read Service. By clicking on an element of the tree view, it is possible to obtain all of the related details. In Figure 4, there is presented an extract of the EntityDescription, which corresponds to "Behavioral therapies" defined in the ADOV1, and is contained in the SOAP message intercepted as a response of the read operation of the Entity Description Read Service. In the details are represented the CTS2 elements that correspond to the OWL elements reported in Figure 3. Figure 5 represents the tree view and the details for the same entity, "Behavioral therapies". It is possible to see, in "Term Info", the OWL elements isDefinedBy and the label "Term Info", and is_entity_used_in and subClassOf in "Term Relations", with the same value as presented in Figure 3. As indicated in Section 2, the OWL element subClassOf "process" represents the parent of "Behavioral therapies", as represented in the tree view. The complete CTS2 EntityDescription "Behavioral therapies", and the other relevant EntityDescriptions, needed to fill the webpage presented in Figure 5, as is reported in the Supplementary Materials.


```xml
<namedEntityDescription about="http://www.healthropy.com/CTS2/test/EntityDescription?id=8636" codeSystemRole="PRIMARY"
entityDescriptionType="NAMED_ENTITY_DESCRIPTION">
    <!-- Element that correspond to "rdfs:isDefinedBy"-->
    <definition>
        <value xmlns="http://www.omg.org/spec/CTS2/1.1/Core">Behaviour therapy or behavioural psychotherapy is an approach to psychotherapy
            in the behaviourism tradition that focuses on the set of methods designed for reinforcing desired and eliminating undesired behaviours
            without concerning itself with the psychoanalytic state of the subject.</value>
    </definition>
    <!-- Property that correspond to "rdfs:label" and to the predicate "label" (See Interaction 4)-->
    <property>
        <predicate uri="http://www.healthropy.com/CTS2/test/EntityDescription?id=6985" xmlns="http://www.omg.org/spec/CTS2/1.1/Core">
            <domain>PREDICATE</domain>
        </predicate>
        <value TargetType="LITERAL" xmlns="http://www.omg.org/spec/CTS2/1.1/Core">
            <literal>
                <value>Behavioral therapy</value>
            </literal>
        </value>
    </property>
    <!-- Property that correspond to 2rdfs:SubClassof.owl:Restriction.owl:onProperty" and to the predicate "is_entity_used_in" (See Interaction 7)-->
    <property>
        <predicate uri="http://www.healthropy.com/CTS2/test/EntityDescription?id=6994" xmlns="http://www.omg.org/spec/CTS2/1.1/Core">
            <domain>PREDICATE</domain>
        </predicate>
        <!-- Element that correspond to the entity "NDOUO:non_pharmacotherapy_treatment_context" (See Interaction 8)-->
        <value TargetType="ENTITY" xmlns="http://www.omg.org/spec/CTS2/1.1/Core">
            <entity uri="http://www.healthropy.com/CTS2/test/EntityDescription?id=10032">
                <name>
                    <namespace>ADOV1</namespace>
                    <name>1494</name>
                </name>
            </entity>
        </value>
    </property>
    <subjectOf>http://www.healthropy.com/CTS2/test/Association?entityIdName=98&amp;entityIdNamespace=ADOV1&amp;type=subject</subjectOf>
    <predicateOf>http://www.healthropy.com/CTS2/test/Association?entityIdName=98&amp;entityIdNamespace=ADOV1&amp;type=predicate</predicateOf>
    <targetOf>http://www.healthropy.com/CTS2/test/Association?entityIdName=98&amp;entityIdNamespace=ADOV1&amp;type=target</targetOf>
    <!-- Element that correspond to "rdfs:SubClassOf"-->
    <parent uri="http://www.healthropy.com/CTS2/test/EntityDescription?id=10089">
        <!-- Element that correspond to the entity "process" (See Interaction 9)-->
        <name xmlns="http://www.omg.org/spec/CTS2/1.1/Core">
            <namespace>ADOV1</namespace>
            <name>1551</name>
        </name>
    </parent>
    <parents>http://www.healthropy.com/CTS2/test/EntityDescription?IdParents[]=14932</parents>
    <ancestors>http://www.healthropy.com/CTS2/test/EntityDescription?IdAncestors[]=14932</ancestors>
    <children>http://www.healthropy.com/CTS2/test/EntityDescription?IdChildren[]=14932</children>
    <descendants>http://www.healthropy.com/CTS2/test/EntityDescription?IdDescendants[]=14932</descendants>    <entityType uri="owl:Named"/>
</namedEntityDescription>
```


Figure 4. An extract from the EntityDescription "Behavioral therapies" defined in the ADOV1 contained in the SOAP message, intercepted as a response of the CTS2 operation Entity Description Read Service/read.

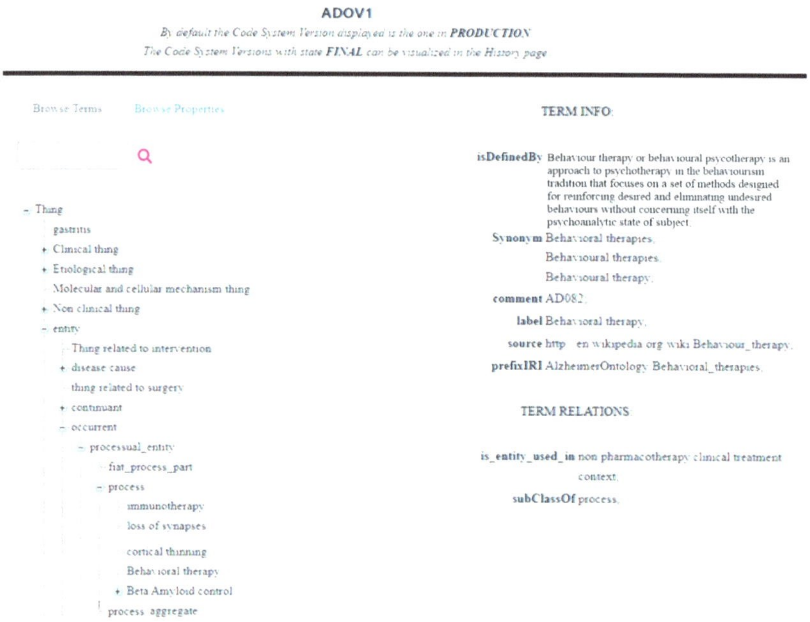

Figure 5. An example of the tree visualization of ADO classes (**left**) and entity details (**right**).

The Query section allows the user to search entities within a CodeSystem stored in HTS. The user can search for entities that contain a specific string in the name or for ones that have a specific property. To execute these searches, the web application calls the CTS2 operations Entity Description Query Service/Restrict and ResolveAsList. An example of a search is presented in Figure 6. All of the resulting entities are presented in the Table "Entity Label", and the user can visualize the details of a specific entity by clicking on "Show Details", which will be presented to the user in the same way as represented in Figure 5.

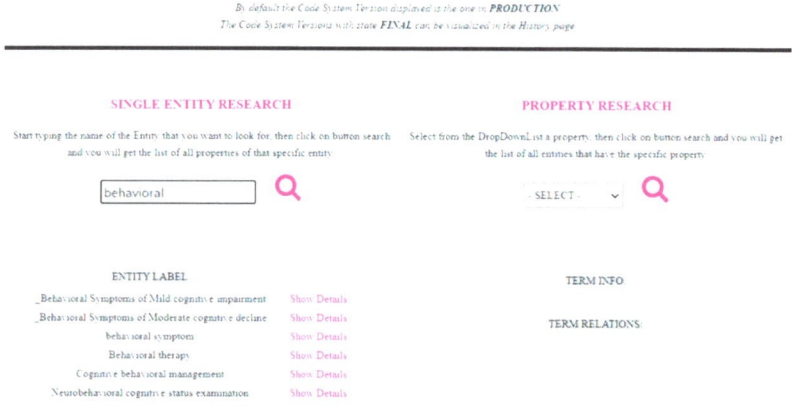

Figure 6. An example of a search for a name.

The Maintenance section allows the user to modify the current CodeSystemVersion (i.e., the version of the CodeSystem in production) in HTS. In detail, the user can update information about the CodeSystemVersion or close it (by calling CTS2 operation Code System Version Maintenance Service/updateCodeSystemVersion) and then open a new one (by calling CTS2 operation Code System Version Catalog Maintenance Service/CreateCodeSystemVersion). He/she can also manage the entity defined in the current version by creating a new entity or by updating or deleting an existing one (by calling CTS2 operation Entity Description Catalog Maintenance Service/CreateEntityDescription and/or UpdateEntityDescription). Figure 7 shows how a user can add information and properties to a new entity by adopting the web application.

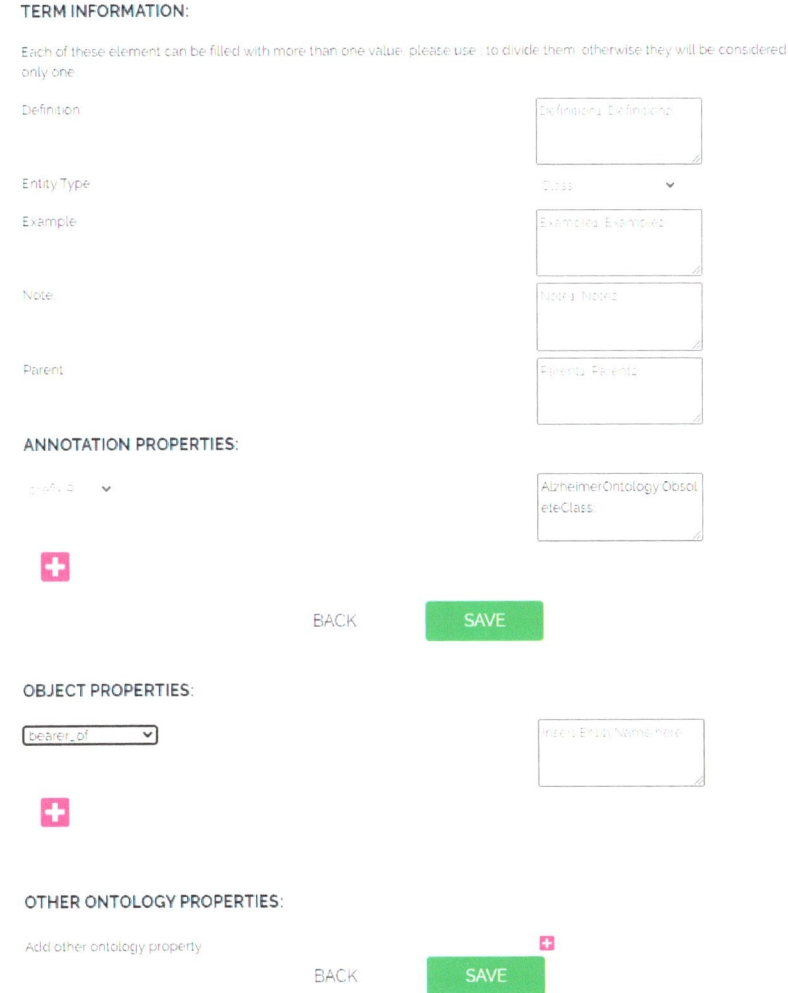

Figure 7. Visualization of term information, annotation properties, and object properties.

The last functionality provided by the web application is the Map section, which allows the user to visualize all existing mappings between the current version of a specific CodeSystem and the current version of another CodeSystem stored in HTS. The client application interacts with HTS to obtain all of the Maps that are defined for the specific source CodeSystem (by calling CTS2 operations Map Catalog Query Service/restrictByCodeSystem and resolveAsList) and propose a list of the target CodeSystems, which correspond to the Maps, to the user on the left side of the webpage in the Ontologies section (Figure 8). The user can select the target CodeSystem, and by clicking on "Show Details", the website interacts with HTS to retrieve all of the MapEntries defined for the current MapVersion (by calling

CTS2 operations Map version Query Service/restrictToCodeSystems and resolveAsList) and present them to the user. Figure 8 shows an example of the three MapEntries defined in the MapCatalogue that correspond to the current version of ADO and AdaLab ontologies.

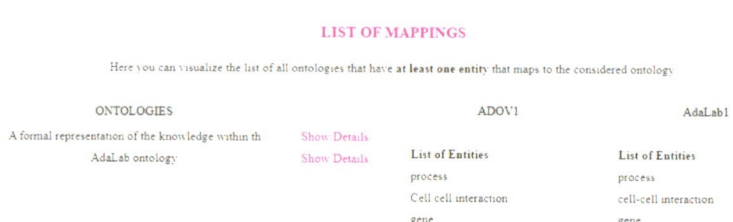

Figure 8. List of all MapEntries belonging to the MapCatalog identified by the two CodeSystems ADO and AdaLab, and more in detail, the two CodeSystemVersions named ADOV1 and AdaLab1.

4. Discussion

Considering the scenario of data integration, the development and usage of standard terminologies obtained a primary role and consistently improved the quality of the resulting outcome. However, it should be considered that terminologies evolve, e.g., the list of terms constantly undergo updates, including insertions and deletions. Therefore, it is necessary to adopt a solution able to track all changes in order to ensure and maintain the integrity of the terminology resource. Following the Chomsky hierarchy of language grammars, we should not forget that an ontological representation is richer and more consistent than a representation at a lower level, such as a terminology (see Figure 1). Therefore, it is inevitable to check the completeness and consistency of mapping two different representation styles using the model and framework of ISO 23903 [3].

OWL represents the most suitable solution to distribute an ontology, but it was not created for the purpose of tracking and visualizing the changes of each concept over the time. For this purpose, the concept of a terminology service was created to indicate a tool that allows us to provide access to terminology content through interfaces to read, query, maintain, and visualize the history of a specific terminology resource. The recent possible standard solution to define a terminology service, Application Programming Interface (API), is represented by the HL7 Fast Healthcare Interoperability Resources (FHIR) Terminology Service, already adopted in the literature [26–29]. The main limitation of the present approach is the possibility of establishing only hierarchical relations between concepts defined in the same code system and those mapped between concepts defined in different code systems. In addition, the FHIR Terminology Service allows us to work on the overall code system, rather than directly on the single entity, making the history of the changes in a single concept difficult to retrieve and visualize. On the contrary, a possible non-standard solution is Protégé (https://protege.stanford.edu/ accessed on 20 June 2024). Specifically, it is an open-source tool aimed at supporting the creation and management of ontologies, and it automatically tracks the changes, made available in the revision history. Its main advantage is that, as it is specifically devised for ontologies, the system is able to deal with all components of an ontology [21,30]. It also presents a main limitation, being that, to the best of our knowledge, at present, there is no API available allowing for a rich set of operations for ontology creation and management. Therefore, users can only use the web interface (Web Protégé) to interact with the database, thus requiring an intense human effort.

In our work, we chose to address the problem of terminology management with a standard solution, specifically the Common Terminology Service Release 2 (CTS2), because it is services-based and we have already used it in several scenarios [13,24–26,31,32]. As a main advantage, the use of CTS2 standard provides specifications useful to implement a set of operations to completely manage all aspects of CTS2 resources. CTS2 has some feature that are suitable for our context of use. First of all, the CTS2 information model for the concept (i.e., Entity Description) provides an indication not only of the direct parents and children, but also for the ancestors and descendants. This is useful to provide an easy navigation in the ontology, as we proposed with a tree view. In addition, the CTS2 information model works at an atomic level (i.e., single concept, Entity Description, and map, MapEntry), making the history of the changes in a single concept and map easy to retrieve and visualize, an important aspect for the authoring of an ontology. For this reason, for a future work, we are planning to implement new functionalities on the web application to visualize the history of the single concept and maps, adopting the operation provided by the CTS2 Entity Description History Service and Map Entry History Service. Other future work will be made on the side of the terminology service and on the client applications. The authors intend to implement the CTS2 Entity Description Transform Service, which is not yet available on HTS, to allow us to transform a concept represented in OWL in the corresponding CTS2 Entity Description. This will allow us to make the translation at the service level instead of at the client level, guaranteeing a more efficient control on the process. Finally, the authors intend to integrate the functionalities provided by the console application to the web application in order to have one tool to perform all of the operations on an ontology.

In personalized medicine, it is essential to accurately describe the situation of a patient at all levels (from macroscopic [22] to molecular [33]) [34,35]. These kinds of systems combine, on the one hand, the analytical nature of ontologies and, on the other hand, the systematic approach and rigor used in standardized tools, such as the CTS2, to preserve the historical evolution of the terminological systems. Therefore, we believe that it can be considered to be one of the enabling tools for the real implementation of the paradigms of medical personalization.

Supplementary Materials: The following supporting information can be downloaded at: https://www.mdpi.com/article/10.3390/jpm14070676/s1, File S1: XML file with the complete CTS2 EntityDescription of "Behavioral therapies".

Author Contributions: Conceptualization, R.G., M.G., S.M. and B.B.; methodology, B.B. and M.G.; software, S.M. and Y.M.; validation, R.G.; formal analysis, B.B. and M.G.; investigation, S.M. and M.G.; resources, M.G.; data curation, S.M. and Y.M.; writing—original draft preparation, S.M.; writing—review and editing, B.B., R.G. and M.G.; visualization, S.M.; supervision, M.G.; project administration, M.G.; funding acquisition, M.G. All authors have read and agreed to the published version of the manuscript.

Funding: This research was funded by European Union's Horizon 2020 research and innovation program, with the Virtual Brain Cloud Project, grant number 826421 and The APC was funded by the project Hub Life Science—Digital Health (LSH-DH) PNC-E3-2022-23683267—DHEAL-COM Project—CUP: D33C22001980001, funded by the Ministry of Health under the National Plan Complementary to the PNRR Innovative Health Ecosystem—UIC: PNC-E.3.

Institutional Review Board Statement: Not applicable.

Informed Consent Statement: Not applicable.

Data Availability Statement: All data is publicly available at: http://www.medinfo.dibris.unige.it/VBC_CTS2/ (accessed on 20 June 2024).

Conflicts of Interest: Roberta Gazzarata is an employee of Healthropy s.r.l. This company produced the CTS2 Service.

References

1. Mora, S.; Blobel, B.; Gazzarata, R.; Giacomini, M. CTS2 OWL: Mapping OWL Ontologies to CTS2 Terminology Resources. In *pHealth 2022—Studies in Health Technology and Informatics*; Blobel, B., Yang, B., Giacomini, M., Eds.; IOS Press: Amsterdam, The Netherlands, 2022; Volume 299, pp. 44–52.
2. Blobel, B.; Oemig, F.; Ruotsalainen, P.; Lopez, D.M. Transformation of Health and Social Care Systems—An Interdisciplinary Approach toward a Foundational Architecture. *Front. Med.* **2022**, *9*, 802487. [CrossRef] [PubMed]
3. *ISO 23903:2021*; Health Informatics—Interoperability and Integration Reference Architecture—Model and Framework. International Organization for Standardization: Geneva, Switzerland, 2021.
4. *ISO/IEC 10746:2009*; Information Technology—Open Distributed Processing (All Parts). International Organization for Standardization: Geneva, Switzerland, 2009.
5. Szolovits, P. *An Overview of OWL, A Language for Knowledge Representation*; Education Resources Information Center: Washington, DC, USA, 1977.
6. Lara, R.; Roman, D.; Polleres, A.; Fensel, D. A Conceptual Comparison of WSMO and OWL-S. In Proceedings of the European Conference on Web Services, Erfurt, Germany, 27–30 September 2004; Springer: Berlin/Heidelberg, Germany, 2004; pp. 254–269.
7. Gore, R.; Diallo, S.; Padilla, J. Conceve: Conceptual Modeling and Formal Validation for Everyone. *ACM Trans. Model. Comput. Simul. TOMACS* **2014**, *24*, 1–17. [CrossRef]
8. Lezcano, L.; Sicilia, M.-A.; Rodríguez-Solano, C. Integrating Reasoning and Clinical Archetypes Using OWL Ontologies and SWRL Rules. *J. Biomed. Inform.* **2011**, *44*, 343–353. [CrossRef] [PubMed]
9. Bagui, S. Mapping OWL to the Entity Relationship and Extended Entity Relationship Models. *Int. J. Knowl. Web Intell.* **2009**, *1*, 125–149. [CrossRef]
10. Schulz, S.; Balkanyi, L.; Cornet, R.; Bodenreider, O. From Concept Representations to Ontologies: A Paradigm Shift in Health Informatics? *Healthc. Inform. Res.* **2013**, *19*, 235. [CrossRef]
11. Cardoso, S.D.; Pruski, C.; Da Silveira, M. Supporting Biomedical Ontology Evolution by Identifying Outdated Concepts and the Required Type of Change. *J. Biomed. Inform.* **2018**, *87*, 1–11. [CrossRef] [PubMed]
12. Han, W.; Han, X.; Zhou, S.; Zhu, Q. The Development History and Research Tendency of Medical Informatics: Topic Evolution Analysis. *JMIR Med. Inform.* **2022**, *10*, e31918. [CrossRef] [PubMed]
13. OMG COMMON TERMINOLOGY SERVICES 2TM (CTS2TM). Available online: https://www.omg.org/cts2/ (accessed on 22 June 2024).
14. Gruber, T. *What Is an Ontology?* Stanford University: Stanford, CA, USA, 1993.
15. Gruber, T.R. Toward Principles for the Design of Ontologies Used Forknowledge Sharing. In Proceedings of the International Workshop on Ontology, Padova, Italy, 17–19 March 1993.
16. W3C—OWL Working Group Web Ontology Language (OWL). Available online: https://www.w3.org/TR/owl2-primer/ (accessed on 22 June 2024).
17. W3C—RDF Working Group Resource Description Framework (RDF). Available online: https://www.w3.org/RDF/ (accessed on 22 June 2024).
18. Robinson, P.N.; Mundlos, S. The Human Phenotype Ontology. *Clin. Genet.* **2010**, *77*, 525–534. [CrossRef] [PubMed]
19. Cowell, L.G.; Smith, B. Infectious Disease Ontology. In *Infectious Disease Informatics*; Sintchenko, V., Ed.; 2010; Available online: https://link.springer.com/book/10.1007/978-1-4419-1327-2 (accessed on 20 June 2024).
20. Sahoo, S.S.; Lhatoo, S.D.; Gupta, D.K.; Cui, L.; Zhao, M.; Jayapandian, C.; Bozorgi, A.; Zhang, G.-Q. Epilepsy and Seizure Ontology: Towards an Epilepsy Informatics Infrastructure for Clinical Research and Patient Care. *J. Am. Med. Inform. Assoc.* **2014**, *21*, 82–89. [CrossRef]
21. *ISO/IEC 21838:2021*; Information Technology—Top-Level Ontologies (TLO). International Organization for Standardization (ISO): Geneve, Switzerland, 2021.
22. Malhotra, A.; Younesi, E.; Gündel, M.; Müller, B.; Heneka, M.T.; Hofmann-Apitius, M. ADO: A Disease Ontology Representing the Domain Knowledge Specific to Alzheimer's Disease. *Alzheimer's Dement.* **2014**, *10*, 238–246. [CrossRef]
23. Coronato, A.; Cuzzocrea, A. An Innovative Risk Assessment Methodology for Medical Information Systems. *IEEE Trans. Knowl. Data Eng.* **2020**, *34*, 3095–3110. [CrossRef]
24. Gazzarata, R.; Monteverde, M.E.; Vio, E.; Saccavini, C.; Gubian, L.; Giacomini, M. A CTS2 Compliant Solution for Semantics Management in Laboratory Reports at Regional Level. *J. Innov. Health Inform.* **2017**, *24*, 127.
25. Gazzarata, R.; Monteverde, M.E.; Vio, E.; Saccavini, C.; Gubian, L.; Borgo, I.; Giacomini, M. A Terminology Service Compliant to CTS2 to Manage Semantics within the Regional HIE. *Eur. J. Biomed. Inform.* **2017**, *13*, 43–50. [CrossRef]
26. Gazzarata, R.; Maggi, N.; Magnoni, L.D.; Monteverde, M.E.; Ruggiero, C.; Giacomini, M. Semantics Management for a Regional Health Information System in Italy by CTS2 and FHIR. In Proceedings of the Applying the FAIR Principles to Accelerate Health Research in Europe in the Post COVID-19 Era: Proceedings of the 2021 EFMI Special Topic Conference; IOS Press: Amsterdam, The Netherlands, 2021; Volume 287, p. 119.
27. Wiedekopf, J.; Drenkhahn, C.; Ulrich, H.; Kock-Schoppenhauer, A.-K.; Ingenerf, J. Providing ART-DECOR ValueSets via FHIR Terminology Servers–A Technical Report. In *German Medical Data Sciences 2021: Digital Medicine: Recognize–Understand–Heal*; IOS Press: Amsterdam, The Netherlands, 2021; pp. 127–135.

28. Saripalle, R.; Runyan, C.; Russell, M. Using HL7 FHIR to Achieve Interoperability in Patient Health Record. *J. Biomed. Inform.* **2019**, *94*, 103188. [CrossRef] [PubMed]
29. Saripalle, R.; Sookhak, M.; Haghparast, M. An Interoperable UMLS Terminology Service Using FHIR. *Future Internet* **2020**, *12*, 199. [CrossRef]
30. Sivakumar, R.; Arivoli, P. V Ontology Visualization PROTÉGÉ Tools—A Review. *Int. J. Adv. Inf. Technol. IJAIT* **2011**, *1*. Available online: https://papers.ssrn.com/sol3/papers.cfm?abstract_id=3429010 (accessed on 20 June 2024).
31. Cardillo, E.; Chiaravalloti, M.T. A CTS2 Based Terminology Service for Managing Semantic Interoperability in the Italian Federated Electronic Health Record. *Int. J. Adv. Life Sci.* **2018**, *10*, 75–89. Available online: https://personales.upv.es/thinkmind/dl/journals/lifsci/lifsci_v10_n12_2018/lifsci_v10_n12_2018_8.pdf (accessed on 20 June 2024).
32. Peterson, K.J.; Jiang, G.; Brue, S.M.; Liu, H. Leveraging Terminology Services for Extract-Transform-Load Processes: A User-Centered Approach. In Proceedings of the AMIA Annual Symposium Proceedings, Chicago, IL, USA, 12–16 November 2016; American Medical Informatics Association: Bethesda, MD, USA, 2016; Volume 2016, p. 1010.
33. Metke-Jimenez, A.; Lawley, M.; Hansen, D. FHIR OWL: Transforming OWL Ontologies into FHIR Terminology Resources. In Proceedings of the AMIA Annual Symposium Proceedings, Washington, DC, USA, 16–20 November 2019; American Medical Informatics Association: Bethesda, MD, USA, 2019; Volume 2019, p. 664.
34. Canepa, S.; Roggerone, S.; Pupella, V.; Gazzarata, R.; Giacomini, M. A Semantically Enriched Architecture for an Italian Laboratory Terminology System. In Proceedings of the XIII Mediterranean Conference on Medical and Biological Engineering and Computing 2013: MEDICON 2013, Seville, Spain, 25–28 September 2013; Springer: Berlin/Heidelberg, Germany, 2014; pp. 1314–1317.
35. Mora, S.; Madan, S.; Gebel, S.; Giacomini, M. Proposal of an Architecture for Terminology Management in a Research Project. In *Digital Personalized Health and Medicine*; IOS Press: Amsterdam, The Netherlands, 2020; pp. 1371–1372.

Disclaimer/Publisher's Note: The statements, opinions and data contained in all publications are solely those of the individual author(s) and contributor(s) and not of MDPI and/or the editor(s). MDPI and/or the editor(s) disclaim responsibility for any injury to people or property resulting from any ideas, methods, instructions or products referred to in the content.

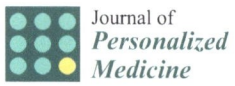

Article

Multidimensional Machine Learning Model to Calculate a COVID-19 Vulnerability Index

Paula Andrea Rosero Perez [1], Juan Sebastián Realpe Gonzalez [1], Ricardo Salazar-Cabrera [1], David Restrepo [1], Diego M. López [1] and Bernd Blobel [2,3,4,*]

1. Research Group in Telematics Engineering, Telematics Department, Universidad del Cauca, Popayán 190002, Colombia; parosero@unicauca.edu.co (P.A.R.P.); jsrealpe@unicauca.edu.co (J.S.R.G.); ricardosalazarc@unicauca.edu.co (R.S.-C.); dsrestrepo@unicauca.edu.co (D.R.); dmlopez@unicauca.ed.co (D.M.L.)
2. Medical Faculty, University of Regensburg, 93053 Regensburg, Germany
3. eHealth Competence Center Bavaria, Deggendorf Institute of Technology, 94469 Deggendorf, Germany
4. First Medical Faculty, Charles University Prague, 12800 Prague, Czech Republic
* Correspondence: bernd.blobel@klinik.uni-regensburg.de

Citation: Rosero Perez, P.A.; Realpe Gonzalez, J.S.; Salazar-Cabrera, R.; Restrepo, D.; López, D.M.; Blobel, B. Multidimensional Machine Learning Model to Calculate a COVID-19 Vulnerability Index. *J. Pers. Med.* 2023, 13, 1141. https://doi.org/10.3390/jpm13071141

Academic Editor: Amir El Assani Hajjam

Received: 28 May 2023
Revised: 4 July 2023
Accepted: 9 July 2023
Published: 15 July 2023

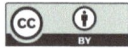

Copyright: © 2023 by the authors. Licensee MDPI, Basel, Switzerland. This article is an open access article distributed under the terms and conditions of the Creative Commons Attribution (CC BY) license (https://creativecommons.org/licenses/by/4.0/).

Abstract: In Colombia, the first case of COVID-19 was confirmed on 6 March 2020. On 13 March 2023, Colombia registered 6,360,780 confirmed positive cases of COVID-19, representing 12.18% of the total population. The National Administrative Department of Statistics (DANE) in Colombia published in 2020 a COVID-19 vulnerability index, which estimates the vulnerability (per city block) of being infected with COVID-19. Unfortunately, DANE did not consider multiple factors that could increase the risk of COVID-19 (in addition to demographic and health), such as environmental and mobility data (found in the related literature). The proposed multidimensional index considers variables of different types (unemployment rate, gross domestic product, citizens' mobility, vaccination data, and climatological and spatial information) in which the incidence of COVID-19 is calculated and compared with the incidence of the COVID-19 vulnerability index provided by DANE. The collection, data preparation, modeling, and evaluation phases of the Cross-Industry Standard Process for Data Mining methodology (CRISP-DM) were considered for constructing the index. The multidimensional index was evaluated using multiple machine learning models to calculate the incidence of COVID-19 cases in the main cities of Colombia. The results showed that the best-performing model to predict the incidence of COVID-19 in Colombia is the Extra Trees Regressor algorithm, obtaining an R-squared of 0.829. This work is the first step toward a multidimensional analysis of COVID-19 risk factors, which has the potential to support decision making in public health programs. The results are also relevant for calculating vulnerability indexes for other viral diseases, such as dengue.

Keywords: COVID-19; dataset; machine learning; vulnerability index

1. Introduction

COVID-19 is a disease caused by a virus called SARS-CoV-2, which was first reported on December 31, 2019, upon warning of a cluster of viral pneumonia cases in Wuhan, China [1]. The first case was confirmed in Colombia on 6 March 2020 [2]. The COVID-19 confirmed testing rates provide critical information to understand the full impact of the pandemic and identify ways to reduce morbidity and mortality.

The National Administrative Department of Statistics (DANE) is responsible for planning, collecting, processing, analyzing, and disseminating official statistics in Colombia. In this context, DANE published in 2020 an index of vulnerability to COVID-19 called the "Index of Vulnerability by Block", using the country demographic variables and comorbidities. The data used were solely obtained from the National Population and Housing Census 2018 (CNPV) and the discharge summaries from the Individual Health Services Register [3]. Climatological, environmental, socioeconomic, and mobility factors, among many others, are variables reported in the literature that were not considered when creating the vulnerability index by DANE. In what follows, the impact of the aforementioned factors will be discussed in more detail.

Several studies have analyzed the impact of climatological and environmental parameters, considering the geographical location of each country and intending to demonstrate the possible relationship between environmental factors and morbidity and mortality due to COVID-19 on the other side [4]. At the global level, there is great evidence on this subject; however, at the national level, there is very little information. In the same direction, other studies have shown that vaccines against COVID-19 effectively protect against the comorbidities associated with this disease, including mortality [5]. Since immunization began worldwide, many countries have performed evaluations of the rates of hospitalization and death from COVID-19 among vaccinated and unvaccinated persons, intending to calculate the effectiveness of vaccination schemes [6]. In this sense, vaccination data can also be useful for determining a vulnerability index. However, DANE did not consider this information, which may be related to the fact that there were not enough vaccination data in Colombia when they calculated their vulnerability index.

Furthermore, the loss of income from work due to unemployment caused by COVID-19 resulted in an increase in poverty rates and income inequality among people in vulnerable conditions, such as informal workers, women and indigenous youth, afro-descendants, and people with disabilities. People in conditions of socioeconomic vulnerability are at greater risk of infection and death from COVID-19 since inequalities are directly related to their ability to protect themselves from infection. A higher incidence of comorbidities is also associated with greater severity of the disease and even death. The percentage of the overcrowded population also plays an important role because areas with a higher proportion of overcrowded people are more affected by COVID-19 [7]. The inclusion of the aforementioned impact factors in the calculation of a new vulnerability index will lead to different results and interpretations, influencing its level of certainty.

Considering the context mentioned above, the following research question arose: how can a COVID-19 vulnerability index for Colombia be determined which considers COVID-19 case data published daily by the National Institute of Health, and other relevant risk factors in addition to those proposed by DANE?

The general objective of this research was to propose a machine-learning (ML) model to calculate a COVID-19 vulnerability index that considers human, environmental, sociodemographic, and socioeconomic risk factors as well as the database of historical cases of COVID-19 in an integrated manner. The outcome can assist decision making in public health programs. For that purpose, we developed a base ML model with information similar to that used by DANE (except for the information on comorbidities, which was not publicly available due to privacy concerns). The aim was to compare how close the base vulnerability index was to the reference vulnerability index obtained by DANE. Then, a multidimensional index, including several risk factors that were not included in the DANE index, was proposed to support the decision-making process of health agencies and make it possible to identify vulnerability to COVID-19 in the country's main cities. The additional data sources taken into account additionally to those of the DANE vulnerability index were COVID-19 data including vaccination data from the Ministry of Health as the main source, unemployment and gross domestic product information from DANE, and mobility, climatological, and spatial information from satellite images. This manuscript is an extended version of the paper published in the IOS SHTI pHealth 2022 Proceedings called "Risk Factors for COVID-19: A Systematic Mapping Study" [8].

The subsequent sections of the document are organized as follows. Section 2 presents the materials and methods used in this research. Section 3 presents the results of the research. Section 4 discusses the results obtained. Finally, Section 5 presents the conclusions and future work.

2. Materials and Methods

This section includes 4 sections: the identification of relevant COVID-19 risk factors; the development of the base model; the development of the multidimensional index; and the evaluation of the proposed multidimensional index.

2.1. Identification of Relevant Risk Factors of COVID-19

A systematic mapping was performed to identify the risk factors of COVID-19, followed by an analysis of the results.

To identify the risk factors, a search for review articles was performed using the Scopus database, which has broad coverage of scientific research, where 1786 related studies were identified and reviewed, of which 564 met the inclusion criteria. As the documents were analyzed, similar characteristics were detected among them, such as the type of review and the factors they covered, so two classifications were generated in the mapping. The first classification was called "type of research" and referred to the type of review conducted. For example, some reviews conducted experimental studies called "Review and experimentation". Some reviews did not conduct studies but fulfilled the objective of a review called "Review". Finally, some reviews did not indicate or follow a systematic review methodology in the abstract. Therefore, they were classified as "Non-formal reviews".

The second classification was called "research context" and referred to the types of factors found and the possible combinations among them. This classification included the following categories:

- Human risk factors. They refer to people's health conditions.
- Sociodemographic and socioeconomic risk factors. These indicate the characteristics of the population.
- Environmental factors. These factors include environmental variables.
- Sociodemographic and socioeconomic risk factors, and human factors.
- Sociodemographic and socioeconomic risk factors, and environmental risk factors.
- Sociodemographic and socioeconomic risk factors, environmental, and human risk factors.

Subsequently, an analysis of the results was performed, in which the risk factors were highlighted. The map of studies obtained in the systematic mapping, presented in Figure 1, allows identifying that the largest number of documents corresponds to the "review" type and just addresses human risk factors. The second largest number of documents, also corresponding to the "review" type, includes studies in the category of sociodemographic, socioeconomic, and human risk factors. The "review and experimental" group is the least dominant on the map. Concerning environmental risk factors, they are the least represented in the documents reviewed. In addition, among all the "type of research" categories, very few results were obtained for papers addressing environmental and human risk factors. The "non-formal review" type presents low dominance in the systematic mapping, and in the research context, human risk factors were the most prevalent ones for this category. Finally, it should be noted that the risk factors with the greatest presence in the documents were comorbidities such as diabetes, hypertension, obesity, and cardiovascular disease, but also age and sex.

Continuing with identifying risk factors, research was conducted on vulnerability indexes developed in the country (Colombia) and internationally to find out what had been done in other studies and the variables that had been considered.

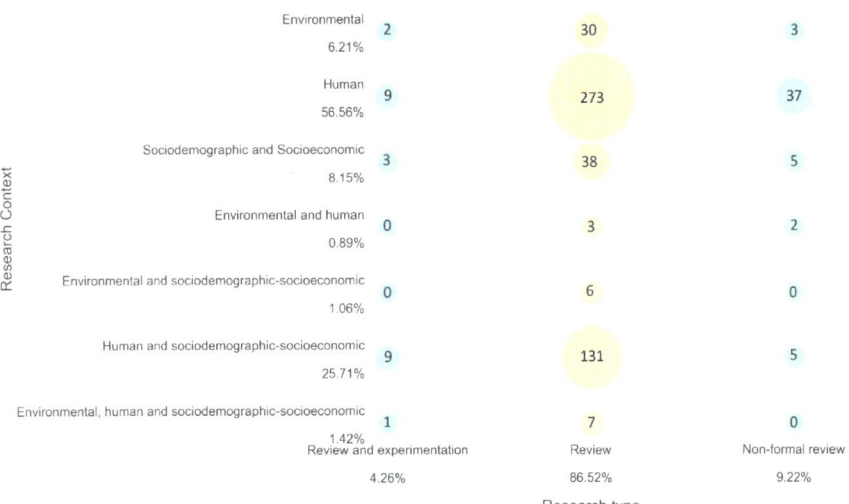

Figure 1. Bubble chart mapping and associating the type of research with the research context. Percentages are calculated for each axis.

Regarding the vulnerability indexes for COVID-19, the most relevant were the following:

- C19VI vulnerability index [9]. This index was developed in the United States by the Center for Disease Control and Prevention (CDC), considering the following variables to calculate the index: socioeconomic status, household composition, disability, minority status and language, type of housing and transportation, and epidemiological and health system factors.
- As a result, a vulnerability map was obtained in which each city was identified with a color according to the level of vulnerability found.
- Vulnerability index of Colombia (DANE) [3]. DANE provided a COVID-19 vulnerability index with a geographic disaggregation level by blocks. The study's objective was to categorize which people, according to the block where they live, have a higher probability of complications in case of infection by COVID-19. For this purpose, demographic characteristics and health conditions were considered. The variables used to calculate the DANE vulnerability index are presented below:
    - Comorbidities: hypertension, diabetes, ischemic heart disease, chronic pulmonary disease, and cancer.
    - Demographic characteristics: identification of people over 60, households in overcrowded rooms and bedrooms, and households at high and medium intergenerational risk per block.

Based on these variables, a series of steps were performed to consolidate a database of 407,277 rows with the columns above. After that, the K-means cluster analysis was applied, allowing the blocks to be grouped according to demographic characteristics and comorbidities.

Finally, the result obtained was the vulnerability map of Colombia, which shows the vulnerability to COVID-19 by block.

Considering the systematic mapping and the search of existing vulnerability indexes, it was found that the index developed by the CDC was the most appropriate reference model to this work. In this sense, a vulnerability index was constructed, called the "Base model", in which variables of the CDC vulnerability index were considered, except those regarding comorbidities, because open access to these data is restricted in Colombia due to confidentiality concerns. The CNPV 2018 datasets, also developed by DANE, were the main data source to construct the index.

2.2. Base Model

The stages suggested by the Cross-Industry Standard Process for Data Mining (CRISP-DM) methodology were followed for constructing the base model. The CRISP-DM stages are business understanding, data understanding, data preparation, modeling, evaluation, and deployment (this last stage was not performed) [10].

First, a dataset was built in which 5 tables of the CNPV 2018 were used (housing, households, deceased, persons, and georeferenced data [11]). The objective of the base dataset was to determine whether it was necessary or not to create a new dataset that considers other types of risk factors and, therefore, to propose a new vulnerability index. These data were in the comma-separated values (CSV) format and classified by department (regional geographical units in which Colombia is divided). There are 32 departments in the country. The variables taken into account were the following: type of housing, number of bedrooms per household, number of deceased per household, the total number of persons in the household, sex of the dead (male or female), age of the deceased, sex of the person, age of the person in five-year groups, ethnic recognition, speaking the native language of his/her people, speaking other native languages, quality of health service provision, literacy, highest educational level achieved, and economic activity performed during the past week (variable focused on asking if the person worked and received income from work). The dataset also includes a variable called "COVID-19 vulnerability," which contains the COVID-19 vulnerability data published by the DANE index aggregated by each municipality in the country (1104 municipalities and 19 special districts). This is a discrete value from 0 to 5, where 0 means no vulnerability, and 5 means high vulnerability. This variable was used as a dependent variable in the ML model evaluation phase to calculate the vulnerability values already calculated by DANE.

The dataset was processed using the Python Pandas library. The data was cleaned and pre-processed to eliminate variables that did not contribute to the objective of the work. The municipalities that did not include a value for vulnerability (output variable) were eliminated, thus resulting in a dataset of 89 columns and 1103 rows. This dataset can be found on Kaggle's web platform as the "Base COVID-19 Dataset" [12].

In the modeling phase of the base index development process, confusion matrices were generated to observe the correlation between the dependent variable (output variable) and the independent variables. For this purpose, Pearson's and Spearman's correlations were considered. Pearson's correlation evaluates the linear relationship between two quantitative variables [13]. Pearson's coefficient indicates the variables' association, and its value can take values between -1 and 1. Therefore, no linear relationship exists when variables show a correlation around zero. Spearman's correlation was applied, because there was a monotonic relationship between the dependent and independent variables [14]. Nevertheless, the correlation between the variables was still close to zero.

Classification algorithms were considered for the CRISP-DM evaluation phase because they allow the prediction of discrete or qualitative outputs [15]. The objective of the base model was to evaluate whether the obtained dataset performs an efficient vulnerability prediction by a municipality. Therefore, classification algorithms were used because the vulnerability values, calculated by the DANE, are discrete variables. The aim was to determine how well these values could be predicted with the created model. The evaluation used two scenarios (dividing the dataset into different percentages for training and testing in each scenario). In scenario 1, 80% of the dataset was taken as training and 20% for testing. In scenario 2, 70% of the dataset was taken as training and 30% for testing. Considering that no correlation was perceived in the confusion matrices, six different models were used for evaluation.

The first model implemented was a linear discriminant analysis (LDA), a supervised classification method where a predictive model is built to determine the group to which it belongs. The second model was a quadratic discriminant analysis (QDA). This model is used when the set of predictor variables to be classified has two or more classes. It is considered the equivalent of non-linear discriminant analysis. The third model was k-nearest neighbors (KNN), where a learning classifier algorithm can be used as a regression or classification algorithm. The fourth model was the decision tree classifier, a supervised learning algorithm mainly used in classification problems. The fifth model was Gaussian Naive Bayes (GNB), a probabilistic ML algorithm typically used as a classifier. Finally, the sixth model used a support vector machine (SVM) algorithm, which can be used for classification and regression. To evaluate the performance of the algorithms, the following metrics were used: F1 (average macro), precision, recall, and accuracy.

The F1 metric considers the number of false positives and false negatives, calculating a weighted average between precision and sensitivity, thus obtaining a single score representing the two variables. The precision metric measures the accuracy of the classifier when predicting positive cases. It is calculated as the ratio between correct predictions and the expected number of correct predictions. The recall metric detects positive instances, also known as sensitivity. It is calculated as the ratio between correct and total positive predictions. The accuracy metric determines the classification accuracy, i.e., the ratio between correct predictions and total predictions [16].

The results of the evaluation of the base dataset are presented in Section 3.

2.3. Multidimensional Index

The multidimensional index was constructed by adding new data from other types of variables to the dataset created for the base model. Thus, the multidimensional index considers sociodemographic, socioeconomic, environmental, and human factors.

The first five stages of the CRISP-DM methodology were also followed for this index (as was done for the base model).

Figure 2 presents a flowchart to facilitate understanding of the construction process of the multidimensional index.

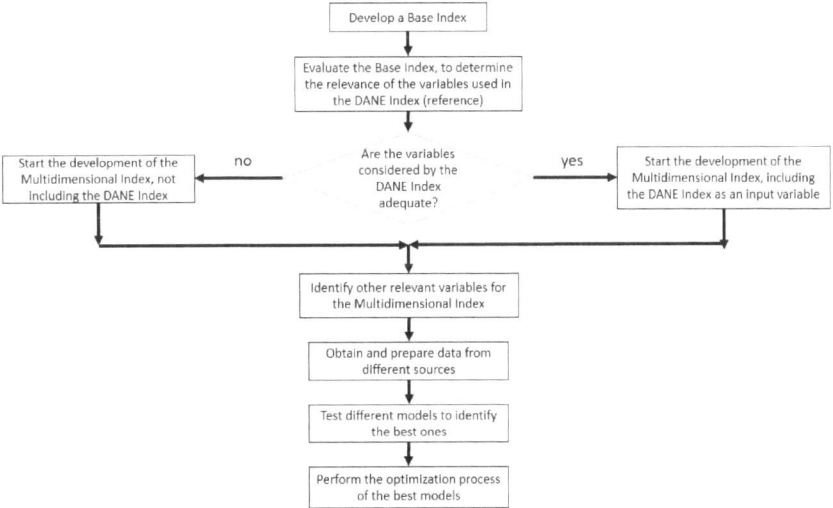

Figure 2. Flowchart of the multidimensional index construction.

The data collection for the construction of this index used open data. The sources found made it possible to unify a target dataset with the following datasets:

- Gross domestic product (GDP). GDP is the standard value-added of producing a country's goods and services during a period [17]. This dataset provides a broader visibility of what each region (department) contributes to the country yearly. Considering the relevant period of the COVID-19 pandemic, data for 2020 and 2021 were considered. This research used GDP at constant prices with an annual periodicity.

- Climatological data. This type of data has been identified as a factor that increases the risk of COVID-19. For this reason, temperature and precipitation data were sought through Google Earth Engine. This platform allows access to these data for all the principal municipalities in Colombia [18] daily.
- Vaccination percentage. For the vaccination data, the information provided by the Ministry of Health was taken into account, which presents a report made in Power BI [19] in which the vaccination percentage curve by the municipality can be visualized.
- Unemployment rate. This dataset was collected from the information published by the Great Integrated Household Survey (named GEIH) conducted by DANE. The survey information is presented for the capitals of 24 departments (out of 32 and one special district) and published quarterly [20].
- Mobility data. This dataset was collected from reports published by Google. These reports allow tracing movement trends over time in different categories of places: grocery and pharmacy, parks, transit stations, retail and recreation, workplace, and residential, taking as a reference the mobility of the 5 weeks between January 3 and February 6, 2020. The increase or decrease percentages of mobility-specific areas were calculated [21].
- COVID-19 vulnerability. Same as the previous index, it contains the COVID-19 vulnerability data published by DANE. Including these data allows having a representative value of the variables already measured with the national index, therefore reflecting data on comorbidities, information on older adults in households, and overcrowding places data.
- COVID-19 case data. This is the output variable, considering that the evaluation of the model was performed using multiple machine learning models to predict the incidence of COVID-19 cases in the main cities of Colombia. Data were obtained from information published by the Ministry of Health, where daily data reported in each of the municipalities of Colombia can be found in the CSV format [22].

Considering the temporal and geographical limitations of some of the data sources, it was determined that a quarterly data periodicity was most appropriate to work for the following cities: Quibdó, Cali, Cúcuta, Armenia, Popayán, Ibagué, Neiva, Florencia, Valledupar, Tunja, Riohacha, Bogotá, Villavicencio, Pereira, Manizales, Medellín, Santa Marta, Sincelejo, Montería, Pasto, Bucaramanga, Barranquilla, Cartagena, and San Andrés. Subsequently, the datasets were cleaned and pre-processed. It was necessary to transform the data into CSV files for the GDP, vaccination, and unemployment rates. Regarding the climatological data, an average was made to find each quarter's temperature and precipitation values. Next, the mobility dataset was cleaned, deleting unnecessary data. Then, an average mobility dataset per municipality was made for each quarter. The complete and integrated dataset can be found on Kaggle's web platform as the "Multidimensional index of COVID-19 Colombia" [23].

In the multidimensional index development modeling phase, confusion matrices were generated to determine the correlation between the independent and dependent variables (output variables). The results section (Section 3) shows the confusion matrices obtained.

Regarding the evaluation of this model, several supervised learning regression algorithms were applied because the output variable (incidence) is continuous [24]. The algorithms used were linear regression, decision trees, KNN, SVM, random forest, and gradient boosting. Two meta-estimators called Extra Trees Regressor and AdaBoost Regressor were also used.

The same two scenarios (presented in the base model) were used to divide the dataset into training and tests. As the output variable was the COVID-19 incidence, the algorithm with the best performance in predicting this variable was evaluated.

The multidimensional model is expected to perform better than the base model in estimating COVID-19 vulnerability. The root means square error (RMSE) and R-squared were used to assess the algorithm's performance. The RMSE metric indicates how close the observed data points are to the predicted values. It can also be interpreted as the standard deviation of the unexplained variance. A low RMSE value indicates a better fit. R-squared suggests the fitness of the model. This metric takes values between 0 and 1, where 0 represents that the proposed model does not improve the prediction over the mean model, and 1 indicates perfect prediction [25]. Negative R-squared values are likely to occur; this situation arises in cases where the model is less fitted than the average [26].

To improve the performance of the multidimensional index models, it was decided to optimize the hyper-parameters of the algorithms with the best results in the first tests. The hyper-parameters' optimization is presented in Appendix A.

2.4. Evaluation of the Multidimensional Index for Predicting the Incidence of COVID-19

To complement the evaluation of the performance of the multidimensional index, the best-performing algorithms were used to predict the incidence of COVID-19 cases in the main cities of Colombia. The results are compared with the results of a reference model trained with the DANE vulnerability index (COVID-19 vulnerability column of the multi-dimensional dataset) as the independent variable and the COVID-19 incidence (COVID-19 case data column of the multidimensional dataset) as the dependent variable. This reference model is called a "Reference predictor". The same algorithms were used to predict the cases in the experiment for the two models (multidimensional and reference predictor), i.e., linear regression, decision trees, k-nearest neighbor (KNN), support vector machine (SVM), random forest, and gradient boosting, as well as the two meta-estimators (Extra Trees Regressor and AdaBoost Regressor). Furthermore, the evaluation was performed with the same scenarios (training and evaluation percentages).

Section 3 presents the results of evaluating the multidimensional index for predicting the incidence of COVID-19.

3. Results

Confusion matrices are analyzed for the used variables in the multidimensional index. Later, the performance evaluation results of the base model and multidimensional indexes are presented.

3.1. Confusion Matrixes for the Multidimensional Index

In the confusion matrix in Figure 3, the green color indicates a high positive correlation between variables, the fuchsia color indicates a high negative correlation, and the white color indicates a low correlation. For example, Figure 3 shows that variables such as GDP and "residential" (mobility) are positively correlated, while temperature and "retail_and_recreation" are negatively correlated. In addition, it is important to mention that the incidence column is the output variable. Figure 4 presents the confusion matrix for Spearman's correlation.

In Figure 4 (similar to Figure 3) the last column shows some shades of green and some fuchsia, indicating these variables have a positive correlation (green) or negative (fuchsia). The high intensity of the green color shows a high correlation. In Figure 4, variables such as GDP, "residential", "grocery and pharmacy", and vaccination percentage have a positive correlation with the incidence variable. At the same time, the variables temperature and "workplaces" (mobility) have a negative correlation. In addition, variables such as precipitation and percentage of unemployment show a fairly low correlation with incidence.

3.2. Base Model Evaluation

For the base model, two scenarios were used: splitting the data into 80% training and 20% testing for the first scenario, and 70% training and 30% testing for the second scenario. However, the performance obtained for this model in predicting the reference DANE vulnerability index (COVID-19 vulnerability variable) was deficient for both scenarios. Therefore, in Table 1, only the scenario with the best performance is reported.

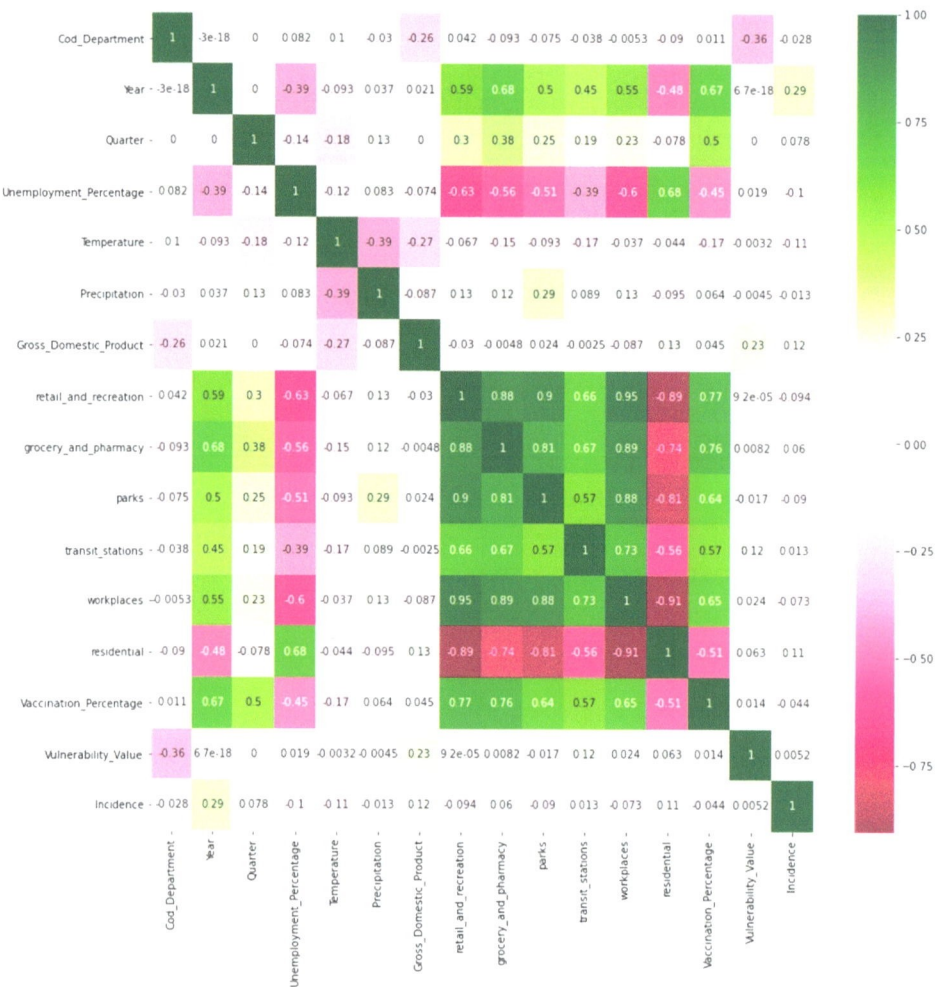

Figure 3. Confusion matrix (Pearson correlation).

Table 1. 70% training and 30% test scenario (base model).

Model	F1 Score	Precision	Recall	Accuracy
LinearDiscriminantAnalysis	0.239	0.226	0.259	0.897
QuadraticDiscriminantAnalysis	0.192	0.185	0.2	0.927
KNeighborsClassifier	0.192	0.185	0.2	0.927
DecisionTreeClassifier	0.429	0.427	0.432	0.873
GaussianNaiveBayes	0.141	0.231	0.504	0.184
SupportVectorMachine	0.192	0.185	0.2	0.927

Table 1 shows that the DecisionTreeClassifier algorithm performs best for the F1 metric. This value was obtained when the dataset was divided into 70% training and 30% test. It can also be noted that the base vulnerability index correctly predicts the vulnerability value by 87.3% among the total predictions. However, the precision and recall values are low, around 43%, indicating that the number of correct predictions compared to all predictions is very low. Because of this, the F1 value in the best performance model is 42.9%.

These results may be due to the lack of comorbidities in the base dataset.

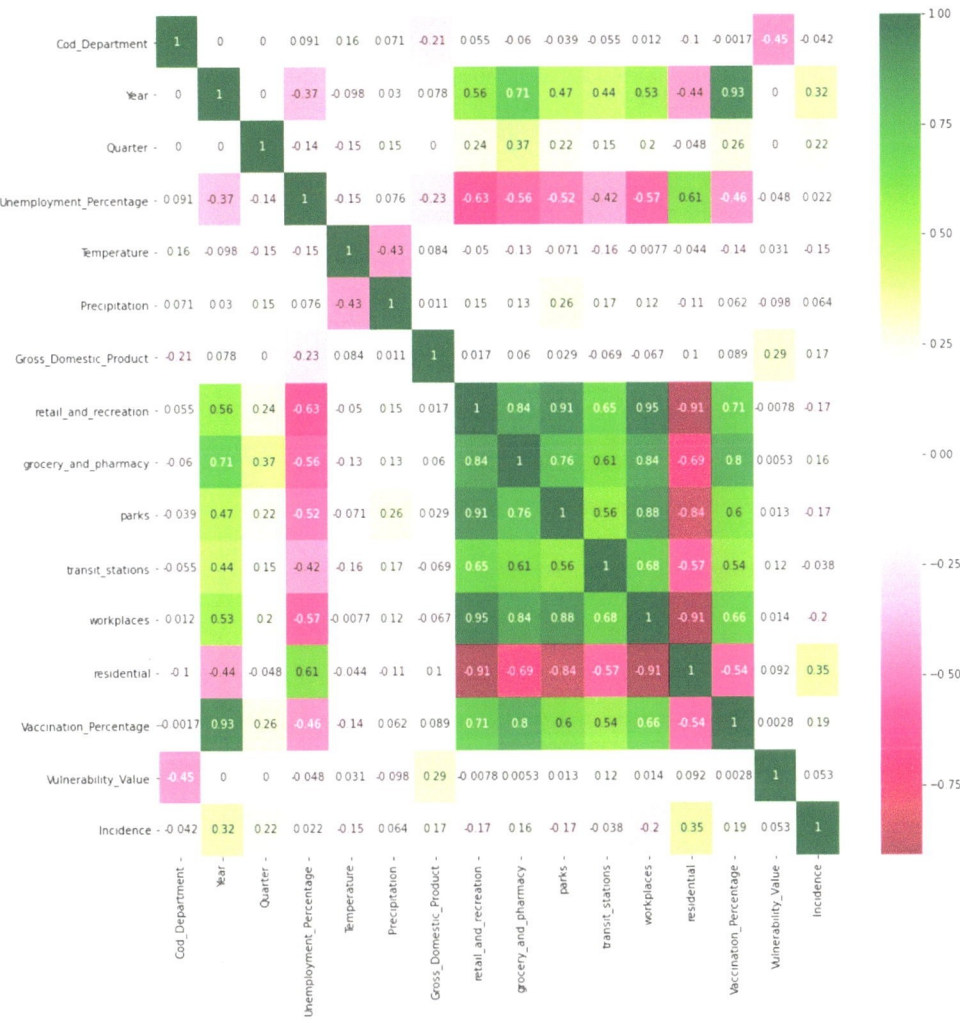

Figure 4. Confusion matrix (Spearman correlation).

3.3. Multidimensional Index Evaluation

The specific variables used in this multidimensional index were the following:

- Gross domestic product (GDP);
- Temperature;
- Precipitation;
- Vaccination percentage;
- Unemployment rate;
- Mobility in grocery and pharmacy;
- Mobility in parks;
- Mobility in transit stations;
- Mobility in retail and recreation;
- Mobility in workplace;
- Mobility in residential;
- COVID-19 vulnerability;
- COVID-19 case data as the output variable.

Table 2 shows the performance for the first scenario (80% training and 20% test) in the multidimensional index for predicting the COVID-19 vulnerability variable of the multidimensional dataset. Table 3 shows the model's performance for this index's second scenario (70% training and 30% test). Table 4 shows the results for the optimized models in this index. The procedure that was followed for the optimization of each model is presented in Appendix A.

Table 2. 80% training and 20% test (multidimensional index).

Model	RMSE	R-Squared
Linear Regression	0.013	0.358
Decision Tree Regressor	0.010	0.611
K-Nearest Neighbor	0.019	−0.207
Support Vector Machine	0.033	−2.697
Random Forest Regressor	0.007	0.790
Gradient Boosting Regressor	0.008	0.758
Extra Trees Regressor	0.007	0.828
AdaBoost Regressor	0.008	0.761

Table 3. 70% training and 30% test (multidimensional index).

Model	RMSE	R-Squared
Linear Regression	0.013	0.319
Decision Tree Regressor	0.012	0.469
K-Nearest Neighbor	0.019	−0.335
Support Vector Machine	0.030	−2.496
Random Forest Regressor	0.008	0.720
Gradient Boosting Regressor	0.009	0.637
Extra Trees Regressor	0.009	0.700
AdaBoost Regressor	0.009	0.683

In Tables 2 and 3, it is possible to observe that the Extra Trees Regressor algorithm presents the best results in each of them, because it has an RMSE level close to 0 and an R-squared value closer to 1. It should be noted that in Table 3 (70% training and 30% test) the RMSE value closest to 0 is that of the Random Forest Regressor algorithm (0.008, while the RMSE value of the Extra Trees Regressor algorithm is 0.009), but the difference in the R-squared value between these two algorithms means that the best option, combined with the two values, is the Extra Trees Regressor algorithm. The best values (RMSE and R-squared) between the two proposed scenarios were obtained for the first scenario of 80% training and 20% test; therefore, this was used in the optimization of hyper-parameters.

In Table 4, in which the results of the algorithms with optimized hyper-parameters are presented, again the Extra Trees Regressor algorithm presents the best results in the optimized values of RMSE and R-squared (0.007 and 0.00829, respectively) using the first scenario (80% training and 20% test).

The extra trees are an extension of the random forest regression model and were proposed by Geurts et al. [27]. The extra trees belong to the class of decision tree-based ensemble learning methods. In decision tree-based ensemble methods, multiple decision trees are used to perform classification and regression tasks. The extra trees are less susceptible to overfitting and report better performance [27].

3.4. Results of the Multidimensional Index for Predicting Incidence of COVID-19

Table 5 shows the performance for the first scenario (80% training and 20% test) of the reference predictor used to estimate the real incidence of COVID-19 cases. Table 6 presents the performance for the second scenario (70% training and 30% test) in the DANE index.

Table 4. Obtained results in the multidimensional index optimized, using 80% training and 20% test.

Model	Hyper-Parameters	Base R-Squared	Base RMSE	R-Squared of the Optimized Model	RMSE of the Optimized Model
Decision Tree Regressor	criterion = 'absolute_error' max_depth = 4 max_features = 'auto' random_state = 329 ccp_alpha = 7.179×10^{-6}	0.611	0.010	0.708	0.009
Random Forest Regressor	max_depth = 13 max_features = 7 n_estimators = 125 random_state = 329	0.790	0.007	0.802	0.007
Gradient Boosting Regressor	learning_rate = 0.5 max_depth = 2 max_features = 'auto' n_estimators = 1000 n_iter_no_change = 5 random_state = 329 subsample = 1	0.758	0.008	0.765	0.008
Hist Gradient Regressor	learning_rate = 0.5 max_depth = 3	Does not apply	Does not apply	0.810	0.007
Extra Trees Regressor	n_estimators = 97 max_features = None random_state = 329	0.828	0.007	0.829	0.007
AdaBoost Regressor *	n_estimators = 247	0.761	0.008	0.811	0.007

* Model works internally with Decision Tree Regressor.

Table 5. 80% training and 20% test (reference predictor).

Model	RMSE	R-Squared
Linear Regression	0.016	0.090
Decision Tree Regressor	0.012	0.517
K-Nearest Neighbor	0.019	−0.287
Support Vector Machine	0.033	−2.697
Random Forest Regressor	0.010	0.608
Gradient Boosting Regressor	0.011	0.546
Extra Trees Regressor	0.011	0.561
AdaBoost Regressor	0.013	0.395

Table 6. 70% training and 30% test (reference predictor).

Model	RMSE	R-Squared
Linear Regression	0.016	0.033
Decision Tree Regressor	0.011	0.474
K-Nearest Neighbor	0.018	−0.220
Support Vector Machine	0.030	−2.496
Random Forest Regressor	0.010	0.596
Gradient Boosting Regressor	0.011	0.480
Extra Trees Regressor	0.011	0.535
AdaBoost Regressor	0.010	0.610

Table 7 presents a comparison between the results obtained in the different models used in the optimized multidimensional index (Table 4) and the results obtained for these same models in the DANE index (reference predictor) use the scenario with the better results 80%–20% (Table 5). It is possible to appreciate that the results obtained in the multidimensional index have better values for the two used metrics (RMSE and R-squared). It should be noted that the values of Tables 2 and 5 are not compared because the models in Table 2 are not optimized, while in Table 4 they correspond to the optimized values explained in Appendix A.

Table 7. Comparison between the models of the reference predictor and multidimensional index (using the best scenario, 80% training and 20% test).

Model	RMSE of Reference Predictor	RMSE of Multidimensional Index	R-Squared of Multidimensional Index	R-Squared of Reference Predictor
Decision Tree Regressor	0.012	0.009	0.708	0.517
Random Forest Regressor	0.010	0.007	0.802	0.608
Gradient Boosting Regressor	0.011	0.008	0.765	0.546
Extra Trees Regressor	0.011	0.007	0.829	0.561
AdaBoost Regressor	0.013	0.007	0.811	0.395

In Tables 2, 3, 5 and 6, some negative values are presented in the R-squared metric. Although it is normal for the values of this metric to be between 0 and 1, this situation can occur in cases where the model is less fitted than the average (as mentioned in [26]).

Next, the models with the best performance (for the multidimensional predictor and reference predictor) were used to predict the incidence of real COVID-19 cases reported by quarters. It is clarified that, when dividing the dataset into training and test, in each execution different data were selected, the common cities were selected in the execution of each model to compare the prediction. Figures 5 and 6 show the results obtained. Figure 7 shows that the values predicted by the multidimensional index are closer to the expected values than those predicted by the DANE index.

Index	City	Year	Quarter	Real_Incidence	DANE_Incidence	Multidimensional_Incidence
0	Valledupar	2020	4	0.015410	0.020321	0.024793
1	Armenia	2021	1	0.025731	0.020944	0.018241
2	Bogota	2020	2	0.003851	0.004024	0.004465
3	Santamarta	2020	3	0.017207	0.020144	0.018831
4	Cartagena	2020	2	0.008119	0.004024	0.005976
5	Neiva	2021	2	0.038239	0.033183	0.028120
6	Cartagena	2021	1	0.013558	0.021089	0.023214
7	Neiva	2020	1	0.000058	0.000597	0.000032
8	Sanandres	2020	2	0.000331	0.004024	0.007598
9	Cali	2020	1	0.000035	0.000034	0.000025
10	Florencia	2021	2	0.012629	0.033183	0.019916
11	Neiva	2020	4	0.044538	0.020321	0.029111
12	Valledupar	2021	2	0.050153	0.033183	0.044783
13	Santamarta	2020	4	0.013797	0.020321	0.028564
14	Medellin	2020	2	0.000825	0.004024	0.003386
15	Bucaramanga	2020	2	0.000250	0.004024	0.003446
16	Sincelejo	2020	4	0.006542	0.029000	0.018318
17	Medellin	2021	3	0.019432	0.012161	0.016081
18	Manizales	2020	2	0.000273	0.004024	0.000875
19	Tunja	2021	1	0.028914	0.021089	0.025863
20	Riohacha	2021	4	0.007358	0.009959	0.005806

Figure 5. Table predicted vs. expected values, part 1.

Index	City	Year	Quarter	Real_Incidence	DANE_Incidence	Multidimensional_Incidence
21	Popayan	2021	4	0.003535	0.009959	0.005252
22	Cartagena	2021	2	0.046409	0.049935	0.059131
23	Monteria	2021	4	0.001464	0.009959	0.002714
24	Pasto	2020	1	0.000005	0.000597	0.000016
25	Ibague	2020	1	0.000017	0.000034	0.000242
26	Ibague	2021	1	0.024407	0.014890	0.020278
27	Sincelejo	2020	1	0.000003	0.002175	0.000121
28	Quibdo	2021	2	0.040171	0.033183	0.028498
29	Manizales	2021	4	0.003040	0.012161	0.010067
30	Riohacha	2020	3	0.015393	0.019812	0.019371
31	Popayan	2020	1	0.000028	0.000591	0.000021
32	Manizales	2021	2	0.063856	0.033183	0.050754
33	Bucaramanga	2021	3	0.020167	0.009959	0.014315
34	Monteria	2020	1	0.000002	0.000591	0.000019
35	Manizales	2020	4	0.044464	0.020321	0.029324
36	Medellin	2020	4	0.033072	0.022291	0.027097
37	Ibague	2020	3	0.016368	0.022960	0.020077
38	Riohacha	2020	1	0.000005	0.000597	0.000015

Figure 6. Table predicted vs. expected values, part 2.

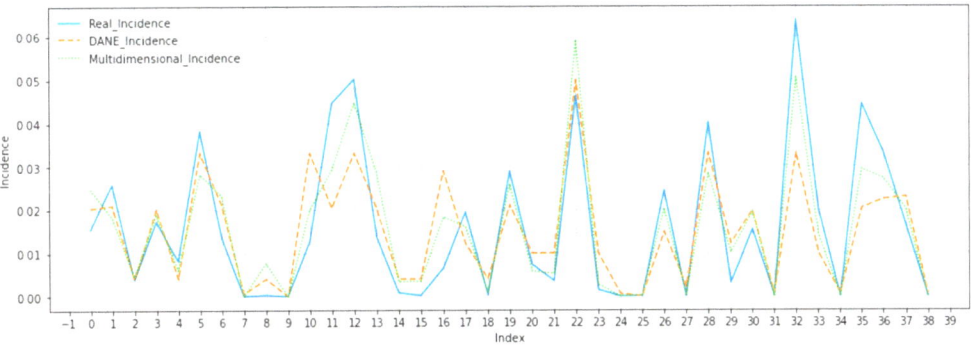

Figure 7. Graph of predicted versus expected values.

4. Discussion

The presented research evaluated the performance of a multidimensional machine-learning model to calculate a COVID-19 vulnerability index that considers human, environmental, sociodemographic, and socioeconomic risk factors in an integrated manner. The vulnerability indexes creation required the evaluation of several ML algorithms to identify which one behaved better in predicting the incidence of COVID. This represents an important differentiation concerning other previous works in the literature in which results of only one algorithm for calculating the index are presented. Another representative difference of this work, concerning the consulted previous works, is the diversity of types of variables used because other works mainly considered human factors.

This research began by creating a base machine learning model with information similar to that used by DANE (except for the information on comorbidities, which was not publicly available due to privacy concerns). The aim was to compare how close the base vulnerability index was to the reference vulnerability obtained by DANE. Regarding the evaluation of the base model, it is important to mention that most of the algorithms used presented a high precision. However, the value of the F1 score metric was very low. This is because the F1 score is the average between the precision and recall metrics. Therefore, correct predictions relative to all predictions were low. In addition, although several sociodemographic and socioeconomic variables were considered for the base model, optimal results were not obtained. This could be because human risk factors, i.e., comorbidities (for which no data were available), which seem quite relevant, were not taken into account.

Therefore, the construction of a multidimensional index of COVID-19 was necessary. The new index added different types of risk factors to improve the performance of the vulnerability index. The proposed multidimensional index, without optimizing and after performing the hyper-parameter optimization, presents a high performance in predicting COVID-19 incidence. After optimization (a process that did not generate significant results), the R-squared and RMSE metrics with the multidimensional index obtained a maximum value of 0.829 and 0.007, respectively, with the Extra Trees Regressor algorithm. This algorithm is a meta-estimator, which calculates the best predictions from various decision trees.

The Decision Tree Regressor algorithm was the one that most improved the value of the R-squared metric after adjusting the hyper-parameters, obtaining a tree in which the number of nodes and leaves was considerably reduced. This algorithm is relevant because, in the regression algorithms, the decision trees present a better behavior for the datasets used in this study.

Through optimization, it was possible to show that the internal CV performed by the GridSearchCV function caused the R-squared metric of the optimized algorithms not to exceed the metric value before optimization. Consequently, it was necessary to perform the evaluations manually to avoid the internal CV of the GridSearchCV function but considering in the evaluation the values of the hyper-parameters that the function returned.

In the case of the multidimensional index, it must be taken into account that although it may have better performance due to the variables added that provide a better context to the model, having a dataset with more characteristics can cause the results to be affected by overfitting. Having a model and dataset that span more dimensions and, therefore, have more variables also require having more samples for training to prevent the model from being more prone to memorizing patterns and, thus, reducing its ability to generalize. In this case, it is suggested to carefully select the most important variables for the model and pre-process them properly in order to have a dataset with the most relevant variables, eliminate possible noise, and reduce the risk of overfitting.

Testing the developed model in different countries, not only in Colombia as was done in the research, may be an interesting option to validate the model created. However, the acquisition of data of all the variables proposed in the model could be a costly process. In addition, it is very likely that the data for some variables cannot be acquired in another country with the same periodicity, or the necessary source is not available. Some data proposed in the model come from national sources, which cannot be obtained in other countries in the region or globally. Although the application of the model in other countries is difficult, exactly as it is proposed, it could be adapted depending on the available sources and the viable variables to use.

In addition, this study used as a reference the index already created in Colombia by DANE in 2020 to compare the performance of the multidimensional index created to predict real COVID-19 cases in the country. The results showed that the metrics obtained by the multidimensional index were better than those of the reference predictor trained with the DANE vulnerability index. The above establishes that the multidimensional index performs a better prediction of the incidence of COVID-19 cases in the country.

For the development of this research, three types of risk factors were determined: human risk factors, sociodemographic and socioeconomic risk factors, and environmental risk factors. Taking the above into account, the classification of the datasets used in the multidimensional index is presented below:

- Vulnerability variable. The variable of this dataset is human and sociodemographic type because it includes vulnerability data already calculated from comorbidities and characteristics of people such as age and overcrowding in homes.
- GDP. The variables of this dataset are sociodemographic and socioeconomic risk factors.

- Percentage of unemployment. The variables of this dataset are sociodemographic and socioeconomic risk factors.
- Vaccination percentage. The variables of this dataset are human risk factors.
- Mobility data. The variables of this dataset are sociodemographic and socioeconomic risk factors.
- Temperature and precipitation. The variables of this dataset are environmental risk factors.

Some limitations should be considered in this study, such as the fact that it was not possible to include the risk factor of comorbidities, which has been used in most of the vulnerability indexes found and has also been characterized in the literature as a risk factor. It is important to mention that due to data policies in Colombia it was not possible to add this variable in the base model. For the multidimensional index, this risk factor is indirectly included in COVID-19 vulnerability index. In addition, it is also worth noting that the multidimensional index does not consider data for 2022, and only handles data for 2020 and 2021. Furthermore, during the data collection phase of the base model, it became evident that access to the data was too limited to calculate an index that could consider various types of risk factors. In addition, the pre-processing and data cleaning required considerable work to implement the ML models. Despite the work done, the lack of access to data on variables resulted in the algorithms obtaining low values for the selected metrics.

It is important to clarify that the proposed model only considered the main cities of Colombia, due to data acquisition limitations that exist for certain variables in cities with a low population in the country. The periodicity of most of the variables considered in the multidimensional index was quarterly; this can generate a certain level of error in the predicted data, considering that a shorter period of time would be ideal.

On the other hand, it should be noted that, in Colombia, no study has considered an index comprising variables that consider different types of risk. Additionally, at the international level, the vast majority of studies do not take into account environmental variables. This study showed that considering variables that belong to different types of risk factors generates an efficient prediction of the incidence of COVID-19. Likewise, the temporality of the data plays a key factor and has not been considered in most of the developed indexes, which handle a static temporality.

In this study, different machine learning algorithms were used to predict the incidence of COVID-19 to know which one performs better according to the dispersion of the data, as opposed to most studies where mathematical methods have been applied or a single machine learning algorithm has been implemented.

Finally, although this study has developed a multidimensional index to predict the incidence of COVID-19 in Colombia, it should be taken into account that the characteristics of the data of the variables in Colombia are not the same as in other countries, so it would imply that the data of each country should be taken into account. However, this study is a valuable contribution to the organizations or entities in Colombia because it can assist in health decision making, predicting the value of the incidence with high values for the metrics.

5. Conclusions

This study shows how using open data sources allows the construction of a multidimensional dataset (a dataset that integrates risk factors of different types). This approach generates a great effort in the pre-processing stage. There may also be a lack of data for some variables selected for different periods. Nevertheless, it is an interesting solution that made it possible to identify and evaluate other factors found in the literature as factors of relevance for calculating a COVID-19 vulnerability index.

This research also included evaluating several ML models implemented with various algorithms. This evaluation was optimized, trying to improve the results. The whole process showed that the model using the Extra Trees Regressor algorithm was the best for predicting the incidence of COVID-19 in 24 Colombian department capitals.

Finally, this research shows the need for comprehensive access to data in Colombia and the protocols for open and anonymized data. This way, different groups or organizations could collect information for research purposes. In addition, delays in data publication and data release in inconsistent formats such as the portable document format (PDF) are common. These problems were addressed in the development of this research by performing manual imputation regarding some variables.

This work is a first step for future research, in which a greater number of variables considered as risk factors for COVID-19 could be regarded in the search for an index that increasingly performs better predictions of the incidence of COVID-19. It is also relevant for calculating vulnerability indexes for other viral diseases, such as dengue.

For future work, other machine learning models could be evaluated, and the index could be extended to other countries. As subsequent work, the adaptation of the model proposed for COVID-19 in other countries is also recommended, considering the review of the acquisition of previously necessary variables in this new context. Another option for future work is related to the application of the proposed model in the same context (Colombia) in a different timeline, which is recommended to be performed in approximately 2 years. Finally, another interesting option for future work is to adjust the model for other types of diseases such as dengue, which would require a greater amount of resources than the previous options since it is necessary to evaluate whether the selected variables are adequate, or if some need to be replaced or removed.

In summary, this work exemplifies the healthcare transformation towards a multidisciplinary, knowledge-based, context-aware ecosystem [28].

Author Contributions: Conceptualization, D.M.L. and R.S.-C.; methodology, D.M.L., D.R. and R.S.-C.; software, P.A.R.P. and J.S.R.G.; validation, P.A.R.P., J.S.R.G. and R.S.-C.; formal analysis, P.A.R.P., J.S.R.G., D.M.L., D.R. and R.S.-C.; investigation, P.A.R.P. and J.S.R.G.; resources, D.M.L., R.S.-C. and B.B.; writing—original draft preparation, P.A.R.P., J.S.R.G. and R.S.-C.; writing—review and editing, D.M.L., D.R., R.S.-C. and B.B.; supervision, D.M.L. and R.S.-C.; funding acquisition, D.M.L. and B.B. All authors have read and agreed to the published version of the manuscript.

Funding: This research received no external funding.

Institutional Review Board Statement: Not applicable.

Informed Consent Statement: Not applicable.

Data Availability Statement: The data presented in this study are available on request from the corresponding author.

Acknowledgments: The authors wish to thank Universidad del Cauca (Telematics Department) and DANE (Colombia).

Conflicts of Interest: The authors declare no conflict of interest.

Appendix A

To improve the performance of the multidimensional index models, it was decided to optimize the hyper-parameters of the algorithms with the best results in the first tests (Decision Tree Regressor, Random Forest Regressor, Gradient Boosting Regressor, and Extra Trees Regressor).

The Decision Tree Regressor was optimized by splitting the data by 80% for training and 20% for testing. The Decision Tree Regressor algorithm deployed the pruning technique, emphasizing the cost complexity parameter (ccp_alpha) to increase the R-squared performance metric. The ccp_alpha seeks a balance between leaf removal and prediction accuracy [29]. Therefore, the GridSearchCV cross-validation (CV) technique evaluated hyper-parameters such as criterion, max_depth, and max_features to obtain the most appropriate values [30]. The model optimization is presented in Figure A1.

```
                    DecisionTreeRegressor
DecisionTreeRegressor(ccp_alpha=7.17948717948718e-06,
                      criterion='absolute_error', max_depth=4,
                      max_features='auto', random_state=329)
```

Figure A1. Optimized model for the Decision Tree Regressor algorithm.

The same data splitting was used to optimize the Random Forest Regressor algorithm (80% training and 20% test). In this case, the parameters that stop tree growth were considered. This algorithm has the advantage that the number of trees (n_estimators) is not a critical parameter; on the contrary, adding trees can improve the result each time, i.e., it does not generate overfitting, but an excess of trees can cause a greater consumption of computational resources [31]. Using GridSearchCV, the hyper-parameters evaluated were n_estimators, max_features, and max_depth. The optimization of the model is presented in Figure A2.

```
                    RandomForestRegressor
RandomForestRegressor(max_depth=13, max_features=7, n_estimators=125,
                      random_state=329)
```

Figure A2. Optimized model for the Random Forest Regressor algorithm.

For the Gradient Boosting Regressor algorithm, the same data splitting was used. The n_estimators parameter was adjusted, because many trees can increase the risk of overfitting [32]. For this case, GridSearchCV was implemented using the early stopping technique, where the number of trees is not included as a hyper-parameter. Within the parameters of the cross-validation technique were learning_rate, max_depth, max_features, and subsample. The optimization of the model is presented in Figure A3.

```
                    GradientBoostingRegressor
GradientBoostingRegressor(learning_rate=0.5, max_depth=2, max_features='auto',
                          n_estimators=1000, n_iter_no_change=5,
                          random_state=329, subsample=1)
```

Figure A3. Optimized model for Gradient Boosting Regressor algorithm.

Specifically, for regression problems, the Hist Gradient Boosting Regressor class can be used, and it works the same way when applying the early stop. Figure A4 presents the used code.

```
                    HistGradientBoostingRegressor
HistGradientBoostingRegressor(early_stopping=True, learning_rate=0.5,
                              max_depth=3, max_iter=1000, random_state=329,
                              tol=1e-05, validation_fraction=0.01)
```

Figure A4. Optimized model for Hist Gradient Boosting Regressor algorithm.

For the Extra Trees Regressor algorithm, the optimal number of trees for the lowest root mean squared error (RMSE) was calculated by dividing the dataset into 80% training and 20% testing [33]. The parameters evaluated for the GridSearchCV cross-validation technique were max_depth, max_features, and n_estimators. Figure A5 presents the code obtained.

```
ExtraTreesRegressor
ExtraTreesRegressor(max_features=None, n_estimators=97, random_state=329)
```

Figure A5. Optimized model for the Extra Trees Regressor algorithm.

The latest algorithm to optimize was the AdaBoost Regressor, which by default works with the Decision Tree Regressor algorithm. The objective was to improve the R-squared metric [34]. Using GridSearchCV, the best value for the parameter n_estimators was sought. Figure A6 presents the code obtained.

```
AdaBoostRegressor
AdaBoostRegressor(base_estimator=DecisionTreeRegressor(ccp_alpha=7.179487e-06,
                                                       criterion='absolute_error',
                                                       max_depth=4,
                                                       max_features='auto',
                                                       random_state=329),
                  n_estimators=247)
    ▸ base_estimator: DecisionTreeRegressor
        ▸ DecisionTreeRegressor
```

Figure A6. Optimized model for AdaBoost Regressor algorithm.

References

1. Información Basíca Sobre la COVID-19. Available online: https://www.who.int/es/news-room/q-a-detail/coronavirus-disease-\protect\unhbox\voidb@x\hbox{COVID-19} (accessed on 12 September 2021).
2. El Coronavirus en Colombia. Available online: https://coronaviruscolombia.gov.co/Covid19/ (accessed on 22 September 2021).
3. Available online: https://www.dane.gov.co/files/comunicados/Nota_metodologica_indice_de_vulnerabilidad.pdf (accessed on 13 June 2023).
4. Pastor-Sierra, K.S.; Peñata-Taborda, A.; Coneo-Pretelt, A.; Jiménez-Vidal, L.; Arteaga-Arroyo, G.; Caldera, D.R.; Salcedo-Arteaga, S.; Galeano-Páez, C.; Espitia-Pérez, P.; Espitia-Pérez, L. Factores ambientales en la transmisión del SARS-CoV-2/COVID 19: Panorama mundial y colombiano. *Salud UIS* **2021**, *53*, 15. [CrossRef] [PubMed]
5. Lo Que Debes Saber Sobre Las Vacunas Contra la COVID-19. Available online: https://www.unicef.org/es/coronavirus/lo-que-debes-saber-sobre-vacuna-covid19 (accessed on 26 February 2023).
6. En Colombia, No Vacunados Tienen de 4 a 9 Veces Más Riesgo de Morir Por COVID-19. Available online: https://www.minsalud.gov.co/Paginas/En-Colombia-no-vacunados-tienen-de-4-a-9-veces-mas-riesgo-de-morir-por-\protect\unhbox\voidb@x\hbox{COVID-19}-.aspx (accessed on 26 February 2023).
7. Economic Commission for Latin America and the Caribbean. *La Prolongación de la Crisis Sanitaria y su Impacto en la Salud, la economía y el Desarrollo Social*; Informes COVID-19 de la CEPAL; United Nations: San Francisco, CA, USA, 2021; ISBN 978-92-1-001637-7.
8. Rosero, P.A.; Realpe, J.S.; Farinango, C.D.; Restrepo, D.S.; Salazar-Cabrera, R.; Lopez, D.M. Risk Factors for COVID-19: A Systematic Mapping Study. In *PHealth 2022: Proceedings of the 19th International Conference on Wearable Micro and Nano Technologies for Personalized Health*; IOS Press: Amsterdam, The Netherlands, 2022; pp. 63–74. [CrossRef]
9. Tiwari, A.; Dadhania, A.V.; Ragunathrao, V.A.B.; Oliveira, E.R.A. Using Machine Learning to Develop a Novel COVID-19 Vulnerability Index (C19VI). *Sci. Total Environ.* **2021**, *773*, 145650. [CrossRef] [PubMed]
10. IBM Docs. Available online: https://prod.ibmdocs-production-dal-6099123ce774e592a519d7c33db8265e-0000.us-south.containers.appdomain.cloud/docs/es/spss-modeler/SaaS?topic=dm-crisp-help-overview (accessed on 23 September 2021).
11. COLOMBIA—Censo Nacional de Población y Vivienda—CNPV—2018—Data Dictionary. Available online: http://microdatos.dane.gov.co/index.php/catalog/643/data_dictionary#page=F9&tab=data-dictionary (accessed on 10 November 2022).
12. Base COVID-19 Dataset. Available online: https://www.kaggle.com/datasets/sebastianrgonzalez/base-dane-covid19-dataset (accessed on 26 February 2023).
13. Una Comparación de los Métodos de Correlación de Pearson y Spearman. Available online: https://support.minitab.com/es-mx/minitab/20/help-and-how-to/statistics/basic-statistics/supporting-topics/correlation-and-covariance/a-comparison-of-the-pearson-and-spearman-correlation-methods/ (accessed on 26 February 2023).
14. Spearman's Rank Correlation: The Definitive Guide to Understand | Simplilearn. Available online: https://www.simplilearn.com/tutorials/statistics-tutorial/spearmans-rank-correlation (accessed on 9 November 2022).

15. Una Guía Para Principiantes Sobre La Regresión Lineal En Python Con Scikit-Learn. Available online: https://www.datasource.ai/es/data-science-articles/view-source:https://www.datasource.ai/es/data-science-articles/una-guia-para-principiantes-sobre-la-regresion-lineal-en-python-con-scikit-learn (accessed on 26 February 2023).
16. Evaluando El Error En Los Modelos de Clasificación—Aprende IA. Available online: https://aprendeia.com/evaluando-el-error-en-los-modelos-de-clasificacion-machine-learning/ (accessed on 13 January 2023).
17. Producto Interno Bruto (PIB) | Banco de La República. Available online: https://www.banrep.gov.co/es/glosario/producto-interno-bruto-pib (accessed on 18 November 2022).
18. Google Earth Engine. Available online: https://earthengine.google.com (accessed on 3 February 2023).
19. Microsoft Power BI. Available online: https://app.powerbi.com/view?r=eyJrIjoiNThmZTJmZWYtOWFhMy00OGE1LWFiNDAtMTJmYjM0NDA5NGY2IiwidCI6ImJmYjdlMTNhLTdmYjctNDAxNi04MzBjLWQzNzE2ZThkZDhiOCJ9 (accessed on 4 February 2023).
20. Empleo y Desempleo. Available online: https://www.dane.gov.co/index.php/estadisticas-por-tema/mercado-laboral/empleo-y-desempleo (accessed on 18 November 2022).
21. COVID-19 Community Mobility Report. Available online: https://www.google.com/covid19/mobility?hl=en (accessed on 18 November 2022).
22. Casos Positivos de COVID-19 en Colombia | Datos Abiertos Colombia. Available online: https://www.datos.gov.co/Salud-y-Protecci-n-Social/Casos-positivos-de-\protect\unhbox\voidb@x\hbox{COVID-19}-en-Colombia/gt2j-8ykr (accessed on 1 December 2022).
23. Multidimensional Index of COVID-19 Colombia. Available online: https://www.kaggle.com/datasets/sebastianrgonzalez/covid19-colombia (accessed on 26 February 2023).
24. Sambangi, S.; Gondi, L. A Machine Learning Approach for DDoS (Distributed Denial of Service) Attack Detection Using Multiple Linear Regression. *Proceedings* **2020**, *63*, 51. [CrossRef]
25. Zach RMSE vs. R-Squared: Which Metric Should You Use? *Statology*. 2021. Available online: https://www.statology.org/rmse-vs-r-squared/ (accessed on 26 February 2023).
26. Explaining Negative R-Squared. Available online: https://towardsdatascience.com/explaining-negative-r-squared-17894ca26321 (accessed on 30 June 2023).
27. John, V.; Liu, Z.; Guo, C.; Mita, S.; Kidono, K. Real-time lane estimation Using Deep features and extra trees regression. In *Lecture Notes in Computer Science (Including Subseries Lecture Notes in Artificial Intelligence and Lecture Notes in Bioinformatics)*; Springer: Berlin/Heidelberg, Germany, 2016; Volume 9431, pp. 721–733. [CrossRef]
28. Blobel, B.; Oemig, F.; Ruotsalainen, P.; Lopez, D.M. Transformation of Health and Social Care Systems—An Interdisciplinary Approach Toward a Foundational Architecture. *Front. Med.* **2022**, *9*, 802487. [CrossRef]
29. Post Pruning Decision Trees with Cost Complexity Pruning. Available online: https://scikit-learn/stable/auto_examples/tree/plot_cost_complexity_pruning.html (accessed on 14 December 2022).
30. sklearn.model_selection.GridSearchCV. Available online: https://scikit-learn/stable/modules/generated/sklearn.model_selection.GridSearchCV.html (accessed on 6 January 2023).
31. Random Forest Python. Available online: https://www.cienciadedatos.net/documentos/py08_random_forest_python.html (accessed on 14 January 2023).
32. Gradient Boosting Con Python. Available online: https://www.cienciadedatos.net/documentos/py09_gradient_boosting_python.html (accessed on 16 January 2023).
33. sklearn.ensemble.ExtraTreesRegressor. Available online: https://scikit-learn/stable/modules/generated/sklearn.ensemble.ExtraTreesRegressor.html (accessed on 13 January 2023).
34. sklearn.ensemble.AdaBoostRegressor. Available online: https://scikit-learn/stable/modules/generated/sklearn.ensemble.AdaBoostRegressor.html (accessed on 13 January 2023).

Disclaimer/Publisher's Note: The statements, opinions and data contained in all publications are solely those of the individual author(s) and contributor(s) and not of MDPI and/or the editor(s). MDPI and/or the editor(s) disclaim responsibility for any injury to people or property resulting from any ideas, methods, instructions or products referred to in the content.

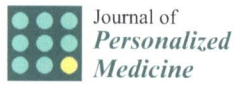

Article

Machine Learning Methods for Pregnancy and Childbirth Risk Management

Georgy Kopanitsa [1,2,*], Oleg Metsker [2] and Sergey Kovalchuk [1]

[1] Faculty of Digital Transformations, ITMO University, 4 Birzhevaya Liniya, 199034 Saint-Petersburg, Russia
[2] Almazov National Medical Research Centre, Ulitsa Akkuratova, 2, 197341 Saint-Petersburg, Russia
* Correspondence: georgy.kopanitsa@gmail.com

Abstract: Machine learning methods enable medical systems to automatically generate data-driven decision support models using real-world data inputs, eliminating the need for explicit rule design. In this research, we investigated the application of machine learning methods in healthcare, specifically focusing on pregnancy and childbirth risks. The timely identification of risk factors during early pregnancy, along with risk management, mitigation, prevention, and adherence management, can significantly reduce adverse perinatal outcomes and complications for both mother and child. Given the existing burden on medical professionals, clinical decision support systems (CDSSs) can play a role in risk management. However, these systems require high-quality decision support models based on validated medical data that are also clinically interpretable. To develop models for predicting childbirth risks and due dates, we conducted a retrospective analysis of electronic health records from the perinatal Center of the Almazov Specialized Medical Center in Saint-Petersburg, Russia. The dataset, which was exported from the medical information system, consisted of structured and semi-structured data, encompassing a total of 73,115 lines for 12,989 female patients. Our proposed approach, which includes a detailed analysis of predictive model performance and interpretability, offers numerous opportunities for decision support in perinatal care provision. The high predictive performance achieved by our models ensures precise support for both individual patient care and overall health organization management.

Keywords: delivery date; childbirth; machine learning; risk factors; prediction

1. Introduction

This paper is an extended version of papers presented in the pHealth 2022 and previous pHealth conferences [1–3].

The timely identification of risk factors in the early stages of pregnancy, along with effective risk management and mitigation [4], prevention strategies [5], and adherence management [6], have the potential to significantly reduce the occurrence of adverse perinatal outcomes and complications for both mother and child [7]. Considering the existing workload of medical professionals, clinical decision support systems (CDSSs) can play a vital role in assisting with risk management. To ensure the effectiveness of CDSSs, it is essential to develop a robust set of high-quality decision support models that rely on validated medical data and offer clinical interpretability [8].

The development of perinatal episodes involves a complex interplay of numerous heterogeneous factors, each contributing differently to the etiology and pathology at various stages. This complexity poses a significant challenge in developing decision support models. In such a scenario, intelligent data analysis and data-driven models [9] can serve as effective foundations for clinical decision support.

For instance, in a review focusing on risk assessment and management to prevent preterm birth, a study was conducted on 47 patients with connective tissue dysplasia and 29 patients without this syndrome [5]. The study utilized data from clinical and laboratory tests, ultrasound, Dopplerometry, Cardiotocography (CTG), the Electrocardiogram (ECG), and echocardiography (ECHO-CG). By analyzing categorical variables related to the history, course, and outcome of pregnancy, the effects of connective tissue dysplasia were evaluated in a sample of 400 pregnant women. The final dataset consisted of 350 features, and the developed model successfully predicted the probability of complications during pregnancy and childbirth.

The forecast generated by the model accurately predicted complications for 32 out of 50 women, with 16 women having more predicted complications and 3 women having fewer predicted complications. Among the patients, approximately 51% experienced complications, with 86% exhibiting chronic fetal hypoxia and 6% experiencing premature detachment of the normally located placenta. These findings align with the results of previous studies [10,11].

The Apgar score serves as a reliable and widely accepted metric for assessing childbirth outcomes due to its comprehensive evaluation of vital signs, including heart rate, respiration, muscle tone, reflex irritability, and color, providing valuable insights into the immediate well-being and overall health of the newborn [12].

Regarding specific metrics, a study utilizing a novel machine learning algorithm [13] aimed to identify clinically significant predictors of neurocognitive development in newborns with perinatal human immunodeficiency virus (HIV). Through multifactor regression with gradient boosting and fivefold cross-validation, the study successfully identified the predictors that have the greatest impact on the neurocognitive stability of newborns. Another study [14] demonstrated the high accuracy of logistic regression models in predicting neonatal mortality. Furthermore, machine learning algorithms were compared with traditional methods for early assessment of adverse risks in pregnant women [15].

In addition to examining individual studies, recent systematic reviews [15–20] have highlighted the limitations of existing models and algorithms in supporting decision-making, particularly in critical situations. The classification and prognosis precision of these models does not exceed 82%, which is considered unsatisfactory. This is primarily attributed to the lack of structured patient data, making it challenging to construct sufficiently accurate mathematical models for pregnancy development. However, the application of machine learning methods has shown promising results in efficient due date prediction based on ultrasound data [21], and artificial neural networks have demonstrated high accuracy in predicting due dates [22]. Thus, despite the experience gained in developing decision-making models and forecasting maternal risks, there is still room for improvement in these models. The further development of such models holds the potential to reduce complications and mortality rates during pregnancy and childbirth.

The goal of this study is to develop real-world-evidence data-driven models based on semi-structured data for pregnancy and childbirth risks prediction. To achieve this goal, we apply machine learning methods to perform a detailed analysis of the importance of predictors for the due date and outcomes to cover the wellbeing of both the mother and children. In this study, we search for the most reliable predictors and identify relationships among them.

2. Materials and Methods

We conducted a retrospective analysis of electronic health records from the perinatal Center of the Almazov specialized medical center in Saint-Petersburg, Russia. The dataset was obtained by exporting data from the medical information system. Dataset A consisted of structured and semi-structured data, comprising a total of 73,115 lines corresponding to 12,989 female patients. This dataset covered the period from 1 January 2015 to 31 December 2019. Additionally, Dataset B included 103,414 lines representing 15,681 newly born patients. Each line in the datasets corresponded to a doctor encounter. To combine the data from the two different health information systems, we used the mother identifier.

2.1. Data Preparation and Preprocessing

In our study, we obtained a substantial dataset, consisting of 73,115 lines, from Dataset A. This dataset encompassed a wide range of information, including 97 structured features and unstructured arrays of additional medical data. Notably, the unstructured data comprised valuable insights from sources such as the electronic health records (EHRs), specifically the mother anamnesis.

The inclusion of unstructured data from the EHR holds significant importance in capturing comprehensive medical information. These unaltered and unanalyzed data directly reflect the recorded details from the healthcare providers, ensuring the authenticity and integrity of the information. By incorporating the unstructured data alongside the structured features, our dataset becomes more comprehensive and allows for a more comprehensive analysis of the perinatal care context.

Figure 1 visually depicts the data flow and acquisition process, illustrating how the unstructured data from the electronic health records were directly integrated into our dataset. The unmodified inclusion of these data ensures that we capture the most accurate and up-to-date information available, enhancing the overall validity and reliability of our analysis.

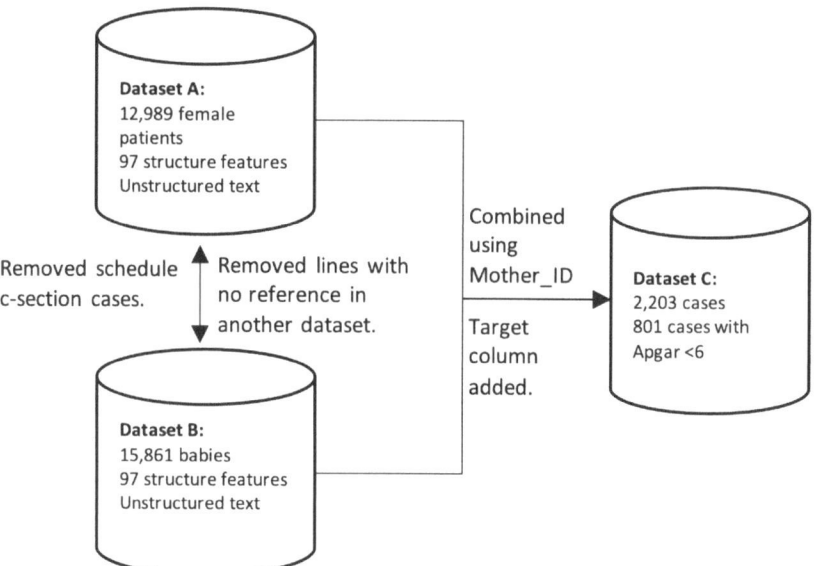

Figure 1. Data preparation process.

The data were taken after the first mandatory screening that takes place between week 11 and 13.

- Mother ID (mother_id) was used as the index to combine two datasets (mothers and newly born).
- All the records from Dataset B that did not have a corresponding mother ID from Dataset A were removed.
- All the lines from Dataset A with no corresponding IDs from Dataset B were removed.
- All the lines that did not contain an Apgar score were removed from the dataset as they were irrelevant for the study.
- All the cases of scheduled C-sections were removed from the datasets.

This resulted in the creation of Dataset C, which comprised 2203 records representing 2203 cases involving both the mother and child. Out of these cases, 801 were identified as having an Apgar score below 6. Any lines in the dataset that did not include the labor date were removed, resulting in 62,734 remaining lines representing an equivalent number of female patients. The target column in the dataset was defined as the length of gestation in days. Additionally, we utilized the Apgar score, ranging from 0 to 10, as a metric for assessing childbirth outcomes [12]. A score of 5 and less was considered as a negative outcome. A target column was added to the dataset: 1 if Apgar score > 5 and 0 if Apgar score < 6.

2.2. Correlation and Feature Importance

In our study, we conducted a correlation analysis to explore the relationships between the predictors and the predicted outcomes. To perform this analysis, we employed the Shapley additive explanations (SHAP) index [23], which is a powerful tool for quantifying the contribution and importance of each feature in the prediction model. The SHAP index provides a valuable insight into the role played by each feature in influencing the predictions made by the model. By quantifying the contribution of individual features, it allows us to identify the most relevant predictors that have a significant impact on the model's predictions.

2.3. Prediction Modeling

2.3.1. Childbirth Risks

In order to effectively classify cases with an Apgar score below 6, which serves as an important indicator of potential health risks in newborns, we designed and conducted an experiment. The foundation of our study was Dataset C, a comprehensive collection of relevant information. To ensure the validity and reliability of our findings, we performed a random split of Dataset C, creating a 70% training set and a 30% test set. For the classification task at hand, we opted to employ the random forest (RF) method, a widely recognized and powerful algorithm in the field of machine learning. The RF method operates by constructing an ensemble of decision tree classifiers, each trained on a distinct subset of the dataset. By utilizing this ensemble approach and leveraging the concept of averaging, RF significantly enhances the predictive accuracy of our classification model while effectively mitigating the risk of overfitting.

2.3.2. Due Date Prediction

Each experiment with Dataset C ran in the setting of stratified 5-fold cross-validation, i.e., a random 70% portion of the training dataset was used for training and a random 30% portion of the training dataset was used for testing (70% random selection from the study dataset). Target class ratios in the folds were preserved. The gradient search parameters were: params = {'min_child_weight':[4,5], 'gamma':[i/10.0 for i in range(3,6)], 'subsample':[i/10.0 for i in range(6,11)], 'colsample_bytree':[i/10.0 for i in range(6,11)], 'max_depth':[2–4]}. We compared Gradient Boosting regression, Random forest regression, Linear regression, and Voting regression. The root-mean-square error was used as a performance metric. After determining the optimal dataset and model parameters, we performed a validation with the testing dataset (30% random selection from the study dataset). The Scikit-learn library was used for the experiment. The Mean Absolute Error (MAE) was used as a performance metric. The best performing regressor was evaluated on the test dataset (30% random selection from the study dataset). For this study, we used Python 3.6.3 and scikit-learn 0.19.1 (https://scikit-learn.org/stable/ accessed date: 9.06.2023) as the basic framework for machine learning models.

2.3.3. Model Evaluation

In our experimental analysis, we evaluated the performance of our model on test datasets, which comprised 30% randomly selected lines from the original dataset. We used commonly used performance metrics, including *Precision*, *Recall*, and *F-measure*, to assess the effectiveness of our model.

Precision measures the accuracy of positive predictions by calculating the proportion of correctly predicted positive instances out of all instances predicted as positive. It indicates the model's ability to minimize false positives.

$$Precision = \frac{true\ positives}{true\ positives + false\ positives}$$

Recall quantifies the model's ability to capture positive instances by calculating the proportion of correctly predicted positive instances out of all actual positive instances. It focuses on minimizing false negatives.

$$Recall = \frac{true\ positives}{true\ positives + false\ negatives}$$

F-measure, the harmonic mean of precision and recall, provides a balanced assessment of the model's performance. It considers both false positives and false negatives, offering a comprehensive evaluation.

$$F-measure = 2 \cdot \frac{recall \cdot precision}{recall + precision}$$

By calculating *Precision*, *Recall*, and *F-measure* on the test datasets, we gain a holistic understanding of our model's effectiveness in accurately identifying positive instances. These metrics allow us to assess precision, recall rates, and the balance between false positives and false negatives.

3. Results

3.1. Due Date Prediction

This section presents predictors (Figure 2) that include well-known factors such as the mother's age, as well as previously less explored predictors such as the child's gender, RH factor, and gastrointestinal diseases. The importance analysis of these features is depicted in Figure 2.

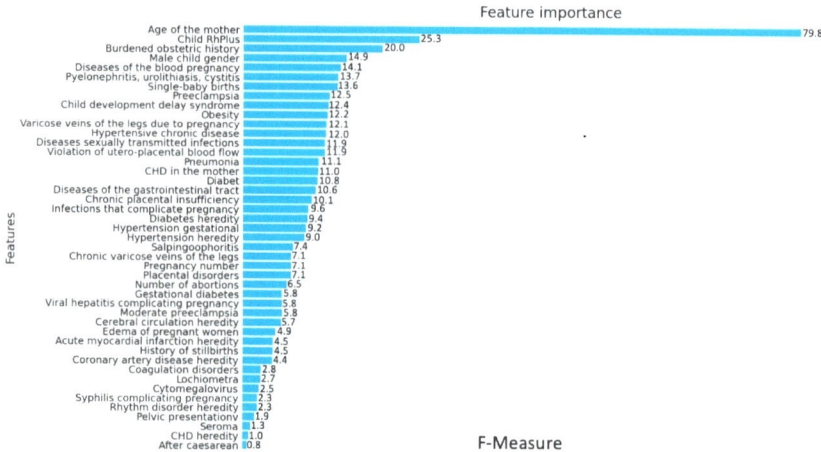

Figure 2. Feature importance for the due date prediction.

Figure 3 and Table 1 present the results of the grid search conducted to find the optimal regression model for due date prediction.

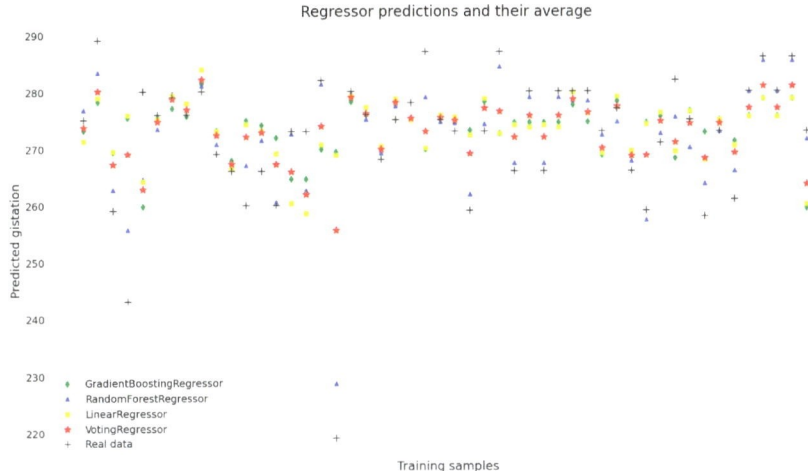

Figure 3. Due date Regression prediction.

Table 1. Prediction efficiency for different regressors.

Regressor	MAE
Random Forrest	3.72
Gradient Boosting	8.02
Linear regression	7.12
Voting regression	6.58

Figure 4 presents a due date prediction biplot for different regressors used in the study.

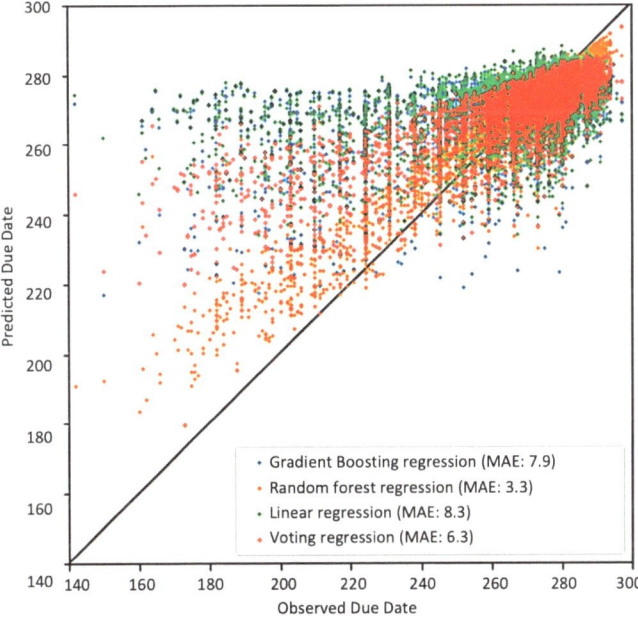

Figure 4. Due date prediction biplot.

The grid search resulted in the optimal grid parameters: {'colsample_bytree':0.9, 'gamma':0.3, 'max_depth':2, 'min_child_weight':4, 'subsample':1.0}. We used the MAE for the delivery due date accuracy assessment. The random forest regression gave the best value of MAE of 3.85 on the test dataset.

3.2. Childbirth Risk Prediction

Correlation and Feature Importance

Top important features for Apgar score < 6 are presented in Figure 5.

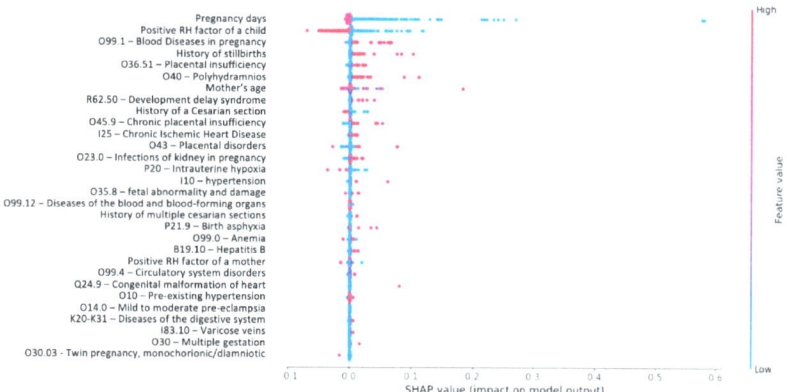

Figure 5. Feature importance for the low APGAR score.

Figure 6 demonstrates that hypoxia has differential contributions to the risk of low Apgar score in boys and girls. Specifically, hypoxia has a lesser impact on the overall risk of negative outcomes in boys compared to girls. Conversely, intrauterine hypoxia in the fetus can result in intrauterine amniotic fluid aspiration, which increases the probability of stillbirth, particularly in boys.

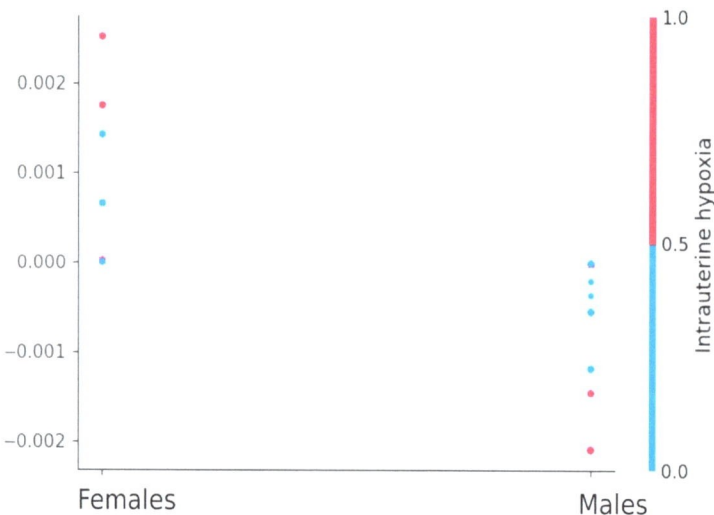

Figure 6. Influence of gender on intrauterine hypoxia.

Figure 7 demonstrates the change in the RH factor influence during the pregnancy.

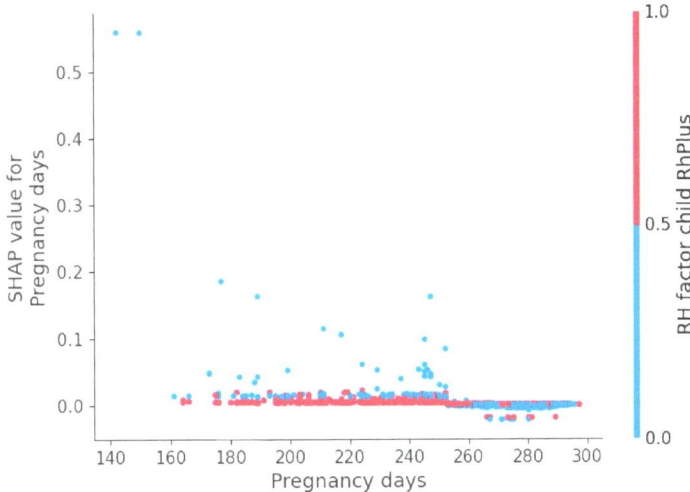

Figure 7. Change in the RH factor influence during the pregnancy.

The Apgar score random forest prediction model achieved a precision of 0.92, indicating a high proportion of correct positive predictions. With a recall of 0.99, it successfully identified the majority of actual positive instances. The F-measure, combining precision and recall, was 0.88, providing an overall assessment of the model's accuracy.

4. Discussion

The findings of our study demonstrate the successful implementation of real-world-evidence data-driven models for the prediction of pregnancy and childbirth risks. By utilizing structured and semi-structured data from electronic health records, this research aimed to develop accurate predictive models that can assist in timely risk identification and improve decision making for medical professionals. We analyzed a comprehensive dataset from a perinatal center, encompassing information from both mothers and newborns, and employed various statistical and machine learning techniques for risk assessment. The results indicate promising outcomes, with the models achieving high precision in predicting adverse childbirth events and due dates. Additionally, the analysis of feature importance revealed clinically significant predictors associated with low Apgar scores, offering valuable insights for early detection and preventive measures. These findings highlight the potential of utilizing data-driven models and real-world evidence to enhance risk management and reduce complications during pregnancy and childbirth.

4.1. Clinical Interpretations and Implications

As observed in Figure 6, a low Apgar score is correlated with stillbirth in the medical history, aggravated obstetric history, the mother's age, presence of uterine scars, and sexually transmitted infections. Complications in the baby are correlated with varicose veins in the legs. Child development delay syndrome is positively correlated with placental insufficiency and fetal growth retardation syndrome, while it is negatively correlated with emergency and spontaneous births.

The male gender of the baby also slightly correlates with newborn complications. Inflammation in the mother can indicate impaired child nutrition, and the development of fetoplacental insufficiency is associated with placental inflammation. Intrauterine intoxication occurs when pyelonephritis affects the kidneys and liver, impairing their function and causing intoxication. Preeclampsia is an indicator that the fetus is suffering, and severe cases may require premature delivery, negatively affecting the fetus. It also disrupts placental blood flow, leading to inadequate nutritional supply. Caesarean sections may be necessary in such cases. Blood diseases, such as anemia, can result in oxygen deficiency and impaired placental oxygen perfusion. When a mother has a blood disease, the child's circulatory system may suffer from hypoxia as the fetus relies on the placenta for nourishment. The prognosis changes from negative to positive when a premature birth or emergency Caesarean section occurs between 33 and 36 weeks of gestation, as the fetus becomes viable and begins to gain weight. Therefore, it is recommended to exclude cases of emergency Caesarean or premature deliveries when analyzing these factors. Risks for the child should be evaluated separately before and after 33 weeks of gestation.

Complications in the perinatal period should be monitored, and children should be followed up until one year of age with regular monthly check-ups and appropriate tests. Hypertensive disease in the mother triggers a similar mechanism to preeclampsia, leading to oxygen deficiency. This can result in either a Caesarean section or earlier natural delivery. Fetal hypoxia can cause premature labor activity, with the baby experiencing increased breathing and potential asphyxiation from inhaling water, leading to a high heart rate. A mismatch of Rh factors may require intrauterine transfusion, which can result in premature births.

Analysis of the Rh factor indicates changes around the 250th day of pregnancy (see Figure 7). This example highlights the importance of analyzing features in relation to gestational time. Exposure to gastrointestinal diseases in the mother is identified as a significant factor for premature births, despite not typically being considered a risk factor. This finding requires further study. Gastrointestinal diseases may affect the absorption of vitamins and nutrients, possibly due to medications taken for ulcers and gastritis. Obesity disrupts vascular function and leads to metabolic syndrome, hyperglycemia, and plaques in blood vessels. This disturbance in the child's diet can result in fetoplacental insufficiency and increased labor activity. Varicose disease can have similar consequences. The number of previous abortions and pregnancies in the medical history are obvious factors indicating data accuracy.

4.2. Models' Performance

This study presents the implementation of predictive models for adverse childbirth events, achieving a higher precision (0.92) compared to most state-of-the-art models. The precision of classification and prognosis in previous studies does not exceed 82%, as indicated in the systematic review [9]. The only available models in the literature that performed better were [14] with a precision of 0.93 and [24] with an accuracy of 99.23%. This can be explained in that both studies worked with very limited datasets (285 children and 322 women, respectively).

This is attributed to the inclusion of unstructured medical data alongside the structured dataset. By identifying the main risk factors through feature importance analysis, clinicians can receive support in early complication analysis and the formulation and implementation of preventive measures. The proposed data-driven model for due date prediction enables highly accurate predictions, facilitating effective resource planning. These models are built upon real-world evidence and can be applied with a limited number of predictors. Furthermore, we have identified the most crucial features for predicting the labor due date, aiding policymakers in establishing appropriate data collection channels to capture essential information in electronic health records.

On the other hand, the detailed analysis reveals distinct error patterns in predictive models between the preterm birth period (37 weeks or earlier) and the normal birth period (later than 37 weeks). This discrepancy can be attributed to several factors. Firstly, the dataset exhibits a high level of imbalance, with the majority of cases resulting in normal birth outcomes. Consequently, the models are primarily trained to reflect this normal scenario. Secondly, the nature of preterm birth differs significantly from normal cases, leading to varied performance among different models (although the random forest model still outperforms others). Considering these factors, we believe that dividing the cases based on a rule-based approach or utilizing classifier-based techniques [24,25] and separately training models, with a potential subsequent combination using ensemble techniques [26], could significantly enhance the performance of the model for preterm delivery prediction. We consider addressing this issue as a crucial avenue for future model improvement, given the substantial impact of preterm birth on both maternal and child health, as well as the management of extensive healthcare services.

Even static features should be analyzed in a multifactorial manner rather than through pairwise analysis. Therefore, it is crucial to evaluate the factors influencing labor outcomes from the perspective of the fetus's gender, as different factors may have contrasting effects on adverse outcomes. Intrauterine hypoxia resulting from intrauterine insufficiency can lead to the aspiration of amniotic fluid, increasing the probability of stillbirth. The intriguing observation that boys are less likely to inhale requires further investigation. Currently, there is limited research that explores the contribution of gender to childbirth outcomes. Our study's findings (Figures 5 and 6) highlight the need for multifactorial analysis, as opposed to traditional two-factor experiments. The prediction and interpretation of Apgar scores show promising results in improving perinatal health services. Analyzing the performance and interpretation of predictive models reveals similar variations in preterm and normal births. Interpretability plays a vital role in the analysis of predictive models, enabling a deeper understanding of the model structure and its outcomes. Feature engineering is a critical aspect of model development, as it allows mapping features to domain-specific concepts, facilitating more comprehensive interpretation and linking with additional information within patients' electronic health records. Moreover, such integration enables the incorporation of flexible decision support into existing regulated healthcare processes, promoting greater trust and readiness for predictive models. [27].

The healthcare system generates a vast amount of medical data, comprising both structured and unstructured formats, with unstructured data being predominant. The digital transformation of healthcare necessitates the utilization of all available medical data. The results of this study demonstrate that applying machine learning methods to unstructured data can enhance the accuracy and precision of predictive models. This presents an opportunity to leverage extensive repositories of clinical data for the development of predictive models that aid healthcare professionals in disease diagnosis and recommending appropriate treatment options for patients.

4.3. Machine Learning for Clinical Decision Support

In real-time continuous applications, ML methods offer immediate and dynamic decision support, enabling timely risk identification and proactive interventions. This capability is particularly valuable in time-sensitive situations such as emergency obstetric care. ML models continuously analyze data, adapt to changing circumstances, and provide real-time recommendations to enhance perinatal care efficiency. On the other hand, ML methods can also serve as powerful tools for developing decision-making tools that are used in a more static manner. By training on large datasets, ML models capture complex patterns and relationships, offering valuable insights and predictions to guide decision making. The practical incorporation of ML results into accessible decision tools for clinicians is crucial. User-friendly interfaces and visualizations can present the model output in a clear and understandable manner. The collaboration between ML experts and healthcare professionals ensures the development of user-friendly decision support tools that align with clinical needs and workflows.

5. Conclusions

The proposed approach offers a range of benefits and opportunities for decision support in perinatal care. One of the key advantages is the high predictive performance achieved by the models. This precision provides valuable support to healthcare services, benefiting both individual patients and health organizations. With accurate predictions, medical professionals can make informed decisions, leading to improved patient outcomes and optimized resource allocation.

Another advantage is the interpretability of the model predictions. This aspect enhances trust and validity, making the technology more suitable for practical use. By understanding the reasoning behind the predictions, healthcare professionals and stakeholders can gain deeper insights into the factors influencing specific outcomes. This transparency fosters trust in the models and facilitates their implementation within clinical settings.

The structured and interpretable nature of the predictive modeling framework also enables further improvements. Researchers can develop even more flexible and interpretable algorithms, expanding the applicability of the approach to diverse scenarios and patient profiles. Additionally, integrating domain-specific knowledge into the models enhances their effectiveness and relevance in perinatal care.

Overall, the results obtained from this study are promising; particularly, they contribute to the overall advancement of a model-based approach with strong predictive performance and clear interpretability. By leveraging these strengths, decision support in perinatal care can be significantly enhanced, leading to improved healthcare outcomes and more efficient resource allocation.

Author Contributions: G.K. was responsible for setting up the concept and methodology of the study, O.M. was responsible for data processing, data analysis, and interpretation, S.K. was responsible for project management and drafting and reviewing of the manuscript. All authors have read and agreed to the published version of the manuscript.

Funding: This research is financially supported by the Ministry of Science and Higher Education, agreement FSER-2021-0012.

Institutional Review Board Statement: Ethical review and approval were waived for this study since all the data used in the study was completely anonymized before the study and no human subjects were involved.

Informed Consent Statement: Patient consent was waived since no patients or data that allowed identification of patients were involved in the study.

Data Availability Statement: The datasets GENERATED and ANALYZED for this study can be requested from the corresponding author.

Conflicts of Interest: The authors declare that the research was conducted in the absence of any commercial or financial relationships that could be construed as a potential conflict of interest.

References

1. Kopanitsa, G.; Kovalchuk, S. Study of the User Behaviour Caused by Automatic Recommendation Systems Call to Action. In Proceedings of the Studies in Health Technology and Informatics, Vienna, Austria, 22–25 May 2022; Volume 299.
2. Metsker, O.; Kopanitsa, G.; Bolgova, E. Prediction of Childbirth Mortality Using Machine Learning. In Proceedings of the Studies in Health Technology and Informatics, Virtual, 14–16 September 2020.
3. Metsker, O.; Kopanitsa, G.; Komlichenko, E.; Yanushanets, M.; Bolgova, E. Prediction of a Due Date Based on the Pregnancy History Data Using Machine Learning. *Stud. Health Technol. Inform.* **2020**, *273*, 104–108. [CrossRef]
4. English, F.A.; Kenny, L.C.; McCarthy, F.P. Risk Factors and Effective Management of Preeclampsia. *Integr. Blood Press. Control* **2015**, *8*, 7–12.
5. Koullali, B.; Oudijk, M.A.; Nijman, T.A.J.; Mol, B.W.J.; Pajkrt, E. Risk Assessment and Management to Prevent Preterm Birth. *Semin. Fetal. Neonatal Med.* **2016**, *21*, 80–88. [CrossRef] [PubMed]
6. Kolkman, D.G.E.; Rijnders, M.E.B.; Wouters, M.G.A.J.; van den Akker-van Marle, M.E.; van der Ploeg, C.P.B.K.; de Groot, C.J.M.; Fleuren, M.A.H. Implementation of a Cost-Effective Strategy to Prevent Neonatal Early-Onset Group B Haemolytic Streptococcus Disease in the Netherlands. *BMC Pregnancy Childbirth* **2013**, *13*, 155. [CrossRef] [PubMed]
7. Hug, L.; Alexander, M.; You, D.; Alkema, L. National, Regional, and Global Levels and Trends in Neonatal Mortality between 1990 and 2017, with Scenario-Based Projections to 2030: A Systematic Analysis. *Lancet Glob. Health* **2019**, *7*, e710–e720. [CrossRef] [PubMed]
8. Krikunov, A.V.; Bolgova, E.V.; Krotov, E.; Abuhay, T.M.; Yakovlev, A.N.; Kovalchuk, S.V. Complex Data-Driven Predictive Modeling in Personalized Clinical Decision Support for Acute Coronary Syndrome Episodes. *Procedia Comput. Sci.* **2016**, *80*, 518–529. [CrossRef]
9. Tsui, K.L.; Chen, N.; Zhou, Q.; Hai, Y.; Wang, W. Prognostics and Health Management: A Review on Data Driven Approaches. *Math. Probl. Eng.* **2015**, *2015*, 793161. [CrossRef]

10. Tezikov, Y.V.; Lipatov, I.S.; Frolova, N.A.; Kutuzova, O.A.; Prikhod'ko, A.V. Methodology of Preventing Major Obstetrical Syndromes. *Vopr. Ginekol. Akuš. Perinatol.* **2016**, *15*, 20–30. [CrossRef]
11. Tezikov, Y.V.; Lipatov, I.S.; Kalinkina, O.B.; Tezikova, T.A.; Rakitina, V.N.; Marthinova, N.V.; Mingalieva, L.K.; Dobrodickaya, A.D. Stratification of Pregnant Women at Risk with the Use Predictive Indexes. *Ultrasound Obstet Gynecol.* **2017**, *58*, 360–368. [CrossRef]
12. Apgar, V. The Newborn (APGAR) Scoring System: Reflections and Advice. *Pediatr. Clin. N. Am.* **1966**, *13*, 645–650. [CrossRef]
13. Paul, R.; Cho, K.; Mellins, C.; Malee, K.; Robbins, R.; Kerr, S.; Sophonphan, J.; Jahanshad, N.; Aurpibul, L.; Thongpibul, K.; et al. Predicting Neurodevelopmental Outcomes in Children with Perinatal HIV Using a Novel Machine Learning Algorithm. *bioRxiv* **2019**, 632273. [CrossRef]
14. Pollack, M.M.; Koch, M.A.; Bartel, D.A.; Rapoport, I.; Dhanireddy, R.; El-Mohandes, A.A.E.; Harkavy, K.; Subramanian, K.N.S. A Comparison of Neonatal Mortality Risk Prediction Models in Very Low Birth Weight Infants. *Pediatrics* **2000**, *105*, 1051–1057. [CrossRef] [PubMed]
15. Aoyama, K.; D'Souza, R.; Pinto, R.; Ray, J.G.; Hill, A.; Scales, D.C.; Lapinsky, S.E.; Seaward, G.R.; Hladunewich, M.; Shah, P.S.; et al. Risk Prediction Models for Maternal Mortality: A Systematic Review and Meta-Analysis. *PLoS ONE* **2018**, *13*, e0208563. [CrossRef] [PubMed]
16. Verstraete, E.H.; Blot, K.; Mahieu, L.; Vogelaers, D.; Blot, S. Prediction Models for Neonatal Health Care-Associated Sepsis: A Meta-Analysis. *Pediatrics* **2015**, *135*, e1002–e1014. [CrossRef]
17. Ukah, U.V.; De Silva, D.A.; Payne, B.; Magee, L.A.; Hutcheon, J.A.; Brown, H.; Ansermino, J.M.; Lee, T.; von Dadelszen, P. Prediction of Adverse Maternal Outcomes from Pre-Eclampsia and Other Hypertensive Disorders of Pregnancy: A Systematic Review. *Pregnancy Hypertens.* **2018**, *11*, 115–123. [CrossRef]
18. Verhagen, T.E.M.; Hendriks, D.J.; Bancsi, L.F.J.M.M.; Mol, B.W.J.; Broekmans, F.J.M. The Accuracy of Multivariate Models Predicting Ovarian Reserve and Pregnancy after in Vitro Fertilization: A Meta-Analysis. *Hum. Reprod. Update* **2008**, *14*, 95–100. [CrossRef] [PubMed]
19. Lamain-De Ruiter, M.; Kwee, A.; Naaktgeboren, C.A.; Franx, A.; Moons, K.G.M.; Koster, M.P.H. Prediction Models for the Risk of Gestational Diabetes: A Systematic Review. *Diagn. Progn. Res.* **2017**, *1*, 3. [CrossRef] [PubMed]
20. Sananès, N.; Langer, B.; Gaudineau, A.; Kutnahorsky, R.; Aissi, G.; Fritz, G.; Boudier, E.; Viville, B.; Nisand, I.; Favre, R. Prediction of Spontaneous Preterm Delivery in Singleton Pregnancies: Where Are We and Where Are We Going? A Review of Literature. *J. Obstet. Gynaecol.* **2014**, *34*, 457–461. [CrossRef]
21. Naimi, A.I.; Platt, R.W.; Larkin, J.C. Machine Learning for Fetal Growth Prediction. *Epidemiology* **2018**, *29*, 290. [CrossRef]
22. Podda, M.; Bacciu, D.; Micheli, A.; Bellù, R.; Placidi, G.; Gagliardi, L. A Machine Learning Approach to Estimating Preterm Infants Survival: Development of the Preterm Infants Survival Assessment (PISA) Predictor. *Sci. Rep.* **2018**, *8*, 13743. [CrossRef]
23. Ogami, C.; Tsuji, Y.; Seki, H.; Kawano, H.; To, H.; Matsumoto, Y.; Hosono, H. An Artificial Neural Network-Pharmacokinetic Model and Its Interpretation Using Shapley Additive Explanations. *CPT Pharmacomet. Syst. Pharmacol.* **2021**, *10*, 760–768. [CrossRef] [PubMed]
24. Despotović, D.; Zec, A.; Mladenović, K.; Radin, N.; Turukalo, T.L. A Machine Learning Approach for an Early Prediction of Preterm Delivery. In Proceedings of the 2018 IEEE 16th International Symposium on Intelligent Systems and Informatics (SISY), Subotica, Serbia, 13–15 September 2018; pp. 265–270.
25. Grzymala-Busse, J.W.; Woolery, L.K. Improving Prediction of Preterm Birth Using a New Classification Scheme and Rule Induction. In Proceedings of the Annual Symposium on Computer Application in Medical Care, Washington, DC, USA, 5–9 November 1994; pp. 730–734.
26. Kovalchuk, S.V.; Boukhanovsky, A.V. Towards Ensemble Simulation of Complex Systems. *Procedia Comput. Sci.* **2015**, *51*, 532–541. [CrossRef]
27. Kovalchuk, S.V.; Kopanitsa, G.D.; Derevitskii, I.V.; Savitskaya, D.A. Three-Stage Intelligent Support of Clinical Decision Making for Higher Trust, Validity, and Explainability. *J. Biomed. Inform.* **2020**, *127*, 104013. [CrossRef] [PubMed]

Disclaimer/Publisher's Note: The statements, opinions and data contained in all publications are solely those of the individual author(s) and contributor(s) and not of MDPI and/or the editor(s). MDPI and/or the editor(s) disclaim responsibility for any injury to people or property resulting from any ideas, methods, instructions or products referred to in the content.

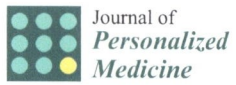

Article

Using EfficientNet-B7 (CNN), Variational Auto Encoder (VAE) and Siamese Twins' Networks to Evaluate Human Exercises as Super Objects in a TSSCI Images

Yoram Segal [1,*], Ofer Hadar [1] and Lenka Lhotska [2]

1. School of Electrical and Computer Engineering, Ben Gurion University of the Negev, Be'er-Sheva 84105001, Israel; hadar@bgu.ac.il
2. Czech Institute of Informatics, Robotics and Cybernetics, Faculty of Biomedical Engineering, Czech Technical University in Prague, 160 00 Prague, Czech Republic; lenka.lhotska@cvut.cz
* Correspondence: yoramse@post.bgu.ac.il

Citation: Segal, Y.; Hadar, O.; Lhotska, L. Using EfficientNet-B7 (CNN), Variational Auto Encoder (VAE) and Siamese Twins' Networks to Evaluate Human Exercises as Super Objects in a TSSCI Images. *J. Pers. Med.* **2023**, *13*, 874. https://doi.org/10.3390/jpm13050874

Academic Editors: Bernd Blobel, Mauro Giacomini and Bian Yang

Received: 7 March 2023
Revised: 16 May 2023
Accepted: 18 May 2023
Published: 22 May 2023

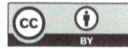

Copyright: © 2023 by the authors. Licensee MDPI, Basel, Switzerland. This article is an open access article distributed under the terms and conditions of the Creative Commons Attribution (CC BY) license (https://creativecommons.org/licenses/by/4.0/).

Abstract: In this article, we introduce a new approach to human movement by defining the movement as a static super object represented by a single two-dimensional image. The described method is applicable in remote healthcare applications, such as physiotherapeutic exercises. It allows researchers to label and describe the entire exercise as a standalone object, isolated from the reference video. This approach allows us to perform various tasks, including detecting similar movements in a video, measuring and comparing movements, generating new similar movements, and defining choreography by controlling specific parameters in the human body skeleton. As a result of the presented approach, we can eliminate the need to label images manually, disregard the problem of finding the start and the end of an exercise, overcome synchronization issues between movements, and perform any deep learning network-based operation that processes super objects in images in general. As part of this article, we will demonstrate two application use cases: one illustrates how to verify and score a fitness exercise. In contrast, the other illustrates how to generate similar movements in the human skeleton space by addressing the challenge of supplying sufficient training data for deep learning applications (DL). A variational auto encoder (VAE) simulator and an EfficientNet-B7 classifier architecture embedded within a Siamese twin neural network are presented in this paper in order to demonstrate the two use cases. These use cases demonstrate the versatility of our innovative concept in measuring, categorizing, inferring human behavior, and generating gestures for other researchers.

Keywords: OpenPose (OP); MediaPipe (MP); rehabilitation; tree structure skeleton image (TSSI); tree structure skeleton color image (TSSCI); variational auto encoder (VAE); Siamese twin neural network; simulator; human body movements; human pose estimation (HPE); computational imagination; computational creativity

1. Introduction

This paper is an extended, updated version of the pHealth 2022 conference publication [1]. It presents a more general and generic approach to the solution based on a super-object model using a TSSCI image. We improved the model by basing it on variational auto-encoder (VAE) for generating human movements instead of the generative adversarial network (GAN) model presented at the pHealth 2022 conference. Additionally, we explain how to control the skeleton choreography movement in the simulation components.

We present a more effective CNN network compared to the CNN network presented at the conference. Furthermore, we expand our explanation of the dataset preparations, pre-processing, data structure, and the meaning of the various database types. We also refer to various practical challenges, such as normalizing the human skeleton, improving the loss function, providing more detailed reference to the movement performance scoring, and adding analysis and explanation of how the network operates using the t-distributed stochastic neighbor embedding (t-SNE) algorithm.

We update and expand our experiment descriptions and present better results than the ones previously presented at the conference. Overall, this article presents a significantly improved and more comprehensive version of the research presented at the conference, with additional details, improvements, and explanations.

2. Literature Review

Remote healthcare utilizes human posture and gait for real-time medical rehabilitation [2,3]. The COVID-19 pandemic demonstrated the importance of remote diagnosis and treatment. This importance of remote healthcare is further emphasized in the introductory paper of the Frontiers in Medicine Research [4]. The comprehensive view presented in this paper underscores the significance of lifestyle factors, including exercising, in healthcare management. By incorporating these principles into remote healthcare practices, healthcare professionals can enhance patient care and optimize treatment outcomes.

In the modern age, it is now possible to utilize a camera video stream to collect, analyze, and interpret human emotions in a remotely located 3D environment by using artificial neural networks [5]. Our objective is to characterize human motion using neural network architectures such as auto-encoder [6] and Siamese twin [7], in conjunction with human pose estimation (HPE) techniques such as real-time multi-person key point detection algorithms such as OpenPose [8] and MediaPipe [9]. Remote therapy may be used when many patients recuperate after movement disorders caused by hip, knee, elbow, or shoulder surgery [10,11]. A variety of non-contact medical treatments might be developed by utilizing a family of neural network designs resulting from this research. This dissertation proposes a solution to enrich and enhance skeletal data veracity, by providing accurate and specific data tailored to research requirements using the VAE deep-learning method [12]. In the articles [13–15], some databases contain video clips of human movements divided into a variety of classes. They start by processing the data using the OpenPose software, translating the video frames into skeletal pose sequences, which are then analyzed. A three-dimensional matrix represents each skeletal pose. To preserve the relationship between the skeletal joints, the authors reordered every pose as part of deep first search (DFS). Our movement generator is based on skeletal data that provide spatial and temporal information. Several studies have investigated the issue of recognizing human movement using skeleton-based neural networks (CNNs) [13,16]. Therefore, deep convolutional generative adversarial networks (DC-GANs) use CNN layers as their generator and discriminator [8]. It is proposed in [13,15,17,18] to use an image format (TSSI—tree structure skeleton image) to generate a tree structure skeleton image based on the collection of N tree structure sequences. Therefore, we utilized deep first search (DFS) to restructure and create tree structure skeletons.

3. Materials and Methods

There are six basic physiotherapy exercises in the database, which have been carefully selected to be suitable for analyzing and processing with a single camera (two-dimensional processing see [3]), as illustrated in Figure 1.

There are approximately 100 participants in our proprietary database, which is now open to the public. Each participant performs six exercises. Ten cycles comprise each exercise (e.g., rotating the right arm). Exercises are performed once with a right tilt and once with a left tilt (for example, once with a right foot rotation and once with a left foot rotation). A total of about 7500 motion cycle videos have been tagged and timed in the database. This study included healthy subjects (volunteers—students) with no disability identified during tests to control postural stability. The subjects group comprised of 4 men and 26 women with an average age of 21.1 (standard deviation (SD) 1.2) years, body weight 64.8 (SD 9.4) kg and body height 170 (SD 9) cm. One single measurement of each subject was taken during the session. The study was performed in accordance with the

Helsinki Declaration and the study protocol was approved by the local Ethical Committee, by the Faculty of Biomedical Engineering, Czech Technical University in Prague. The entire database has been encoded as skeletons—a skeleton in every frame (see Figure 2).

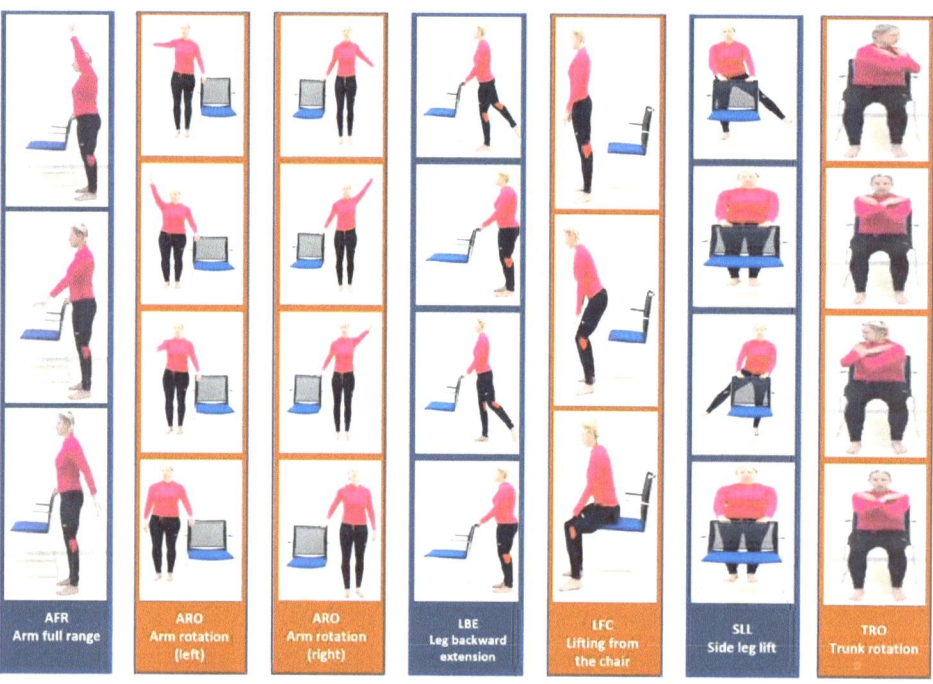

Figure 1. Six basic physiotherapy exercises that we developed and recorded.

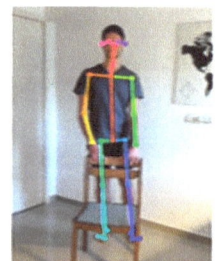 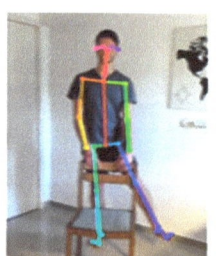 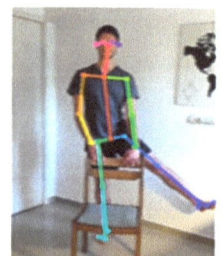 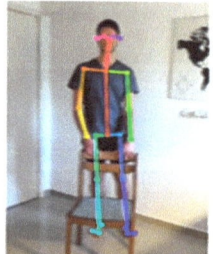

Figure 2. Database has been encoded as skeletons—a skeleton per frame.

Performing exercises creates skeletal structures. The human body is represented by 25 vertices in each skeleton. The vertex has three components: Coordinate X, coordinate Y, and coordinate C, which indicates the level of certainty about each point in the skeleton on a scale from 0 to 1 (1—absolute certainty, 0 absolute uncertainty). Collecting data for training a deep learning model requires careful consideration of various factors that could potentially affect the quality and reliability of the data. The fact that the students at Ben Gurion University were photographed independently in their homes simulates a real-world scenario but also introduces data variability and quality challenges. The difference in resolution and orientation of the photographs is a significant concern as it can impact the performance of the deep learning model. The four different orientations observed—head touching the upper edge of the monitor, a skeleton lying on the right side, upside down, and a skeleton lying on the left—could potentially affect the accuracy of the model predictions (see TRO exercise as example in Figure 3). To mitigate this issue, we had to perform data pre-processing by rotating the skeletons to a standard orientation (0 degrees).

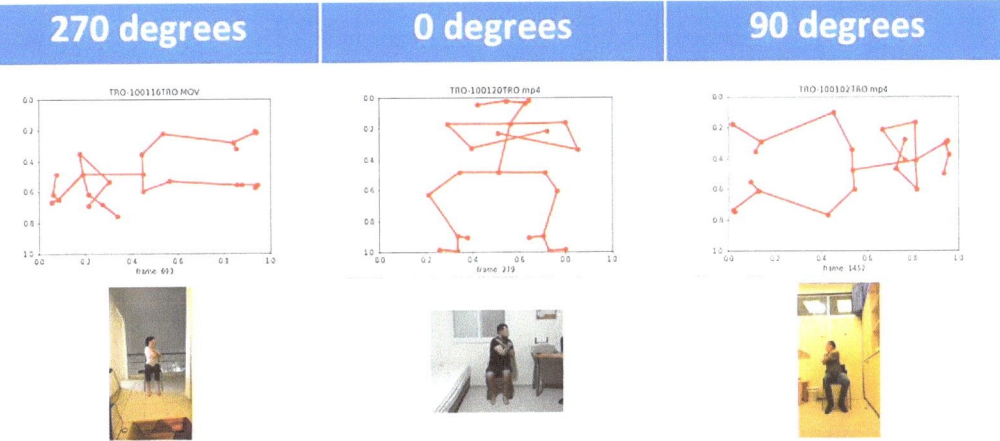

Figure 3. Homemade photoshoot challenges due to camera orientation.

Skeleton Rotation

We extract n key points per skeleton from a single video frame. The frame may contain more than one skeleton, but we always use the first skeleton.

For the i'th key point Vi = (x_i, y_i), let x_i be the Vi, X component.

The following formula can be used to normalize coordinates to the range -0.5 to $+0.5$

$$x_{ni} = \frac{x_i}{(M_{axX} - M_{inX})} - \frac{M_{axX} + M_{inX}}{2(M_{axX} - M_{inX})} \quad (1)$$

where:

M_{axX}—max(x_i) for $i \in \mathbb{Z}, 0 \leq i \leq n$
M_{inX}—min(x_i) for $i \in \mathbb{Z}, 0 \leq i \leq n$
x_{ni}—The normalized value of the skeleton's X component key points $x_{ni} \in \mathbb{R}, 0 \leq i \leq n$

The second step is rotation of 90°, 180°, or 270°. Let Vi be the original 2D key point vector with x_i, y_i components, which indicates the position of the key point prior to rotation. Based on the angle of rotation, we can use the following formulas to rotate a 2D vector: 90 degrees counterclockwise rotation: Ki = (y_i, $-x_i$); 180 degrees counterclockwise rotation: Ki = ($-x_i$, $-y_i$); 270 degrees counterclockwise rotation: Ki = ($-y_i$, x_i), where Ki is the rotated vector and x_i and y_i are the original components of the vector Vi. The third step is restoring the original coordinates. It is important to note that the frame is rectangular. Therefore, in a rotation of 270 degrees, X is the long side of the rectangle before the rotation, while Y is the long side after the rotation:

$$x_{Ri} = (M_{axX} - M_{inX})x_n + \frac{M_{axX} + M_{inX}}{2} \quad (2)$$

where x_{Ri} is the restored coordinates after rotation.

The Y-axis of the skeleton should be similarly adjusted.

Another challenge introduced by data collection was camera vibrations and movement during training. As a result, we obtained a blurry or unstable image, affecting the performance of the deep learning model. To minimize the difficulties arising from unsupervised photography in the patient's home environment, we recommended ensuring that the cameras used for data collection are stable and that the physiotherapist instructs the patients to minimize camera movement during data collection. In conclusion, collecting high-quality data is crucial for the success of deep learning models in physical therapy applications. Careful consideration of resolution, orientation, and camera stability are essential to ensure that the model's predictions are accurate and reliable.

4. Human Movement as a Static Super Object

4.1. Review of Existing Technics to Describe Human Movements

We can use recorded series of human body positions using motion capture to represent a series of human body positions. Motion capture refers to recording a person's movement while wearing a marker or sensor and then using those data to produce an animation of that person's movement (the animation shows the movement of specific dots on the human body). The animation result may either be a single image or a series of images. Pose estimation is another method for representing the successions of human body postures at a specific time, which involves identifying and tracking the body parts and joints of a person in a video or sequence of pictures and encoding that information as a single image or a group of images. Motion representation is the representation of the motion of an object or a succession of moving objects in a meaningful and compact manner. Here are some examples:

- Optical flow describes the mobility of pixels or points in an image series by estimating their displacement between consecutive frames [19];
- Researchers use Euler angles and quaternions to represent an object's orientation in 3D space by establishing rotation angles around the x, y, and z axes [20];
- By charting an object's position in space at different points in time, researchers can use a trajectory to describe an object's passage through time [21];
- In motion fields, researchers store the velocities and accelerations of each point on the object to represent an object's motion over time [22].

4.2. Our New Approach-Movement as a Static Super Object

Research literature analyzes the movement as an object in motion, meaning a sequence of objects' positions, orientations, and sizes that change over time and space. Our innovative approach combines objects and represents the entire movement as a single static super object. Our original approach provides a fresh perspective on human movement. To begin with, we treat a tree structure skeleton image (TSSI) as a color image (TSSCI), then generalize movement to a color image as an object. For example, if there are several objects in the picture (such as three cats in a typical picture), then in our model there are three movements, and therefore there are three objects within the TSSCI image. By applying this approach, an object can be small, meaning the object begins and ends simultaneously within the image. In our representation a small object indicates fast motion as opposed to a large object, which describes slower motion. As a result of adjusting two object sizes, we can sync them up. We can locate the object in a specific place in the TSSCI image while identifying all other pixels as the background. The places where the object does not exist in the image indicate no movement or an idle movement period before and after the exercise of interest. Using this concept, we can automatically determine when a movement starts and ends, and therefore we can use automatic editing to extract specific movements from long videos. Neural networks can extract unique attributes of objects in the latent space, thus allowing the network to differentiate between objects in the same way that describing the movement as a super object allows extracting movement characteristics.

4.3. Generic Neural Network Implementations with TSSCI

We can use TSSCI images as inputs to all neural networks capable of analyzing and processing images. For example, a CNN classification network can label objects within a color image, such as tagging cats. Inserting a TSSCI image into the CNN, the network can identify and tag different movements. We can generate TSSCI images using variational auto-encoder (VAE) networks containing new super objects, i.e., simulating new fake movements. Using the VAE network, TSSCI allows the generation of objects, such as faces. In addition, the VAE network allows the combination of objects (faces). In order to produce objects A and B together, one can take a picture of a bald man without glasses (object A) and combine it with another picture of a man wearing glasses and hair (object B). Thus, it is possible to produce the man (object A) with hair and glasses that we take from object B. In the same way, we can take a TSSCI image of a periodic movement of raising hands up and down (object A) as well as a TSSCI image of a periodic movement of raising a leg (object B) and then generate a fake combination that describes a skeleton raising its hands as well as its legs.

4.4. How to Define and Label Specific Movement as a Super Object

Our article has explained the concept of representing motion as a static object within a TSSCI image. Next, we will examine how super objects are defined and labeled. It is not easy to classify movements. For example, how do we describe the physical exercise of raising and lowering hands? Is there one movement for raising and one for lowering a hand? Could the super object be a combination of two movements? In general, what does a super object look like? Can we even distinguish it or describe it in the TSSCI image? The first advantage of our approach is that we can define super objects for each partial movement and even connect them. However, movement classification and labeling is a subjective process as opposed to ordinary objects such as cats, which are generally agreed upon and, therefore, can be labeled. Moreover, the abstract nature of the TSSCI image makes it difficult to identify, locate, or define an object within the image as a human. For the same movement, we can obtain many different labels. In order to overcome this problem, we utilize the motion time domain, that is, by tagging the movement within a movie before converting it into TSSCI format. In other words, each individual will label the videos based on their understanding and objectives. We convert these tagged videos into TSSCI images. Thus, we have a labeled TSSCI image containing a super object that describes movement. Despite the difficulty of understanding the super object in TSSCI images, it is not necessary since the neural network can identify it. In summary, the user or the researcher determined the nature of super objects. Given a video that the user tagged, we converted it into a TSSCI image, and then we succeeded to tag specific super objects in the TSSCI domain. After collecting TSSCI images representing a motion or a collection of motions, it is possible to train the network to perform tasks such as motion tagging, generating new motions, or other options that the neural networks offer us.

4.5. TSSCI Use Cases Examples Base on Super Objects

For clarity and to demonstrate how extensively relevant our approach is to studying human body movements, we provide multiple interpretations for referring to the human movement as a super object using TSSCI. Table 1 illustrates how classical and advanced neural networks, commonly used for various image processing applications, can be applied to TSSCI images representing movement as a static super object.

By taking a novel approach to human motion, we show in Table 1 that deep learning networks can process the TSSCI and have a wide range of practical applications.

Table 1. TSSCI Applications.

Neural Network	Regular Image	TSSCI Application
EfficientNet-B7	Object classifier	A system for classifying and labeling movements
UNET	Semantic segmentation	Colors and marks the super object inside the TSSCI image. Allows extrapolation between two movements.
YOLO	Object detection and tracking	Locating a particular movement in a film. Includes the option to extract specific movements.
ESRGAN	Super-resolution	Enhancing motion captured at a low frame rate to a higher frame rate.
DAE or DnCNN	Denoising auto-encoder or a denoising convolutional neural network	Restoration of the skeleton's missing key points
NST	Transfer the style of one image to the content of another image	Changing dance style from hip-hop to ballet while maintaining the original movements
DC-GAN	Generating fake images	Creating fake movements
VAE-based Image Composition	Generate new images that combine features from the two images	Combining two different movements, such as jumping and clapping, to create a new movement
Transformer-XH	Predict the next frame in a video	Predict the next movement in a sport game
Grid-CNN	Predict a 3D model from 2D images (stereo reconstruction)	Create a 3D model of the skeleton from a 2D skeleton (stereo reconstruction)
DALL-E	Generate images from natural language descriptions	Create an all-encompassing choreography based on natural language descriptions

4.6. Comments Regarding Table 1

- This table presents a proposal for using existing architectures, but some modifications may be necessary, such as changing the dimensions of the input image. A TSSCI image typically has smaller dimensions than a typical image input. As an example, in the examples we present later in this article, the dimensions of the TSSCI image are $49 \times 49 \times 3$, thus using the VGG network for classification was not appropriate since the image dimensions at the VGG entrance are $240 \times 240 \times 3$, and the depth of the network exceeds our database size. Therefore, overfitting occurred. For this reason, we used an EfficientNet-B7 image classification CNN network. Similarly, particular adaptations will be required to use the architectures listed in the table. We recommend selecting most suitable networks for performing the desirable task and scaling the TSSCI dimensions;
- A few propositions require practical proof because they are theoretically logical inferences. We must train the network extensively with diverse TSSCI images tagged with various texts to formulate a choreography in which DALL-E uses a ritual to control human skeleton movements;
- We recommend using this table to develop additional ideas based on existing architectures, using the super object method for human movement description.

5. Convert a Sequence of Human Skeleton Movements into a TSSI Single Image

Paper [14] presents a method for recognizing human actions in video sequences using a combination of spatial-temporal visual attention and skeleton image processing. In the paper, the authors introduce the concept of converting the skeleton image sequences into tree structure skeleton images, which they refer to as "TSSI" images. TSSI images are a type of abstract image representation that captures a person's skeletal structure in a video sequence and can be used to analyze and recognize human actions (see Figure 4).

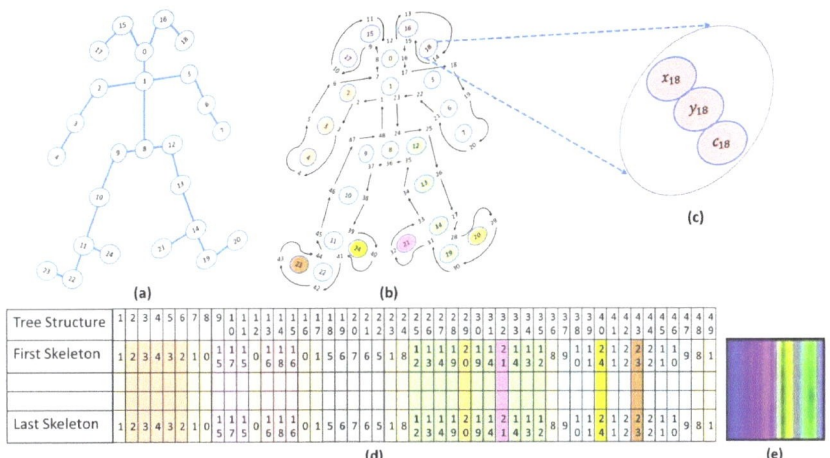

Figure 4. OpenPose Tree structure skeleton to TSSCI: (**a**) OpenPose skeleton; (**b**) Skeleton tree for TSSI or TSSCI generating; (**c**) Visualizing key points: A 3D representation; (**d**) A collection of tree structures: pose patterns are tabulated row by row; (**e**) Visualizing key point locations and confidence Levels: TSSCI-RGB Image.

The authors show that TSSI images are a more efficient and effective representation of human actions compared to traditional video or image data, as they capture the critical aspects of movement and can be processed more efficiently. To recognize actions in TSSI image sequences, the authors propose a method that combines spatiotemporal visual attention with a convolutional neural network (CNN) for classification. They used the visual attention mechanism to focus on relevant parts of the TSSI image sequence and the CNN to recognize the exercise performed by the athletes. In contrast to the traditional TSSI perspective, in which TSSI represents a movement within an image, our TSSCI (tree structure skeleton color image) method first converts the key points into RGB color images (we normalize the skeleton coordinate values to be between 0 to 1). Converting skeleton key points to RGB-colored TSSCI images allows for representing multiple human movements as one super object. X, Y, and confidence level—C coordinates represent each key point in the skeleton. We grouped the skeletons in three dimensions array. We convert the 3D array into RGB channels by taking the red color channel to represent the X coordinates, the green color channel to represent the Y coordinates, and the blue color channel to represent the C coordinates. We refer to the colored TSSI as TSSCI, which represents the composition of the exercise from start to finish as an abstracted color image.

5.1. TSSCI Needs a Buffer to Convert Temporal-Spatial Data into Spatial Data

With no prejudice to generality, TSSCI contains a sequence of our human skeletons, initially presented as time series (e.g., each video frame might contain one or more skeletons). To convert video into a TSSCI image, we need a frame buffer containing frames with or without skeletons. The buffer contains a time mark for the first and last frames. As a result, when processing skeletons, we have complete information about the entire movement from beginning to end. Several factors determine the buffer size: the degree of latency we are willing to accept between real-time (the last frame in the buffer) and how much historical information we require (the first frame). Image resolution is also a factor. Our column resolution component is determined by how many key points are in our skeleton, which we enlarge by the TSSCI skeleton tree. (For example, the OpenPose body model contains 25 key points. By duplicating some key points following the skeleton tree scheme, we obtain 49 key points, which constitute 49 columns.). The row resolution component is determined by how fast the frame rate is and how long the movement (or submovement) is. We can break apart any length movement (or submovement) into slices using our super object approach. Furthermore, with our super object concept, we can process each sub-super object separately and then concatenate them to form one super object. This approach can also accelerate the processing speed leveraging GPU parallel processing.

5.2. Methods for Normalizing Skeleton Coordinates for the Implementation as TSSCI Pixels

As explained in the previous section, we have a buffer that contains all the movement of the skeletons from the beginning to the end. In order to prevent discontinuities of the skeletons between frames as a result of normalization, we will simultaneously normalize the entire buffered group of skeletons. Several normalization methods are described in the literature. For TSSCI, we can simultaneously measure the reference points of all the buffered skeletons using any of the following methods.

- Mean and standard deviation: Normalizing the coordinates by calculating their mean and standard deviation [23];
- Min-Max normalization: We can use it to scale coordinates so that they fall within a specified range, such as (0, 1). The minimum and maximum values of the coordinates must be determined first, and then the coordinates must be scaled using the following formula: (x − min)/(max − min) [24];
- Zero-mean normalization: Center the data around zero by subtracting the mean from each coordinate. This method helps remove any bias in the data [25];
- Root mean square normalization (RMSE): To ensure that subsequent analyses are not affected by the scale of the coordinates, this method scales the coordinates so that the root mean square (RMS) is equal to one [26];
- Scaling to unit norm: Scaling coordinates in this manner ensures that the L2 norm of the coordinates is equal to one. It ensures that scale does not affect the results of subsequent analyses [27].

We present several examples of using the super object method in this article. For the results presented in this article, we used the Min-Max normalization method. We followed the following formulas:

If i is the row index in the TSSCI and j is the column index in the TSSCI and the $C_{ij} \geq threshold$ (if the confidence level is low then the x, y coordinates are considered as noise):

$$x_{max} = max(max(x_{ij}))$$
$$x_{min} = min(min(x_{ij})) \quad (3)$$
$$x_L = x_{max} - x_{min}$$

$$\hat{x}_{ij} = \frac{x_{ij}}{x_L} \quad (4)$$

In the same way we calculate the normalized y component:

$$\hat{y}_{ij} = \frac{y_{ij}}{y_L} \quad (5)$$

The normalized key point $\widehat{kp}_{ij}$ is defined as:

$$\widehat{kp}_{ij} = (\hat{x}_{ij}, \hat{y}_{ij}, c_{ij}) \quad (6)$$

which used as our TSSCI pixel.

5.3. TSSCI Dataset Augmentation

The limited amount of video data in our database posed a challenge for training neural networks effectively. To address this, we applied dataset augmentation techniques to the videos. The videos were sampled at 30 frames per second, with a 33-millisecond interval between consecutive frames. This short time frame made it difficult to capture significant differences in movement from one frame to the next. Each video in the database had a typical length of 100 s. To ensure that our method for measuring and labeling movements based on TSSCI was effective, we selected a sample of 49 frames (approximately two seconds of separate consecutive frames), to obtain meaningful information between frames. We employed two modeling methods. The first method involved randomly selecting 49 frames out of the total number of frames, allowing for acceleration and deceleration within the exercise. The second method involved dividing the total number of frames into 49 equal segments and randomly selecting one frame from each segment. This method smoothed out fluctuations and internal accelerations within the exercise.

5.4. CNN-Based Automatic and Manual Video Editing

In order to improve the accuracy of the initial training of movements, it was necessary to eliminate unnecessary frames at the beginning and end of each video. To achieve this, we manually edited the videos and marked the frame numbers for the start and end of each movement in a separate CSV file. We also demonstrated that the TSSCI method is robust against the specific start and end location of the movement, as convolutional neural networks (CNNs) have the ability to identify the movement regardless of its location or size in the video, in much the same way as a CNN can identify a cat in an image despite its location or size within the image. To accommodate both approaches, we developed a code that allows the user to either work with the entire video without editing or with edited videos by specifying the start and end points using the CSV file, resulting in more accurate results.

5.5. Treatment of Low Confidence Level Key Points (Missing Key Points)

In some cases, the skeleton key point extraction software may fail to locate a key point with sufficient accuracy. This can be due to various reasons such as a person being photographed in profile, where one shoulder is visible while the other is obscured, or poor lighting conditions that deteriorate image processing quality. To address these missing key points, we implemented in our algorithm a method termed "complementing from the left". This method replaces missing key points with their closest neighbors on the left. This results in an unrealistic representation of the skeleton where body parts appear to be suspended in the air without any connections. For example, if the elbow key point is missing, the algorithm will only show the skeleton up to the shoulder, resulting in a floating palm detached from the shoulder. Suppose there is a sequence of key points according to TSSCI description, for example 0, 1, 5, 6, 7, 6, 5, 1, 8, 12..., and key point 6 is missing (its confidence level is below a given threshold of 0.3). According to the left completion method, the sequence would be 0, 1, 5, 5, 7, 7, 5, 1, 8, 12... where 5 replaced the missing 6 and then 7 replaced the missing 6.

6. Movements Classification with Google CNN EfficientNet

We have explored our novel approach to analyzing human movements—the super object method. This method aims to provide a generic solution for a wide range of human movement analysis problems. To validate our theory, we experimented with demonstrating the effectiveness of the super object method. We used a convolutional neural network (CNN) optimized for small images with a resolution of 49×49. We used for our CNN classification model the EfficientNet-B7 classifier architecture, which has achieved state-of-the-art results in image classification tasks. EfficientNet is a new method for scaling CNNs that considers both the depth and width of the network and the resolution of the input image. This method balances the trade-offs between accuracy, computational cost, and the amount of data required, making it a promising approach for improving the performance of CNNs in various tasks. We employed several techniques to improve our model learning and prediction performance, including data augmentation and transfer learning. In the transfer learning approach, we trained only the last layers of the EfficientNet network while freezing the first three layers. It allowed us to achieve improved performance while minimizing the risk of overfitting to the limited data available. We set the final model to have six classes corresponding to the six different human movements that we have in our dataset: "AFR," "ARO," "LBE," "LFC," "SLL," and "TRO." We present, in Figure 5, the results of the classification and the training progress. Part A and Part B show the progression of the loss function and accuracy function, respectively, as a function of the number of epochs. Using a pre-trained network and a clean data set significantly contributed to fast and accurate learning. The rapid decline of the loss function and the steady increase in the accuracy function demonstrate the effectiveness of the super object method in human movement analysis. We summarized the classification results in the confusion matrix illustrated in Figure 5 The results of our experiment provide evidence that the super object method is a viable and practical approach to analyzing human movements.

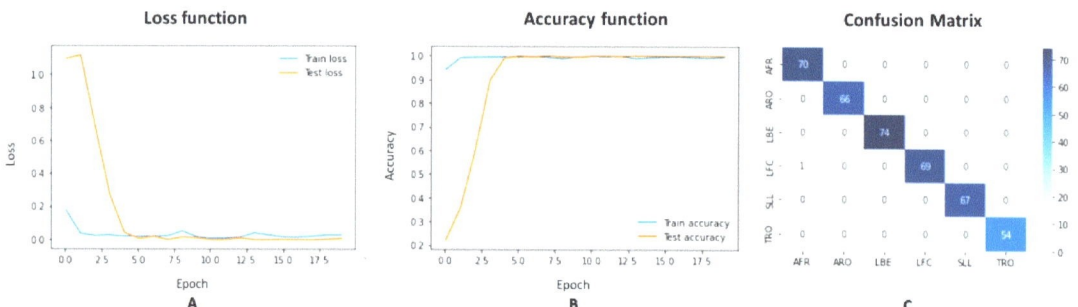

Figure 5. Classification with Google CNN EfficientNet results: (**A**) Loss function; (**B**) Accuracy function; (**C**) Confusion matrix.

As a final note, it is essential to highlight that for simplicity, we used only the dataset of the Czech students in this experiment. These students made exercise recordings in a controlled manner and under laboratory conditions, providing a clean and consistent data set for demonstration purposes. The goal was to demonstrate the principle of operation using the super object method and not to focus on extreme cases that may require more training and possibly use more complex architectures. Using the Czech students data set allowed for a clear and straightforward demonstration of the super object method and its potential for human movement analysis.

7. Variational Auto Encoder (VAE)

A variational auto-encoder (VAE) is a non-supervised artificial neural network (see Figure 6). We design VAEs to learn a compressed representation of high-dimensional data, such as images or audio, and then utilize it to generate new data samples. As a generative model, VAEs can generate new instances of the input data distribution that they were trained on. In paper [12] Kingma and Welling describe the VAE framework as a Bayesian way to learn latent variable models. They offer a way to train the VAE by combining the encoder-decoder network with a variational inference objective.

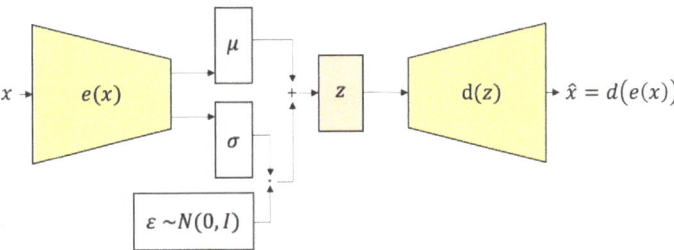

Figure 6. Structure of the variational auto-encoder (VAE).

The encoder network takes a sample as input and creates parameters that determine a probability distribution over the latent space. The decoder network takes a sample from this distribution and builds an output similar to the original input. The goal of variational inference is to find the parameters of the encoder and decoder networks so that the distribution in the latent space matches a distribution from before and the reconstructed output matches the original input. Another benefit of VAEs is that we can use the learned distribution over the latent space to generate new samples. By taking samples from the distribution it has learned, the VAE may be able to make new outputs that are identical to the original data. The ability of VAEs to generate new samples from the learned distribution makes them an efficient tool for creating images and sounds. Another feature of VAEs is their ability to learn deconstructed representations of incoming data. The fact that each dimension of the latent space corresponds to an essential feature of the input data, such as the position of an object in a photograph, demonstrates the usefulness of VAEs. This property makes VAEs useful for data compression and visualization applications. VAEs can learn compressed representations of high-dimensional data, generate new samples of the input distribution, and learn unconfused representations of the input distribution. Because of its capacity to combine encoder and decoder networks with a variational inference objective, the architecture presented in Kingma and Welling's study [12] has become a popular method for training VAEs.

8. Demonstration of How to Measure Gesture Mimics Via Siamese Twin Neural Network

The neural network chosen for this project is the Siamese twin neural network [7]. The reason for selecting the Siamese twin network is its one-shot learning capability. The result is that once the network has been properly trained, it is possible to classify a new image into a class that was not included in the initial training. Using TSSCI technique, we managed to capture the entire motion of the human body in one image as a super object. It is not necessary to use all of the frames within a time window to create a good representation of TSSCI. We conclude that different gestures require different time windows for optimal TSSCI representation.

The input to the network (see Figure 7) consists of a pair of TSSCIs with dimensions of 49×49 pixels each. Inputs are fed into the same convolutional and pooling layers and the output is a tensor with 4096 elements for each input, which can be considered as a type of code or latent of the TSSCI. For the CNN block in the Siamese twin model we have used the EfficientNet-B7 [28] classifier architecture embedded within a Siamese twin neural network. "EfficientNet-B7 achieves state-of-the-art 84.4% top-1/97.1% top-5 accuracy on ImageNet, while being 8.4× smaller and 6.1× faster on inference than the best existing ConvNet." [28]. These latent codes are fed into the differentiation layer, which computes their L_1 distance.

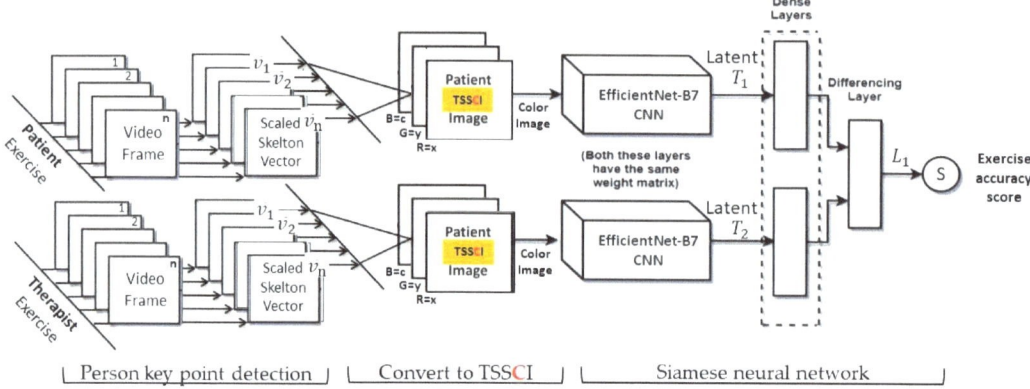

Figure 7. Siamese twin network layout.

EfficientNet Transfer Learning

To improve the learning and prediction performance of our model with limited data, we employed several methods. One method was data augmentation. Another method was taking advantage of the pre-trained EfficientNet network for image classification by performing transfer learning. In our approach, we kept the parameters of the first three layers of the network, as we considered that these layers are responsible for learning the background information of the objects, which is common across different object types. This allowed us to focus the training on the last layers, which were tasked with learning the specific features of our motion object. By doing this, we aimed to achieve improved performance while minimizing the risk of overfitting to the limited data available. We can train the Siamese twin neural network using two different methods. The first is a complete training of the entire network from start to finish, which is suitable for adding a new movement to the database that does not require any relation or connection to other movements. The second method is a particular case of the first, which we term the partial Siamese twin network. This method calculates an accuracy score when comparing a reference movement (performed by a trainer/therapist) to the patient movement. The Siamese twin network is a classic approach to measuring similarity between a pair of images, and this is an unsupervised problem, as the training is based solely on labeling similar and dissimilar movements. The second method is a classic supervised problem, where the movements are known in advance and labeled according to the recognized movement the patient is performing. In this case, we only train the CNN as a closed classification system to classify the known movements.

$$L_1 = D = flatten(|T_1 - T_2|) \tag{7}$$

where T_1, T_2 are the tensors obtained from the convolutional and pooling layers (latent feature vectors), respectively. There is only one neuron in the final dense layer that has a sigmoid activation function. We can model this layer mathematically:

$$L_1 = \sigma(bias + \sum_i (w_i C_i))$$
$$Loss = (1-Y)\tfrac{1}{2}(D_w)^2 + (Y)\tfrac{1}{2}\{\max(0, m - D_w)\}^2 \tag{8}$$

where:

- σ is the sigmoid function:

$$\sigma(x) = \frac{1}{1 + e^{-x}} \tag{9}$$

- C_i is the i'th element of the input vector $C = Concat(T_1, T_2) = [T_1, T_2]$;
- w_i is the corresponding i'th weight.

$$Loss = (1-Y)\frac{1}{2}(D_w)^2 + (Y)\frac{1}{2}\{\max(0, m - D_w)\}^2 \qquad (10)$$

where:

- *Loss*: overall loss that the model incurs in making predictions for a binary classification problem;
- *Y*: label for a particular data point. It takes a value of 0 or 1 depending on whether the data point belongs to class 0 or class 1;
- D_w: difference between the predicted value and the actual label. It represents how well the model is performing on a particular data point;
- $(1 - Y)$: error incurred by the model when it predicts the negative class;
- $(D_w)^2$: square of the difference between the predicted value and the actual label. It is used to penalize larger differences;
- (Y): error incurred by the model when it predicts the positive class;
- $\max(0, m - D_w)$: margin between the predicted value and the actual label. The max function ensures that this value is always non-negative;
- $(1/2)$: term used to normalize the loss.

Accordingly, the output of the network is a number between 0 and 1, which correlates to the degree of similarity between the two inputted TSSCIs. The closer the output value is to zero, the higher the level of similarity predicted. Our Siamese twin network output termed L_1, ranges from 0 to plus infinity. Therefore we converted the L_1 into an accuracy score S, which ranges from 0 to 1, with 0 being a complete mismatch and 1 being an exact match. We used the following formula to normalize the L_1 score to the S score:

$$S = 1 - L_1 / \|T_2\| \qquad (11)$$

where:

- $\|T_2\|$ is the therapist's latent norm, our reference movement that the CNN converts from the TSSCI exercise image into a latent vector.

9. Results

9.1. Creating the Extended Database Using Normalization and Augmentation

We utilized the EfficientNet-B7 network to classify six pre-defined movements from a database containing 100 students, each performing six movements. We used OpenPose to extract the skeleton vectors from the video frames into NumPy arrays (the skeleton key points vector extracted from a video frame is a line in the array) and performed a centering operation to place the skeleton in the center of the frame. The x and y coordinates were normalized to values between 0 and 1, while the level of confidence c remained between 0 and 1. Due to the low confidence level values for some key points, we could not rely on the position evaluation values provided by OpenPose. Instead, we used the "complementing from the left" algorithm. For instance, if the elbow key point were missing, the algorithm would only display the skeleton up to the shoulder, resulting in a floating palm in the air separate from the body. We selected 49 random lines from each normalized NumPy file for augmentation. Those 49 lines are equivalent to 49 frames with an interval between frames of approximately two seconds. We used them to create a TSSCI tensor, an RGB color image where the red channel represents x values, the blue channel represents y values, and the green channel represents the confidence level c. We repeated this operation 2004 times to generate a total of 2004 tagged TSSCI images. We used 1603 images for training (80%) and the remaining 401 (20%) for evaluation. Figure 8 contains some examples from our extended dataset using normalization and augmentation. The following table shows TSSCI and one of its single skeletons. We took the examples provided here from the videos of the physiotherapist. The expert is our source of reference when performing a correct exercise.

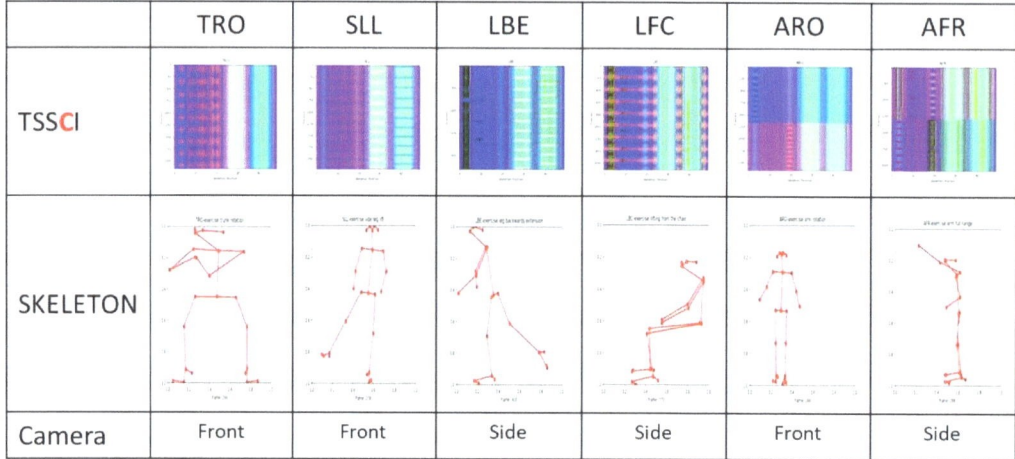

Figure 8. Extended database using normalization and augmentation.

Figure 8 shows TSSCI images for six exercises: TRO—trunk rotation; SLL—side leg lift; LBE—backward leg extension; LFC—lifting from the chair; ARO—arm rotation; AFR—arm full range; In TSSCI images that describe exercises ARO and AFR, there is a central contrast line. There is a separation of tones between the upper and lower portions of the image. This is due to the fact that the movements in these two exercises are performed in two parts: the first involves exercising the right side of the body cyclically, while the second involves exercising the left side of the body cyclically. There are 10 consecutive movements cycles in each part.

9.2. Train and Evaluate the EfficientNet-B7 Model on TSSCI Images

We utilized the pre-trained EfficientNet-B7 network for image classification by performing Transfer Learning. We set the network to have six outputs corresponding to the six movements, with an evaluation set that contains: 70 images for AFR, 66 images for ARO, 74 images for LBE, 70 images for LFC, 67 images for SLL, and 54 images for TRO. The EfficientNet-B7 network yielded a probability vector with six components for each movement, summarized into one (100%). We converted a movement video into a TSSCI image to perform the movement detection, which was then input into the trained EfficientNet-B7 network. We determined the predicted movement label by selecting the output with the highest probability. The classification performance was measured using an evaluation set of 401 samples. The results were presented in a confusion matrix, as shown in Figure 9.

We conducted classification of a noisy data set consisting of exercises performed by students from Ben Gurion University in a home environment. The BGU students recorded these exercises under challenging conditions with varying cameras, shooting distances, camera movement, and lighting. We did not edit the BGU student videos; therefore, each exercise starts and ends at different times. We evaluated the results by presenting them in a confusion matrix, which summarizes the network predictions for each exercise (see Figure 10). The network output is a probability vector for each of the six exercises, and the chosen exercise has the highest probability. The diagonal of the matrix shows how many times the network correctly predicted the exercise. Despite the difficult conditions and although each exercise begins and ends in a different frame, the results show that the network was able to classify the exercises successfully since the diagonal of the matrix is dominant. When using the super object method, we treat the movement as an object, allowing the network to classify movements effectively even in diverse shooting conditions.

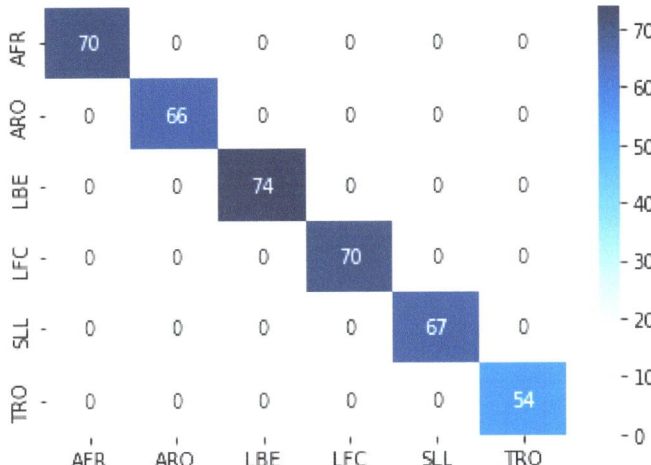

Figure 9. Evaluate the EfficientNet-B7 model on TSSCI images via confusion matrix.

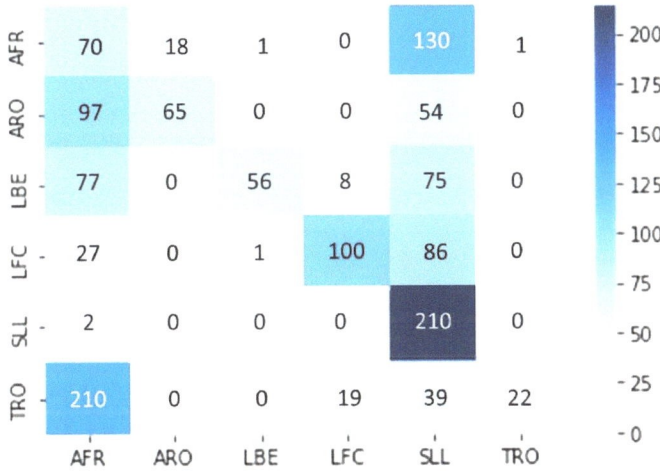

Figure 10. Classifying exercises with the super object under challenging conditions.

While it is possible to continue training and improving the network to achieve better results, that is beyond the scope of this article. The goal is to demonstrate the effectiveness of the super object method in referring to movement.

9.3. Results with Variational Auto Encoder

As a demonstration that our method is general and does not depend on the algorithm of a particular generator, we are presenting results from another movement generator, this time using variational auto-encoder (VAE). The results prove that our method is general and does not depend on the algorithm of a particular generator. This architecture was presented by Kingma and Welling in their paper [12]. The authors describe VAE as a generative model trained using variational principles, which presents an unsupervised learning approach. There are two main components to the VAE architecture: an encoder and a decoder. It is possible to illustrate the architecture using diagrams, as shown in Figure 6: The encoder converts input data into a latent representation, and the decoder converts that latent representation back into the original data space. With our TSSCI images dataset, we trained the VAE and generated several fake TSSCI images (see Figure 11).

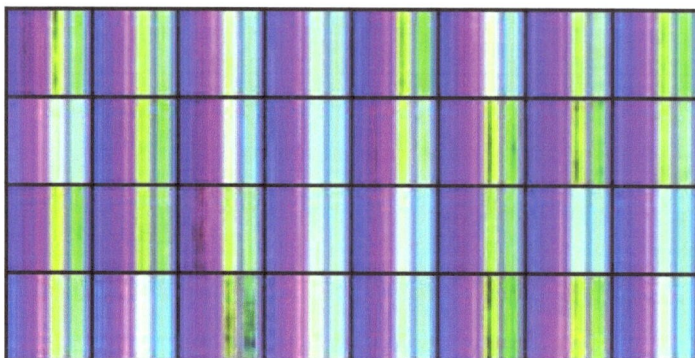

Figure 11. 32 Fake TSSCI images that were generated with AVE.

Using the VAE, we were able to produce 32 TSSCI images (Figure 11). Out of 32 images, we randomly selected three (see Figures 12–14). We converted the three images back into the time domain to reproduce the skeleton movement generated by the network. In Figures 15–17, we present a frame sample containing one skeleton from each TSSCI. We converted each skeleton vector (each line in the TSSCI image) into a video frame sequence that contained one skeleton. In each one of the three pictures we preset one frame from the movement sequence. In Figure 15, we see a small skeleton performing two hand movements over a sequence of frames. Each TSSCI generated by the network is essentially another exercise that describes skeletal movement over a sequence of frames. In Figure 16 we can observe a tall skeleton performing a right-hand movement, and in Figure 17 another tall skeleton performing a hands-up movement. According to the method of representing the skeletons based on the tree structure skeleton image, some key points in the skeleton appear more than once in the vector representing the skeleton. As a result of applying the TSSCI method, some key points appear twice when compared to the original 25 OpenPose key points skeleton. This results in a skeleton vector consisting of 49 key points instead of the original 25 OpenPose key points skeleton. This structure is designed to ensure the connections between the points and preserve a structure of the logical human movement. In our case, we generate new TSSCI images; therefore, we generate new key points, but although initially some of the points are duplicated and identical, in our fake images, we obtain differences between the location of the identical points. As can be seen in the photos Figures 15–17, the differences are minor. We can combine key points into one point, as we showed in VAE products (see [1]), but we chose to emphasize this point for the explanation.

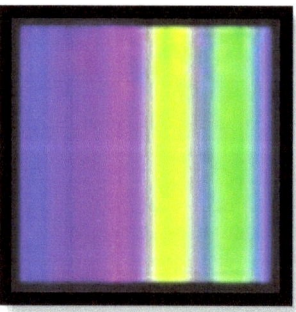

Figure 12. The display of TSSCI A image out of 32 generated by VAE.

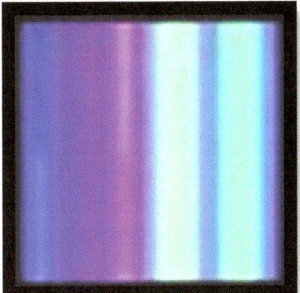

Figure 13. The display of TSSCI B image out of 32 generated by VAE.

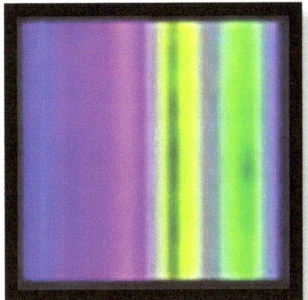

Figure 14. The display of TSSCI C image out of 32 generated by VAE.

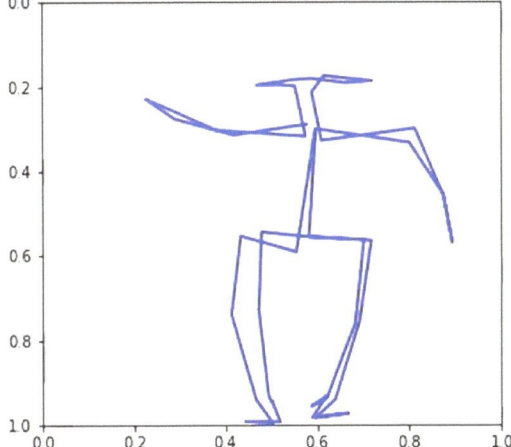

Figure 15. A small skeleton performs movement A (two hands).

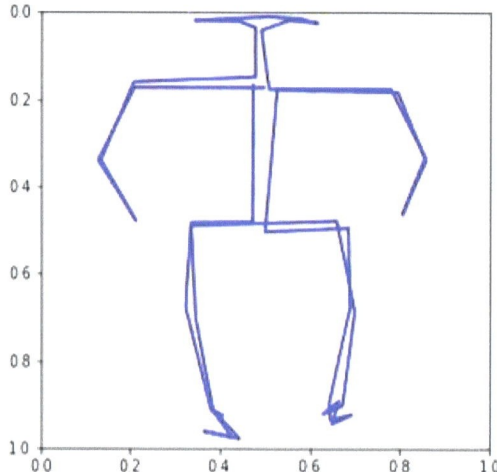

Figure 16. A tall skeleton performs movement B (right hand movement).

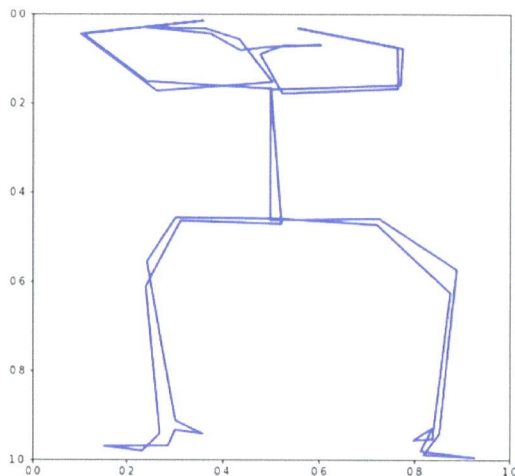

Figure 17. A tall skeleton performs movement C (hands up).

We show, for instance, how we can fix the same key points if we treat the motion in the image as an object (see Figures 18 and 19).

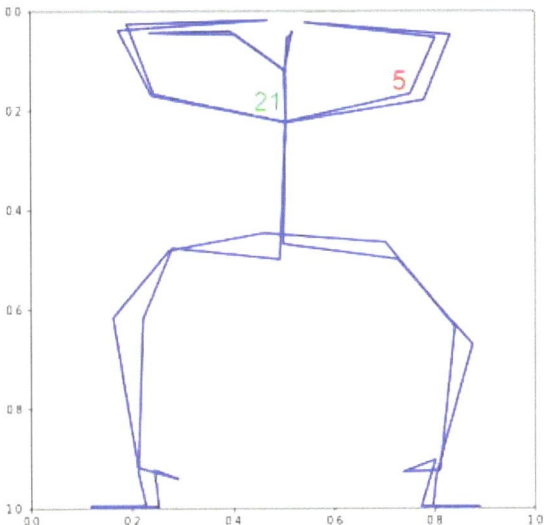

Figure 18. Merge only key point 21 while key point 5 remains unmerged.

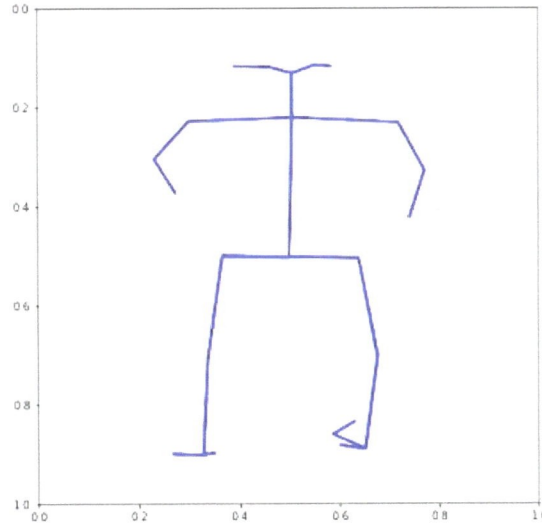

Figure 19. By adding the KPMSE to the loss function, key points are combined.

Since we consider human motion an object in the image, we can use the loss function to constrain the network during training. In the VAE network, the loss function is composed of two components: the mean squared error (MSE) and the distance between the distribution of the training group and a normal distribution with mean 0 and variation 1, which we call the DKL.

$$Loss = MSE + \beta DKL \tag{12}$$

Noting that a key point is a vector of three components (a 3D vector). It contains the coordinates X, Y, and confidence level C.

$$\overline{v}_i = (x_i, y_i, c_i) \tag{13}$$

It is, therefore, possible to determine a vector distance between two key points in the skeleton, particularly between two key points that are supposed to be identical. A KPMSE is the sum of distances between key points in TSSCI images that are assumed to have identical values. We calculate the KPMSE as follows:

$$KPMSE = \sum_{r=1}^{row} \sum_{i=1}^{col} \sum_{j=1}^{ide} (x_{ri} - x_{rj})^2 + (y_{ri} - y_{rj})^2 + (c_{ri} - c_{rj})^2 \tag{14}$$

where:

row—Number of rows in the TSSCI image;
col—Number of columns in the TSSCI image;
ide—Number of identical key points in TSSCI.

It is decided to add the KPMSE to the original VAE loss function while using alpha and beta as weights to achieve a balance between the loss function components. Our new loss function, which helps to merge identical key points, is described in the formula below:

$$Loss = MSE + \beta DKL + \alpha KPMSE \quad \text{where } 0 \leq \alpha, \beta \leq 1 \tag{15}$$

The VAE training loss progress is illustrated in Figure 20.

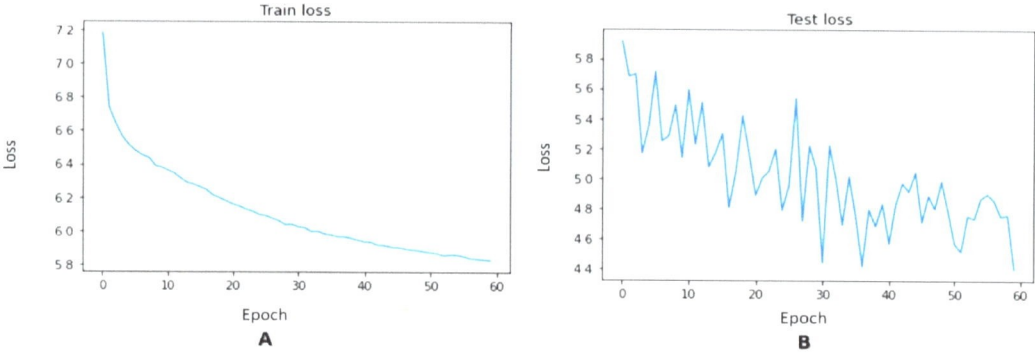

Figure 20. VAE training loss progress ((**A**) train loss, (**B**) test loss).

Figure 21 shows an example of restoring a TSSCI image by compressing until we obtain a latent vector (encoding) and then reconstructing (decoding) the vector back into a TSSCI image.

Our goal is to create synthetic motions similar to the six movements found in our TSSCI picture database, which contains 2004 photos labeled with one of the six movements. We used the TSSCI pictures to train a VAE to recreate each movement. The VAE produces a latent vector for each TSSCI picture, yielding a probabilistic space of latent vectors. We describe the probabilistic space as a cloud of points in an N-dimensional space as a spherical distribution, with a mean of 0 at the center and a standard deviation radius of 1. This spherical distribution encompasses the six motions, and because the TSSCI pictures were successfully separated, we wish to represent the probabilistic space in a two-dimensional graph to demonstrate the apparent distinction between the movements. We used the dimensionality reduction approach t-SNE (t-distributed stochastic neighbor embedding) [29] to visualize and explore high-dimensional data. t-SNE is very good for depicting complicated, non-linear interactions between data points. The t-SNE algorithm maps high-dimensional data points to a lower-dimensional space (usually 2D or 3D) while keeping data point commonalities. The method achieves this by generating a probability distribution over the data points in the high-dimensional space and then mapping the points to the lower-dimensional space while preserving as many similarities as feasible. In more detail, t-SNE starts by computing the pairwise similarities between all the data points in the high-dimensional space (the latent space dimension in our case). We use these similarities to define a probability distribution over the data points, where the probability of a selected point is proportional to the similarity with its neighbors. The algorithm then maps the data points to the lower-dimensional space by optimizing a cost function that measures the difference between the high- and lower-dimensional space probabilities.

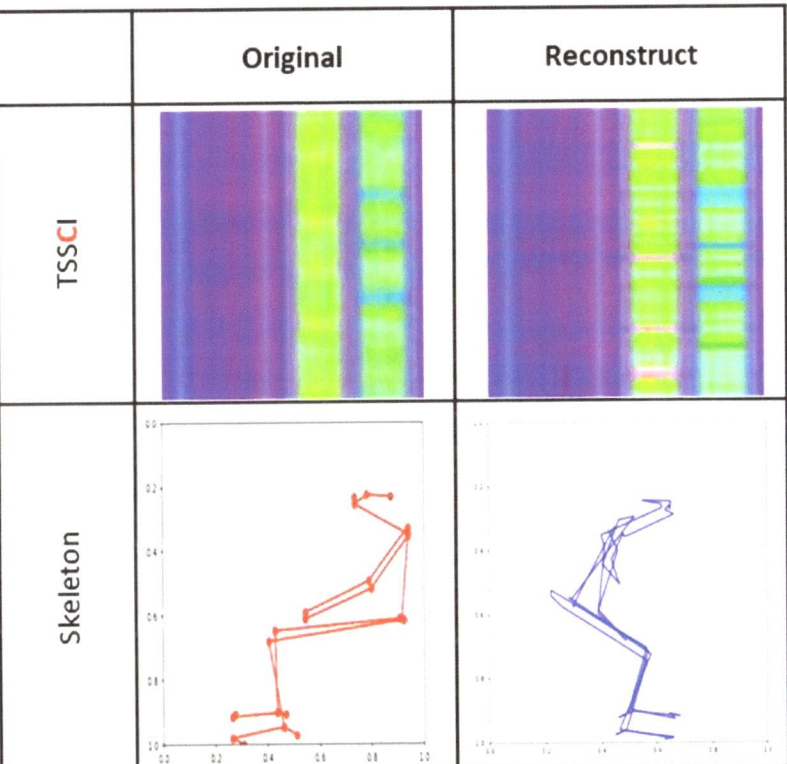

Figure 21. TSSCI encoding and decoding using VAE t-SNE (t-distributed stochastic neighbor embedding) to visualize and explore high-dimensional data.

As demonstrated in Figure 22, the probability space of the latent vectors representing the characteristics of human movements, or TSSCI image properties, exhibits excellent separation. The separation is centered around the origin, resulting in a symmetrical distribution. This indicates that the VAE has generated a probability space that resembles a normal distribution. Therefore, we can extract a vector from a normal distribution, pass it through the VAE, and obtain a novel movement.

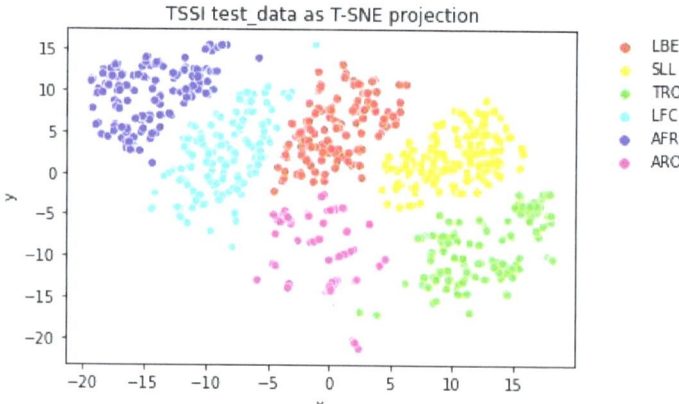

Figure 22. Analyzing the ability to generate similar synthetic movements by using a two-dimensional representation of t-SNE.

9.3.1. Synthesizes a New Movement by Combining Two Foreign Movements TRO + SLL

After employing t-SNE to visualize the distributions of six exercise groups, we seek to showcase the effectiveness of using a super object, specifically TSSCI, to merge two distinct movements into a single, combined motion. Our demonstration involves merging the SLL and TRO movements, which we can characterize by leg and hand-to-chest movement, respectively. Recall that the latent vectors representing the dominant characteristics of each object, in this case, a super object describing a movement, are crucial to our method. Each TSSCI image is transformed into a latent vector using VAE, with each vector serving as a point in an N-dimensional space, where in our example N is 16. VAE converts the distribution of the latent vectors to a normal distribution, meaning that it maps each original latent vector to an equivalent point in a normal distribution. We then choose a latent N-dimensional vector from the normal distribution space belonging to the SLL movement $\bar{v}_{SLL-i}$ and one from the TRO movement $\bar{v}_{TRO-j}$. We create a vector origin between them (the average of the two vectors) and obtain a new synthetic vector $\bar{v}_{merge}$ in the normal distribution space (see Figure 23). This vector represents the combined motion we want to generate. We then inject this vector into the VAE decoder and use it to reconstruct a new movement—the joint movement—which combines the hand and leg movements of the SLL and TRO movements, respectively.

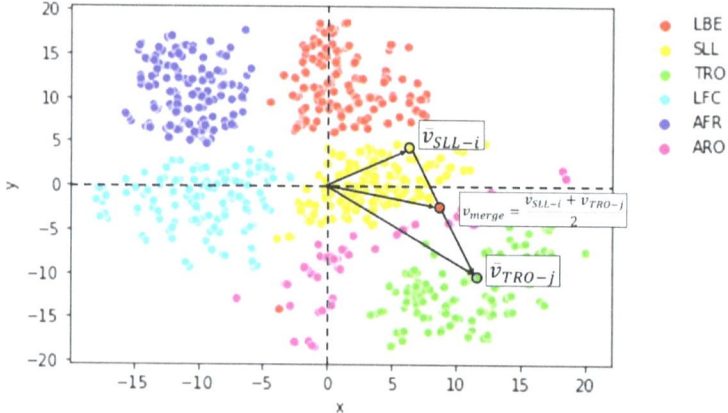

Figure 23. A visual representation of how movement latent vectors merge in the t-SNE dimension.

Using t-SNE, TSSCI, and VAE allows us to merge the distinct characteristics of two movements and generate a new, unique synthetic movement (see Figure 24).

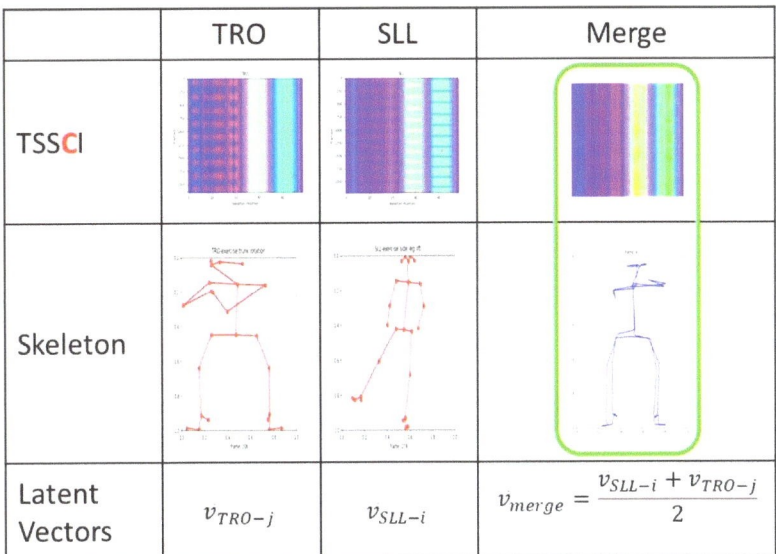

Figure 24. Merging the distinct characteristics of two movements, TRO, and SLL.

9.3.2. Generator of Synthetic Movements for Specific Types Using Super Object Method

Our previous demonstrations have showcased the power of the super object method in classifying, compressing, reproducing, and merging movements. We introduce a new capability: a generator that creates a specific type of movement from the six pre-defined movements. The generator operates by converting the latent vector distribution to a normal distribution. Each subgroup of movements has a different mean and variance, and to produce a new movement of a specific type we create a sub-distribution corresponding to the requested subgroup. We then generate a series of latent vectors from each sub-distribution and pass them through the VAE Decoder to obtain a new TSSCI image depicting a sequence of skeletons in certain positions, which, when played in order, produce a new synthetic skeleton movement of the requested type.

Figure 25 showcases our ability to generate a new AFR (arm full rotate) movement using the super object method. Notably, the TSSCI image features a dividing line in its center, which reflects the combined performance of the exercise, with the right arm working in the first half and the left arm in the second half. However, our reconstruction only includes the right-arm movement. Hence there is no line in the center. As a reminder, we opted to play the synthetic movement in a mirror image of the original to distinguish between the two. The TSSCI image used to generate the synthetic movement describes a skeleton using 49 points, while the original skeleton uses 25 points. We preserved this format to demonstrate the refinement and authenticity of the synthetic reconstruction using VAE on the TSSCI image. We previously demonstrated how to train the network to generate a skeleton of only 25 points by adding a constraint to the loss function. It provides further evidence of the authenticity of our synthetic movements and their potential applicability in real-world settings.

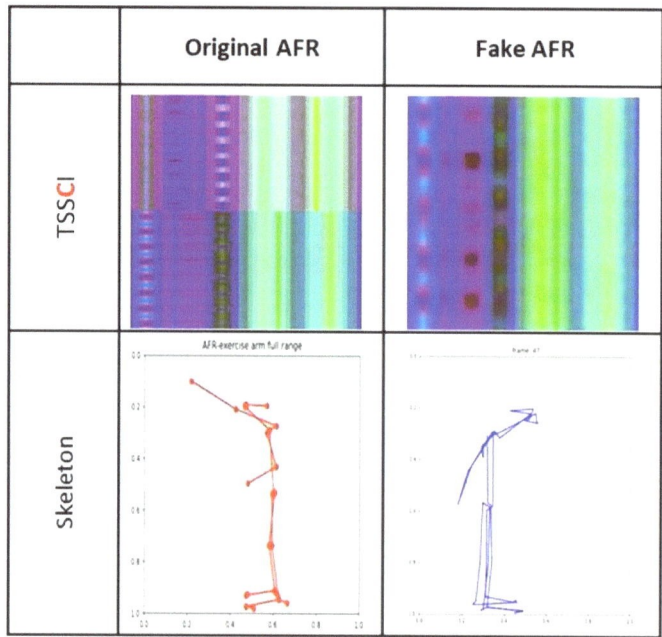

Figure 25. Generator of synthetic AFR movements using super object method.

We pass the synthetic movements through an EfficientNet-B7 CNN network-based movement classifier to validate the generator effectiveness and present a confusion matrix (see Figure 26). The matrix diagonal clearly illustrates the classifier near-perfect success in classifying all the new fake movements. Overall, this new capability of the super object method allows us to enrich our dataset with more tagged movements of the same type, which is an advanced form of augmentation. Additionally, we can use the movement merging algorithm to create a new set of movements different from the original six.

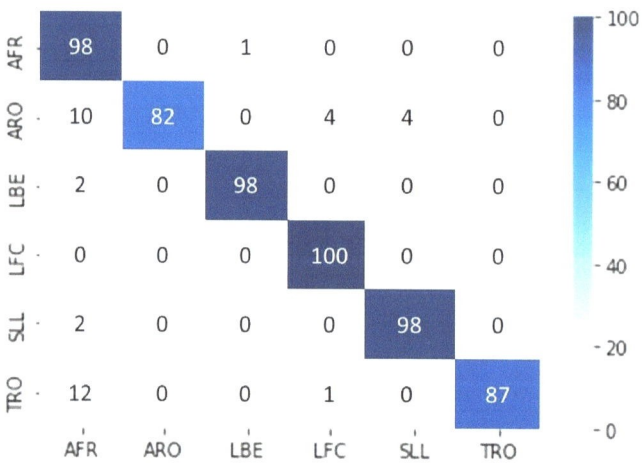

Figure 26. Analyze the quality of creation of 6 movements using a confusion matrix.

9.3.3. Utilizing a Siamese Twin Neural Network to Score the Quality of Physical Therapy Exercises Performed by Student Relative to Expert Physical Therapists

In this section, we highlight the effectiveness of the super object via the TSSCI method in providing a score for the quality of exercise performance compared to an expert physiotherapist. Given that our research framework focuses on demonstrating the effectiveness of the super object method, our dataset consists solely of examples from healthy individuals and does not include patients with movement disorders. To validate the effectiveness of our method, we rely on a set of exercises performed by an expert physiotherapist as a reference point. We developed a Siamese twin network based on the EfficientNet network to provide a score for exercise performance. This network features two channels: a reference channel that receives the specialist TSSCI and an identical parallel channel that receives the TSSCIs of all students performing a mix of exercises. Each channel produces a latent vector, and we measure the Euclidean distance between the vectors of the expert and the student performing a particular exercise. The smaller the distance between the vectors, the higher the score, with a score of 100 indicating a perfect mimicked exercise (performing similar movements). Conversely, the greater the distance, the lower the score, with 0 indicating completely different exercise movements.

For scoring we define the variable f as follow:

$$f = \alpha \frac{100}{D} \tag{16}$$

where:

D—Euclidean distance between the reference and student latent vectors
α—Scaling factor alpha; we empirically chose alpha as 30.

Finally we obtain a score between 0 and 100 by the following formula:

$$s = \begin{cases} f & \text{if } f < 100 \\ 100 & \text{if } f \geq 100 \end{cases} \tag{17}$$

where:

s—score, where $0 \leq s \leq 100$

The Euclidean distance method, commonly used for measuring the similarity between two vectors, suffers from the challenge of an unlimited maximum distance, making it difficult to define a final scale between 0 and 100. To address this challenge, we developed an empirical scoring method that demonstrates the effectiveness of using the super object method rather than focus on providing an accurate score. Our empirical method involves using the inverse of the Euclidean distance and setting a threshold for the maximum value beyond which any similarity score would be considered 100. Specifically, we define a threshold distance of 100, such that any inverse Euclidean distance between the reference and student vectors greater than or equal to 100 is capped at a score of 100. Conversely, any distance less than 100 is multiplied by a scaling factor alpha (in our case, we empirically chose alpha as 30) to obtain a score between 0 and 100. Using this method, we can provide a qualitative score that effectively demonstrates the advantages of the super object method while accommodating the upper unbounded limit challenges of the Euclidean distance method.

To validate the effectiveness of our method, we consider an incorrect movement as one that differs from the reference movement performed by the expert physiotherapist. Specifically, we compare the performance of each student movement to the reference movement of the AFR exercise and expect to obtain a high score for those who accurately perform the AFR exercise and a low score for those who perform a different exercise from the expert. To achieve this, we repeat this process six times, using each of the six reference movements performed by the expert as the reference channel. We compare each student movement to the corresponding reference movement and calculate the score using our empirical scoring method. We summarize the scoring results in a confusion matrix, which provides an overview of the accuracy of each type of exercise the students perform (see Figure 27). The matrix rows represent the reference exercise performed by the expert physiotherapist, while the columns represent the type of exercise performed by the students. In each cell, we present the average score obtained for each type of exercise, enabling us to evaluate the effectiveness of our method in accurately classifying different types of movements. The effectiveness of our method is evident from the confusion matrix, which shows that the average score is high for most exercises, except for the LBE exercise. Interestingly, the LBE and the SLL exercises, for which the average score was also lower, share a common characteristic: the dominant movement is related to leg motion. In the LBE exercise, the leg motion is backward, while in the SLL exercise, it is sideways, which explains the system confusion during the scoring process. To address this limitation, we can continue the training process or explore alternative methods, such as using the EfficientNet network as a whole classifier to output a vector of probabilities for each student exercise. We can use this vector of probabilities as a score for the movement or calculate the Euclidean distance between the probability vectors of the expert and the student. However, since our study aims to demonstrate the effectiveness of the super object method for human movement classification, we believe that our empirical scoring method is sufficient to prove the effectiveness of our approach.

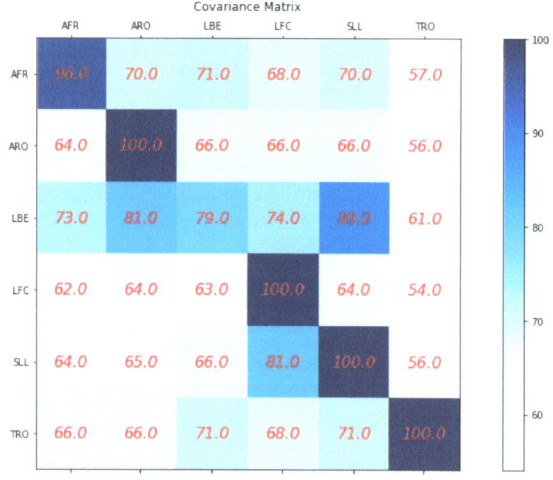

Figure 27. Score of the quality of physical therapy exercises performed by students relative to expert physical therapists.

9.3.4. Comparing the Quality of Synthetic Exercise Generated by VAE to That Provided by Experts Using a Siamese Twin Neural Network

We repeat the scoring process to complete our evaluation using the synthetic exercises we created with VAE. It enables us to demonstrate the quality of the synthetic movements and the effectiveness of our scoring method based on Siamese twin networks. Siamese twin networks have proven efficient for measuring the similarity between images and objects in various contexts. We aim to illustrate that any existing algorithm designed for analyzing the content of an image, particularly object recognition, can be used for analyzing movements based on the super object method. It shows the versatility and applicability of our approach beyond the scope of movement classification.

The effectiveness of our method is evident from the confusion matrix presented in Figure 28, which shows that the average score is high for most exercises in the diagonal as expected.

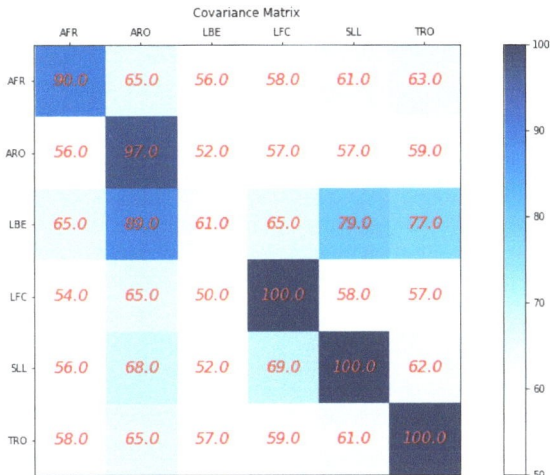

Figure 28. Comparing the quality of synthetic exercise generated by VAE to that provided by experts.

Please note that the majority of the outcomes detailed in this chapter were achieved using Python code, which is available in the Supplementary Materials section of this article.

10. Discussion

Our method enables the representation of a series of human movements as one object by converting multi-person key point detection algorithms to RGB-colored TSSCI images. X, Y, and confidence level—C coordinates are used to represent each of the 25 key points in the skeleton. All skeletons are grouped together in three dimensions (3D arrays—x, y, and confidence level c), obtained by multiplying the number of frames by the number of key points. In order to represent the array in RGB, it is converted into the red color channel, which represents the X coordinates, the green color channel, which represents the Y coordinates, and the blue color channel, which represents the C coordinates. Thus, the TSSCI represents the composition of the exercise from beginning to end as an abstracted color image. This new approach allows us to consider a human exercise as an object within a TSSCI image. As an example, in a typical image containing a cat object, a CNN network trained to tag cats will successfully tag most of the cats in a set of images, regardless of where they are within the image, how large they are, and whether they are rotated. In most cases, the video clip of the therapist will contain the entire exercise from the beginning to the end. As a result, the exercise (which is our super object) takes the entire TSSCI (every raw in the image belongs to this exercise), as if the image contained a large cat. In order to prepare for and repeat the exercise, patients normally prepare themselves prior to and after the actual exercise. The TSSCI image reflects this as an object (exercise) situated in the image center, whereas the top and bottom of the image are irrelevant (similar to a background in a typical image). As a result of this mode, the cat appears small and in the center of the picture, while the rest of the image contains mostly background, as if it were taken from a distance. CNNs extract feature vectors (latent vectors) that are representative of the properties of the object being classified, while filtering out other objects and backgrounds and disregarding the dimensions or orientation of the object. Using this new approach of treating the human motion as an object in a TSSCI image, we are able to use a CNN network to extract the latent vector of the human motion. By extracting a latent vector, which distills the characteristics of a movement into a one-dimensional vector, a variety of actions can be accomplished. The latent vector can be injected into a fully connected network, allowing us to classify and label movements. Another option is to inject the latent vector into a Siamese twin network, allowing us to compare therapist and patient and score the patient exercise relative to the therapist. We can create a probabilistic space of various latent vectors by using a CNN network with many patients who try to mimic the same exercise. Keeping in mind that a vector is by definition a point in an N-dimensional space, our latent vector is also a point in an N-dimensional space. As a result, creating multiple latent vectors from many patients produces a cloud of points in the N-dimensional space that represents our probability space of a specific exercise. While the number of points in the probability space for this specific movement is infinite, we have created only a finite collection of points. These points are referred to as "existence points" or "existence," whereas the probability space between the existing points is referred to as "nothing." Using the VAE network, we are able to add synthetically virtual existence points to the "nothing" based on the "existence" points. The creation of the new virtual points allows us to create a completely new fake TSSCI image from each new point utilizing VAE generator, thus enriching the number of points in our probabilistic space for this particular exercise. Therefore, we can generate from the faked TSSCI image a video showing the movement of skeletons, describing the movement performed by a fake person, which will increase our dataset for training other neural networks able to perform more complex tasks.

10.1. Dataset

We divided our dataset into three parts. The division of it into three parts provides a comprehensive understanding of the different types of environments. The exercises performed by students from the University of Prague under laboratory conditions provide a controlled environment for evaluating the performance of the exercises. It allows for a clear understanding of the effect of the exercises on the students and provides a sterile environment baseline for comparison. On the other hand, the exercises performed by students from Ben Gurion University in an uncontrolled environment provide a real-world scenario of how patients may perform the exercises in the home environment. It provides valuable insights into the practicality and effectiveness of the exercises in a more natural setting. Finally, the exercises the expert physiotherapist performs under controlled laboratory conditions serve as the ground truth, allowing for comparing and measuring the other exercises performed. It provides a benchmark for evaluating the performance of the exercises and allows for a thorough understanding of the efficacy of the exercises. Dividing the dataset into these three parts provides a comprehensive and well-rounded understanding of the exercises and their performance in different scenarios. We felt it appropriate to expand a little beyond the scope of the discussion of this paper and point out that "existence," "nonexistence," or "nothing" are central philosophical themes. According to Plato, non-physical ideas, or Forms ("nothing"), are more real than the physical world we perceive ("existence"). According to him, physical objects (in our case, actual movements) are imperfect copies of these non-physical Forms (movements performed by a fake person or merely fake movements), and that the Forms are eternal and unchanging. This technique of creating virtual points within the space of "nothing" by using the points of "existence" could be called "computational imagination" or " computational creativity".

10.2. Efficient TSSCI Processing with Negligible Resource Consumption

The low resource consumption of TSSCI is a significant advantage that can have a notable impact on human movements analysis. The technique efficiently combines a series of frames into one image, which can be also processed by programs such as OpenPose and MediaPipe that extract the skeletons from the video. These programs typically process 30 frames per second. An average human exercise consists of thousands of frames, say 1000, for this discussion. From the tests we conducted, the TSSCI image processing time using the EfficientNet network is approximately 20 milliseconds. In comparison with a video frame, which has at least 512×512 pixels, TSSCI has a small image size of 49×49 pixels. Additionally, the abstract structure and image orientation, primarily in the y direction, can enhance network convergence. Assuming the time required to extract a skeleton from a frame is T, according to our measurements the TSSCI calculation time is only a quarter of T. We need to process only one TSSCI per exercise. Consequently, for an exercise, it would take 1000T to extract all the skeletons and only a quarter of T to process TSSCI with a neural network. It is worth mentioning that the creation of TSSCI is insignificant as it only aggregates skeletal data into a single array. In summary, using TSSCI as a super object approach has a negligible impact on the total processing time, accounting for only 0.025% of the total processing time compared to the time required to extract the exercise skeletons. It highlights the efficiency and potential of TSSCI to enhance human body movement analysis while minimizing resource consumption. Our results are promising and have implications for various sectors, such as healthcare and fitness, where efficient video analysis can make a significant difference.

11. Conclusions

In this work, we presented a novel and versatile approach to reference human movements, based on super object in the form of a TSSCI image. Our solution provides a generic method for analyzing and processing human movements, using standard deep learning network architectures, allowing for a variety of tasks such as classification, measurement, prediction, completion, and improvement of movements. To demonstrate the effectiveness of our method, we utilized the open-source code from OpenPose [8] and MediaPipe [9], generously provided by the respective authors. This code enabled us to extract a human skeleton graph from a video and consolidate the results into a TSSCI image. We focused on measuring physiotherapy exercises using a dataset of approximately 100 students who performed six physical therapy exercises prescribed by an expert physiotherapist. The data set was divided into three types: exercises performed by an expert, exercises performed in a controlled environment and under laboratory conditions, and a third group who performed the exercises freestyle at home. We demonstrated the versatility of our approach by injecting identical TSSCI images into three different networks (EfficientNet, variational auto-encoder, and Siamese twin networks) for performing different tasks. We successfully classified human movements performed under laboratory conditions and with high accuracy for movements performed under uncontrolled, noisy conditions, except for cases where there were not enough examples for training. Furthermore, we demonstrated the use of a VAE architecture to generate new synthetic skeletons and even merged different movements to create a unique synthetic movement. We explained the VAE architecture using the t-SNE algorithm to present the N-dimensional distribution space of the latent vectors in two dimensions. Finally, we presented the use of the TSSCI method in assessing the performance of physical therapy exercises compared to a specialist physiotherapist using a Siamese twin network. We proposed an empirical scoring method for the quality of the exercise performance and summarized the results in two confusion matrices. Our experiments demonstrate the effectiveness of our super object method in human movement analysis. In conclusion, the combination of convolutional neural networks (CNNs), OpenPose, and MediaPipe can be effectively utilized to evaluate physical therapy exercises performed by patients in a home setting relative to the performance of a remote therapist. The study demonstrates the potential of computer vision techniques in physical therapy and the significance of precise and timely evaluations in enhancing patient results. The super object method was shown to be a practical approach to analyzing human movements, and the Siamese twin network based on the EfficientNet network provided a score for exercise performance. The results of the experiment provide evidence of the method viability and effectiveness, as demonstrated by the confusion matrix. The study can be used as a basis for further research and development in computer vision and physical therapy. Careful consideration of resolution, orientation, and camera stability is essential to ensure that model predictions are accurate and reliable.

Supplementary Materials: The following supporting python code examples and some general explanations can be downloaded from: https://github.com/yoramse/TSSCI.git, https://bit.ly/bgu_pyhton_code_example and from https://bit.ly/BGU_Extra_Info, (accessed on 6 March 2023).

Author Contributions: Conceptualization, Y.S. and O.H.; methodology, Y.S.; software, Y.S.; validation, L.L. and O.H.; formal analysis, L.L.; investigation, Y.S.; resources, Y.S.; data curation, Y.S.; writing—original draft preparation, Y.S.; writing—review and editing, L.L.; visualization, L.L.; supervision, O.H.; project administration, Y.S.; funding acquisition, O.H. and L.L. All authors have read and agreed to the published version of the manuscript.

Funding: This research was supported by a grant from the Ministry of Science Technology, Israel and The Ministry of Education, Youth and Sports of the Czech Republic. The described research was supported by the project No. LTAIZ19008 (Czech) and No. 8773451 (Israel) Enhancing Robotic Physiotherapeutic Treatment using Machine Learning awarded in frame of the Czech–Israeli cooperative scientific research program (Inter-Excellence MEYS CR and MOST Israel).

Institutional Review Board Statement: The study was conducted in accordance with the Declaration of Helsinki and approved by the Ethics Committee of the Faculty of Physical Education and Sports of the Charles University. (protocol code 167/2020 and date of approval 28 August 2020.

Informed Consent Statement: Informed consent was obtained from all subjects involved in the study.

Data Availability Statement: Link to publicly archived datasets analyzed and generated during the study: https://bit.ly/bgu_anonymous_dataset, accessed on 6 March 2023.

Acknowledgments: It is our pleasure to acknowledge the many students who participated in recording the movements from Israel and the Czech Republic. We would also like to thank the members of the Czech research team who contributed to the collection, cleaning, and editing of the database. In particular, we wish to thank Jindrich Adolf from the Czech Institute of Informatics, Robotics and Cybernetics at Czech Technical University in Prague, Czech Republic, who assisted us in pre-processing and converting the data into an anonymous vectors dataset. Physiotherapy exercises were defined by Matyas Turna, Tereza Novakova from the Faculty of Physical Education and Sport, Charles University, Prague, Czech Republic, who added insights from the field of physiotherapy. A photography lab was set up including synchronized photography from several cameras and allowed the exercises to take place, thanks to Jaromir Dolezal, Jan Hejda, and Patrik Kutilek from the Czech Technical University in Prague, Kladno, Czech Republic Faculty of Biomedical Engineering. We wish to express our heartfelt gratitude to Raz Birman for his invaluable English language proficiency and critical thinking. Eliraz Orfaig's exceptional programming skills, specifically in neural networks, were invaluable. Dan Gahokidze's meticulous organization of the database was essential.

Conflicts of Interest: The authors declare no conflict of interest. The funders had no role in the design of the study; in the collection, analyses, or interpretation of data; in the writing of the manuscript; or in the decision to publish the results.

References

1. Segal, Y.; Hadar, O.; Lhotska, L. Assessing Human Mobility by Constructing a Skeletal Database and Augmenting it Using a Generative Adversarial Network (GAN) Simulator. In *PHealth 2022*; IOS Press: Amsterdam, The Netherlands, 2022; pp. 97–103. [CrossRef]
2. Segal, Y.; Yona, Y.; Danan, O.; Birman, R.; Hadar, O.; Kutilek, P.; Hejda, J.; Hourova, M.; Kral, P.; Lhotska, L.; et al. Camera Setup and OpenPose software without GPU for calibration and recording in telerehabilitation. In *IEEE E-Health and Bioengineering*; IEEE E-Health and Bioengineering: Lasi, Romania, 2021.
3. Kutilek, P.; Hejda, J.; Lhotska, L.; Adolf, J.; Dolezal, J.; Hourova, M.; Kral, P.; Segal, Y.; Birman, R.; Hadar, O. Camera System for Efficient non-contact Measurement in Distance Medicine. In Proceedings of the Prague: 2020 19th International Conference on Mechatronics—Mechatronika (ME), Prague, Czech Republic, 2–4 December 2020; pp. 1–6.
4. Blobel, B.; Oemig, F.; Ruotsalainen, P.; Lopez, D.M. Transformation of Health and Social Care Systems—An Interdisciplinary Approach Toward a Foundational Architecture. *Front. Med.* **2022**, *9*, 802487. Available online: https://www.frontiersin.org/articles/10.3389/fmed.2022.802487 (accessed on 6 May 2023). [CrossRef] [PubMed]
5. Adolf, J.; Dolezal, J.; Macas, M.; Lhotska, L. Remote Physical Therapy: Requirements for a Single RGB Camera Motion Sensing. In Proceedings of the 2021 International Conference on Applied Electronics (AE), Pilsen, Czechoslovakia, 7–8 September 2021; pp. 1–4. [CrossRef]
6. Carissimi, N.; Rota, P.; Beyan, C.; Murino, V. Filling the Gaps: Predicting Missing Joints of Human Poses Using Denoising Autoencoders. In *Computer Vision—ECCV 2018 Workshops*; Leal-Taixé, L., Roth, S., Eds.; Lecture Notes in Computer Science; Springer International Publishing: Cham, Switzerland, 2019; Volume 11130, pp. 364–379. [CrossRef]

7. Koch, G. Siamese Neural Networks for One-Shot Image Recognition. Master's Thesis, Graduate Department of Computer Science, University of Toronto, Toronto, ON, Canada, 2015. Available online: http://www.cs.toronto.edu/~gkoch/files/msc-thesis.pdf (accessed on 6 May 2023).
8. Cao, Z.; Hidalgo, G.; Simon, T.; Wei, S.-E.; Sheikh, Y. OpenPose: Realtime Multi-Person 2D Pose. *IEEE Conf. Comput. Vis. Pattern Recognit. CVPR* **2017**, *43*, 7291–7299.
9. Lugaresi, C.; Tang, J.; Nash, H.; McClanahan, C.; Uboweja, E.; Hays, M.; Zhang, F.; Chang, C.L.; Yong, M.; Lee, J.; et al. MediaPipe: A Framework for Perceiving and Processing Reality. Third Workshop on Computer Vision for AR/VR at IEEE Computer Vision and Pattern Recognition (CVPR). 2019. Available online: https://mixedreality.cs.cornell.edu/s/NewTitle_May1_MediaPipe_CVPR_CV4ARVR_Workshop_2019.pdf (accessed on 6 March 2023).
10. Adolf, J.; Dolezal, J.; Kutilek, P.; Hejda, J.; Lhotska, L. Single Camera-Based Remote Physical Therapy: Verification on a Large Video Dataset. *Appl. Sci.* **2022**, *12*, 799. [CrossRef]
11. Liao, Y.; Vakanski, A.; Xian, M. A Deep Learning Framework for Assessing Physical Rehabilitation Exercises. *IEEE Trans. Neural Syst. Rehabil. Eng.* **2020**, *28*, 468–477. [CrossRef] [PubMed]
12. Kingma, D.P.; Welling, M. Auto-Encoding Variational Bayes. *arXiv* **2022**, arXiv:1312.6114.
13. Xi, W.; Devineau, G.; Moutarde, F.; Yang, J. Generative Model for Skeletal Human Movements Based on Conditional DC-GAN Applied to Pseudo-Images. *Algorithms* **2020**, *13*, 319. [CrossRef]
14. Yang, Z.; Li, Y.; Yang, J.; Luo, J. Action Recognition With Spatio–Temporal Visual Attention on Skeleton Image Sequences. *IEEE Trans. Circuits Syst. Video Technol.* **2019**, *29*, 2405–2415. [CrossRef]
15. Caetano, C.; Sena, J.; Brémond, F.; Santos, J.A.D.; Schwartz, W.R. SkeleMotion: A New Representation of Skeleton Joint Sequences Based on Motion Information for 3D Action Recognition. *arXiv* **1907**, arXiv:1907.13025.
16. Ren, B.; Liu, M.; Ding, R.; Liu, H. A Survey on 3D Skeleton-Based Action Recognition Using Learning Method. *arXiv* **2020**, arXiv:2002.05907.
17. Ma, L.; Jia, X.; Sun, Q.; Schiele, B.; Tuytelaars, T.; Gool, L.V. Pose Guided Person Image Generation. *arXiv* **2018**, arXiv:1705.09368.
18. Caetano, C.; Brémond, F.; Schwartz, W.R. Skeleton Image Representation for 3D Action Recognition based on Tree Structure and Reference Joints. *arXiv* **2019**, arXiv:1909.05704.
19. Barron, J.L.; Fleet, D.J.; Beauchemin, S.S.; Burkitt, T.A. Performance of Optical Flow Techniques. *Int. J. Comput. Vis.* **1994**, *12*, 43–77. [CrossRef]
20. Kuipers, J.B. *Quaternions and Rotation Sequences: A Primer with Applications to Orbits, Aerospace and Virtual Reality*; Princeton University Press: Princeton, NJ, USA, 2002.
21. LaValle, S.M. *Planning Algorithms*; Cambridge University Press: Cambridge, UK, 2006.
22. Visual Reconstruction, MIT Press. Available online: https://mitpress.mit.edu/9780262524063/visual-reconstruction/ (accessed on 20 January 2023).
23. Osokin, D. Real-time 2D Multi-Person Pose Estimation on CPU: Lightweight OpenPose. *arXiv* **2018**, arXiv:1811.12004.
24. Brownlee, J. How to Normalize and Standardize Time Series Data in Python. *MachineLearningMastery.com*. 11 December 2016. Available online: https://machinelearningmastery.com/normalize-standardize-time-series-data-python/ (accessed on 21 January 2023).
25. Normalization, Codecademy. Available online: https://www.codecademy.com/article/normalization (accessed on 21 January 2023).
26. How to Normalize the RMSE. Available online: https://www.marinedatascience.co/blog/2019/01/07/normalizing-the-rmse// (accessed on 21 January 2023).
27. Boudreau, E. Unit-Length Scaling: The Ultimate In Continuous Feature-Scaling? *Medium*, 27 July 2020. Available online: https://towardsdatascience.com/unit-length-scaling-the-ultimate-in-continuous-feature-scaling-c5db0b0dab57 (accessed on 21 January 2023).
28. Tan, M.; Le, Q. EfficientNet: Rethinking Model Scaling for Convolutional Neural Networks. In Proceedings of the 36th International Conference on Machine Learning, PMLR, Long Beach, CA, USA, 9–15 June 2019; pp. 6105–6114. Available online: https://proceedings.mlr.press/v97/tan19a.html (accessed on 18 January 2023).
29. van der Maaten, L. Visualizing Data using t-SNE. *J. Mach. Learn. Res.* **2008**, *9*, 2579–2605.

Disclaimer/Publisher's Note: The statements, opinions and data contained in all publications are solely those of the individual author(s) and contributor(s) and not of MDPI and/or the editor(s). MDPI and/or the editor(s) disclaim responsibility for any injury to people or property resulting from any ideas, methods, instructions or products referred to in the content.

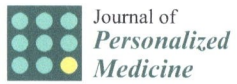

Article

Analysis of Prevalence and Clinical Features of Aortic Stenosis in Patients with and without Bicuspid Aortic Valve Using Machine Learning Methods

Olga Irtyuga [1], Mary Babakekhyan [1], Anna Kostareva [1], Vladimir Uspensky [1], Michail Gordeev [1], Giuseppe Faggian [2], Anna Malashicheva [1], Oleg Metsker [1], Evgeny Shlyakhto [1] and Georgy Kopanitsa [1,*]

1. Almazov National Medical Research Centre, 197341 Saint-Petersburg, Russia; irtyuga_ob@almazovcentre.ru (O.I.); babakekhyan_mv@almazovcentre.ru (M.B.); kostareva_aa@almazovcentre.ru (A.K.); uspenskiy_ve@almazovcentre.ru (V.U.); gordeev_ml@almazovcentre.ru (M.G.); malashicheva_ab@almazovcentre.ru (A.M.); metsker_og@almazovcentre.ru (O.M.); shlyakhto_ev@almazovcentre.ru (E.S.)
2. Department of Cardiac Surgery, University of Verona Medical School, 37134 Verona, Italy; giuseppe.faggian@univr.it
* Correspondence: georgy.kopanitsa@gmail.com

Abstract: Aortic stenosis (AS) is the most commonly diagnosed valvular heart disease, and its prevalence increases with the aging of the general population. However, AS is often diagnosed at a severe stage, necessitating surgical treatment, due to its long asymptomatic period. The objective of this study was to analyze the frequency of AS in a population of cardiovascular patients using echocardiography (ECHO) and to identify clinical factors and features associated with these patient groups. We utilized machine learning methods to analyze 84,851 echocardiograms performed between 2010 and 2018 at the National Medical Research Center named after V.A. Almazov. The primary indications for ECHO were coronary artery disease (CAD) and hypertension (HP), accounting for 33.5% and 14.2% of the cases, respectively. The frequency of AS was found to be 13.26% among the patients (n = 11,252). Within our study, 1544 patients had a bicuspid aortic valve (BAV), while 83,316 patients had a tricuspid aortic valve (TAV). BAV patients were observed to be younger compared to TAV patients. AS was more prevalent in the BAV group (59%) compared to the TAV group (12%), with a p-value of <0.0001. By employing a machine learning algorithm, we randomly identified significant features present in AS patients, including age, hypertension (HP), aortic regurgitation (AR), ascending aortic dilatation (AscAD), and BAV. These findings could serve as additional indications for earlier observation and more frequent ECHO in specific patient groups for the earlier detection of developing AS.

Keywords: machine learning; aortic stenosis; predictors; retrospective study; clinical features

1. Introduction

This paper is an extension of the paper presented in the pHealth 2021 Conference [1]. AS is the most common acquired valvular heart disease [2–5], and the prevalence of moderate or severe valvular disease increases with age, which poses a burden on healthcare systems in developed countries [2–4]. Bicuspid aortic valve (BAV) holds a significant position within the population affected by aortic stenosis [6,7], and it is recognized as one of the most prevalent congenital heart defects [8]. The detectability of BAV in the general population varies between 0.5% and 2%, often associated with aortic pathology [8–10]. Recent studies have revealed a lower diagnosis rate of AS in women compared to men, suggesting an important imbalance given the associated lower survival rates [11]. Further investigations into sex-related differences in AS, regardless of its severity, are warranted [12,13].

The formation of aortic stenosis remains a topic without a unified consensus. The question of early diagnosis and its impact on disease progression, aiming to reduce the need for surgical treatment, remains unanswered. Our knowledge regarding predictors of symptom development and adverse outcomes primarily focuses on data concerning asymptomatic severe AS, with a lack of information regarding the natural history of AS. Numerous studies aim to identify factors influencing the rate, timing, and extent of aortic stenosis, regardless of its morphology [4,14]. This field of research may help refine the indications for earlier echocardiographic screening in specific populations. Currently, echocardiography is recommended for patients with an unexplained systolic noise on the aortic valve, second heart sound, a history of BAV, or symptoms that may be attributed to AS [7]. Few studies have explored the role of risk factors in the onset and progression of AS, with functional status being one of the few indicators investigated [13]. No significant differences have been observed for age, sex, cause of aortic stenosis, comorbid diseases, smoking history, or coexisting coronary artery disease (CAD). Some population-based studies have indicated that higher body mass index and obesity correlate with the occurrence of aortic stenosis, although these findings are specific to certain races and geographical locations [15,16]. Limited data are available regarding predictors of AS development in mild and moderate cases, although indicators such as the degree of aortic valve calcification and the presence of CAD have been associated with progression and prognosis [14,17].

Echocardiography is the key diagnostic method for AS [3,6], and there are currently no medical therapies known to influence the natural history of aortic stenosis, as per the recent ESC guidelines [3]. Large medical centers have the capacity to collect, store, and analyze substantial amounts of information [18]. This wealth of data can be utilized for statistical analysis and machine learning methods to uncover new relationships between risk factors and the development of asymptomatic diseases. Consequently, our study enables the evaluation of a specific population's prevalence of AS and its associations with various predictors.

The goal of this study is to identify the most important risk factors in the development of aortic stenosis, focusing on their prognostic significance. To attain this objective, we thoroughly analyze the importance of various predictors and distinguish between risk factors associated with aortic stenosis and those that predict the occurrence of ascending aortic aneurysms.

2. Materials and Methods

The research plan received authorization from the ethics committee at the Almazov National Medical Research Centre in Saint Petersburg, Russian Federation, following the guidelines specified in the Declaration of Helsinki before the study was initiated.

2.1. Study Cohort

To identify patients with aortic stenosis (AS) and different valve morphologies (bicuspid aortic valve—BAV, and tricuspid aortic valve—TAV), we conducted a retrospective analysis of the ECHO database at the Almazov National Medical Research Centre. The database encompassed 145,454 echocardiograms from both outpatients and hospitalized patients who received observation and treatment at the center between January 2010 and November 2018. It is important to note that the patient cohort used in this analysis is the same as the one utilized in our previous study [1]. Please see Table 1.

Table 1. Clinical and demographic characteristics of male patients.

Features	BAV, n = 983 Median; Quartiles			TAV, n = 39,703 Median; Quartiles		
	With AS, n = 536	Without AS, n = 447	p	With AS, n = 4423	Without AS, n = 35,280	p
Age, years (median and bounds)	50 (34; 60)	29 (21; 46)	<0.0001	66 (57; 74)	57 (46; 65)	<0.0001
Aortic diameter at the sinus of the Valsalva, mm	37 (34; 41)	37 (33; 41)	<0.05	36 (34; 39)	36 (33; 39)	<0.0001

Table 1. *Cont.*

Features	BAV, n = 983 Median; Quartiles			TAV, n = 39,703 Median; Quartiles		
	With AS, n = 536	Without AS, n = 447	p	With AS, n = 4423	Without AS, n = 35,280	p
Aortic diameter at the proximal ascending aorta, mm	39 (35; 44)	24.8 (21.8; 27.8)	<0.0001	37 (34; 40)	34 (31; 37)	<0.0001
BMI, kg/m^2	26.3 (23.9; 30)	24.8 (21.8; 27.8)	<0.0001	27.3 (24.5; 30.3)	27.4 (24.5; 30.6)	0.48
AS dpmax, mmHg	29 (20; 50)	10 (7; 12)	<0.0001	30 (20; 53)	6 (5; 8)	<0.0001
EF LV (%)	63.8 (57.4; 69)	64.2 (59.5; 69.7)	0.04	62.4 (53.4; 68)	60.9 (51.5; 67)	<0.0001
SBP office, mmHg	135 (124; 142)	130 (120; 140)	0.12	140 (129; 150)	130 (120; 140)	<0.0001
DBP office, mmHg	80 (75; 85)	80 (80; 85)	0.86	80 (80; 88)	80 (80; 87)	0.46
AR, n (%)	123 (22.95)	118 (26.46)	0.20	778 (17.59)	1286 (3.65)	<0.0001
Hypertension, n (%)	316 (58.95)	268 (59.96)	0.5	2803 (63.37)	25,532 (72.37)	<0.001
Diabetes mellitus, n (%)	31 (5.78)	17 (3.80)	0.15	451 (10.20)	3204 (9.08)	0.2
CAD, n (%)	127 (23.69)	46 (10.29)	<0.001	1818 (41.10)	14,222 (40.31)	0.31
COPD, n (%)	58 (10.82)	23 (5.15)	0.001	460 (10.40)	3687 (10.45)	0.92
Asthma, n (%)	22 (4.10)	9 (2.01)	0.06	88 (1.99)	732 (2.07)	0.71
Obesity, (BMI > 30), n (%)	61 (11.3)	19 (4.25)	<0.0001	394 (8.9)	3005 (8.52)	0.15
Hyperlipidemia, n (%)	135 (25.19)	56 (12.53)	<0.0001	1170 (26.45)	9061 (25.68)	0.27
Heart failure, n (%)	320 (59.70)	156 (34.90)	<0.0001	2332 (52.72)	14,770 (41.87)	<0.001

BMI—body mass index; SBP—systolic blood pressure; DBP—diastolic blood pressure; AS dpmax—antegrade gradient across the narrowed aortic valve; EF LV—left ventricular ejection fraction, AR—aortic regurgitation; COPD—chronic obstructive pulmonary disease; CAD—coronary artery disease.

We used the following criteria in the process of data collection (Figure 1):

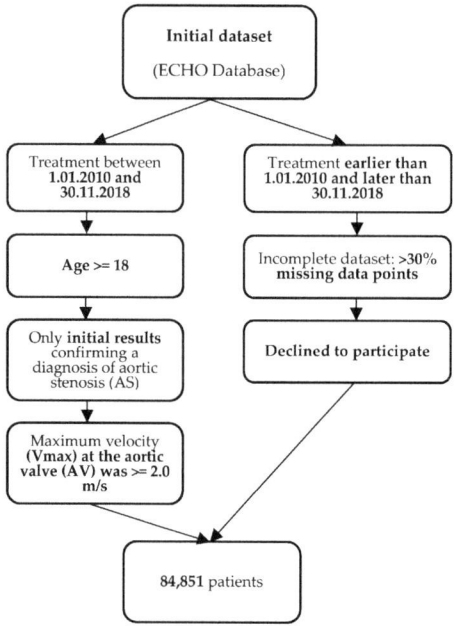

Figure 1. Inclusion and exclusion criteria.

2.1.1. Inclusion Criteria

1. Patients from the ECHO database who initiated treatment between 1 January 2010 and 30 November 2018;
2. For patients who underwent multiple ECHO examinations during this period, only the initial results confirming a diagnosis of aortic stenosis (AS) were considered for the study. ECHO examinations were primarily conducted in the following clinical scenarios: suspected cardiac etiology based on symptoms, signs, or other tests, as well as evaluation and follow-up of individuals with cardiovascular disease;
3. The age of the patients was equal to or greater than 18 years;
4. Patients were included in the study if the maximum velocity (Vmax) at the aortic valve (AV) was equal to or greater than 2.0 m/s, based on the definition of AS outlined in the 2020 ACC/AHA Guideline for the Management of Patients with Valvular Heart Disease [6].

2.1.2. Exclusion Criteria

1. Patients whose treatment started before 1 January 2010 or ended after 30 November 2018;
2. Patients who had incomplete datasets;
3. Patients who declined to participate in the study.

To confirm AS we also considered the mean aortic transvalvular pressure gradient and aortic valve area. The AV velocity served as the cutoff point for further analysis. Additionally, the average gradient on the AV and the size of the AV orifice were considered. However, it is worth noting that not all conclusions included these features. The presence of AS was confirmed through its mentioning in the electronic medical record diagnosis and was defined using the International Classification of Diseases, 10th Revision, Clinical Modification (ICD-10-CM) codes I35.0 (Aortic (valve) stenosis), I35.1 (Nonrheumatic aortic (valve) insufficiency), I35.2 (Aortic (valve) stenosis with insufficiency), I35.8 (Other nonrheumatic aortic valve disorders), and I35.9 (Nonrheumatic aortic valve disorder, unspecified).

The initial dataset contained 51 features, but for 25 of them, we had less than 30% of data points available. After removing these features, we ended with a dataset with 26 features. The resulting dataset contained 26 predictors: age, gender, aorta maximum diameter (max aorta), aortic diameter at the sinus of the Valsalva (max aorta sinus), systolic blood pressure (SPB), diastolic blood pressure (DBP), pulse blood pressure (SBP), AR, BAV, HP, CAD, heart failure, congenital heart disease (CHD), atrial fibrillation (AF), thoracic aortic aneurysm (TAO), hyperlipidemia, diabetes mellitus (DM), obesity, ulcer disease, chronic obstructive pulmonary disease (COPD), cholecystitis, stroke, asthma, cholelithiasis, goiter, and thyroid disorders. All drugs taken by patients were combined into two groups: antihypertensive and lipid-lowering.

A retrospective analysis was conducted on a total of 84,851 cases that satisfied the predetermined inclusion and exclusion criteria. All patients were categorized into two subgroups: those with tricuspid aortic valve (TAV) (n = 83,316) and those with bicuspid aortic valve (BAV) (n = 1544).

All patients underwent comprehensive two-dimensional and Doppler transthoracic echocardiography, following the latest echocardiography guidelines. The Vivid 7.0 system (GE, Philadelphia, PA, USA) was employed for the echocardiographic examinations [6,19].

Aortic diameters, ventricular sizes, ventricular function, and valve performance measurements were conducted in accordance with the current recommendations for echocardiography [6,19]. The maximal aortic diameter was indexed to the body surface area to obtain an absolute value.

The diagnosis of bicuspid aortic valve (BAV) was established through short-axis imaging of the aortic valve (AV), which revealed the presence of only two commissures, delineating two AV cusps.

Additionally, for each echocardiography case, an analysis was performed to determine the reason for ordering the echocardiogram. In 33.5% of cases, echocardiography was performed for patients with coronary artery disease (CAD), while in 14.2% of cases, it was conducted for patients with hypertension (HP).

Tables 1 and 2 present the clinical and demographic characteristics of the patient groups, respectively.

Table 2. Clinical and demographic characteristics of female patients.

Variables	BAV, n = 541 Median; Quartiles			TAV, n = 43,613 Median; Quartiles		
	With AS, n = 365	Without AS, n = 185	p	With AS, n = 5928	Without AS, n = 40,925	p
Age, years (median and bounds)	49 (31; 61)	31 (26; 49);	<0.0001	71 (62; 77)	58 (41; 68);	<0.0001
Aortic diameter at the sinus of the Valsalva, mm	32 (30; 35)	32 (29; 36)	0.89	32 (30; 35)	32 (30; 34)	<0.0001
Aortic diameter at the proximal ascending aorta, mm	36 (32; 40)	33 (29; 39)	<0.0001	34 (31; 37)	31 (28; 34)	<0.0001
BMI, kg/m^2	25.6 (22.6; 29.9)	24.6 (21.7; 26.9)	0.01	28.8 (25.2; 32.6)	27.1 (23.5; 31.2)	<0.0001
AS dpmax, mmHg	32 (22; 56)	10 (8; 13)	<0.0001	31 (20; 60)	7 (5; 9)	<0.0001
EF LV (%)	66.9 (61.8; 71.4)	66 (61; 70)	0.15	65.9 (60.7; 70)	65.7 (60.6; 70)	0.34
SBP office, mmHg	120 (120; 140)	120 (110; 127.5)	0.13	140 (130; 150)	130 (120; 140)	<0.0001
DBP office, mmHg	80 (70; 80)	80 (70; 80)	0.61	80 (80; 90)	80 (75; 85)	<0.0001
AR, n (%)	64 (17.53)	27 (14.59)	0.38	814 (13.74)	1284 (3.14)	<0.0001
Hypertension, n (%)	177 (48.5)	99 (53.5)	0.1	3589 (60.5)	26,923 (65.78)	0.3
Diabetes mellitus, n (%)	20 (5.48)	9 (4.86)	0.76	824 (13.9)	3870 (9.45)	0.1
CAD, n (%)	58 (15.89)	18 (9.73)	0.05	2183 (36.83)	9968 (26.45)	<0.0001
COPD, n (%)	15 (4.11)	5 (2.70)	0.40	426 (7.19)	2144 (5.69)	0.5
Asthma, n (%)	10 (2.74)	5 (2.70)	0.98	208 (3.51)	1133 (3.01)	0.8
Obesity, (BMI > 30), n (%)	47 (12.8)	5 (2.70)	0.0002	862 (14.54)	4026 (9.83)	<0.0001
Hyperlipidemia, n (%)	94 (25.75)	19 (10.27)	<0.0001	1661 (28.02)	8888 (23.59)	<0.0001
Heart failure, n (%)	213 (58.36)	60 (32.43)	<0.0001	3221 (54.34)	14,120 (37.47)	<0.0001

BMI—body mass index; SBP—systolic blood pressure; DBP—diastolic blood pressure; AS dpmax—antegrade gradient across the narrowed aortic valve; EF LV—left ventricular ejection fraction, AR—aortic regurgitation; COPD—chronic obstructive pulmonary disease; CAD—coronary artery disease.

2.2. Statistical Methods

The statistical analysis was conducted using STATISTICA v. 10.0 (StatSoft Inc., Tulsa, OK, USA). The baseline characteristics of the study population were presented as percentages for qualitative variables and as medians and quartiles for quantitative variables that were not normally distributed, as deemed appropriate. The *p*-test was utilized to determine the probability of the distribution of characteristic values between different groups of patients with bicuspid aortic valve (BAV) compared to those with tricuspid aortic valve (TAV). Notably, due to the significant differences observed between sexes in terms of demographic characteristics, all analyses were separately reported for men and women.

2.3. Data Preprocessing

To filter out obvious outliers, we eliminated 1% of values with the highest z-scores. Subsequently, we applied min–max normalization to the remaining values.

2.4. Classification Model Grid Search and Features Importance

To determine the best performance model among Artificial Neural Network (ANN), Support Vector Machine (SVM), Decision Tree (DT), and Random Forest (RF), each experiment ran in the setting of stratified 5-fold cross-validation, i.e., a random 80% of the training dataset was used for training and a random 20% of the training dataset for testing. Target class ratios in the folds were preserved. For the performance assessment of SVM and DT classifiers, we ran it 100 times; 100 × 5-fold cross-validation resulted in 500 predictions. All the measurements were performed separately per dataset and per model parameter value to determine the best parameters for classifiers as well as optimal data preprocessing. After determining the optimal dataset and model parameters, we performed a validation with the testing dataset. As an additional performance assessment score, we used the AUC of the ROC, which represents the trade-off between the sensitivity and specificity of the model. We used a series of classification models available within scikit-learn as a pool for the selection of the best predictive methods to be applied within the proposed scheme. A summary of the required model parameters is presented in Table 3. The algorithm was implemented in Python 3.6.3 with the scikit-learn 0.19.1 library (https://scikit-learn.org/stable/ accessed on 20 October 2023).

Table 3. Performance evaluation with comorbidities.

	Precision	Recall	F1 Score	Accuracy	AUC
ANN	**0.83**	0.72	0.77	0.81	0.78
SVM	0.77	0.78	0.78	0.80	0.79
Decision Tree	0.79	0.81	0.78	0.82	0.79
Random Forest	0.79	0.81	0.80	0.83	0.80

A Random Forest (RF) is an ensemble of machine-learning algorithms that combines multiple tree predictors. Each tree in the forest relies on values from a randomly sampled vector, independently and with the same distribution for all trees.

Feature importance measurements were performed with the RF model as the best-performing model for our settings.

The p-value was calculated using different methods. For categorical features, the chi-square criterion was applied, while for continuous features, the Kolmogorov-Smirnov test was utilized.

Python 3 packages, including scikit-learn [20] and Catboost [21], were employed for implementing machine-learning models, seaborn [22] and matplotlib [23] for data visualization, SMOTE [24] for dataset balancing, and SHapley Additive exPlanations (SHAP) [25] for interpreting black-box results. The discrimination of the models was evaluated using ROC curves.

The Shapley value for each feature was calculated as the average contribution it makes across all possible combinations of features, with different permutations of features getting equal weight. Shapley values provide a way to fairly distribute the value (in this case, the prediction) among the features in a predictive model. Shapley values offer a more comprehensive and fair understanding of how each feature contributes to the model's predictions.

3. Results

The study included a population of 84,851 patients who underwent screening by echocardiography (ECHO). The primary indications for performing ECHO included the presence of coronary artery disease (CAD), hypertension (HP), known valvular heart disease (VHD), various forms of arrhythmia, as well as other reasons (refer to Figure 2 for details). The article on the clinical characteristics of ascending aortic dilatation in patients with and without bicuspid aortic valve (BAV) [16] provides a comprehensive description of the patients' referral reasons.

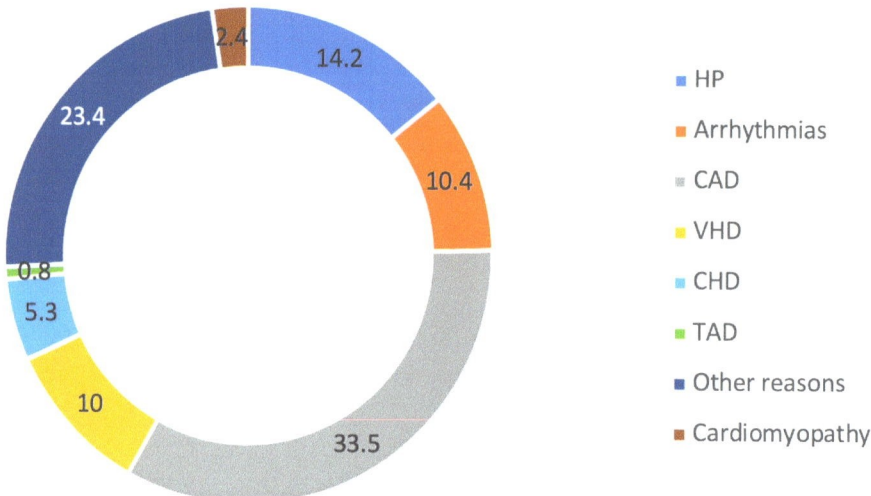

Figure 2. Study population characteristics.

BAV was detected in 1544 patients, according to ECHO, while TAV was detected in 83,316 patients. AS was diagnosed in 11,252 (13.26%) patients. At the same time AS was more frequent in the group of patients with BAV (n = 901, 58.7%): 59.5% (n = 536) in men and 40.5% (n = 365) in women than in the group of TAV (n = 10,351, 12.42%): 42.7% (n = 4423) in men and 57.3% (n = 5928) in women ($p < 0.0001$).

The results showed that both male and female patients with AS were significantly older, had heart failure more often, and had wider diameter of ascending aorta and higher Vmax, regardless of AV morphology (Table 1, $p < 0.0001$). Patients with AS and BAV had hyperlipidemia, CAD, COPD, increased weight, and obesity more often in comparison to patients without AS ($p < 0.01$). Higher blood pressure (both systolic and diastolic blood pressure) was registered in the TAV group. Patients without BAV but with AS had diagnoses of aortic regurgitation more often ($p < 0.0001$). Also, female patients without BAV but with AS had more common diagnoses of hyperlipidemia, CAD, and obesity ($p < 0.01$) (Tables 1 and 2).

The grid search results are presented in Table 3 with Random Forest showing the best overall performance.

In AS patients, diabetes mellitus, obesity, ulcers, COPD, and cholecystitis appeared as less important predictors (Figure 3). The area under the curve (AUC) of the receiver operating characteristic (ROC) was calculated to be 0.80. The corresponding ROC curve is depicted in Figure 4.

Figure 5 shows that gender changes its influence on the AS at 60. Women younger than 60 have higher chances of getting AS than men of the same age. This reverses after a cross point at 60 years old.

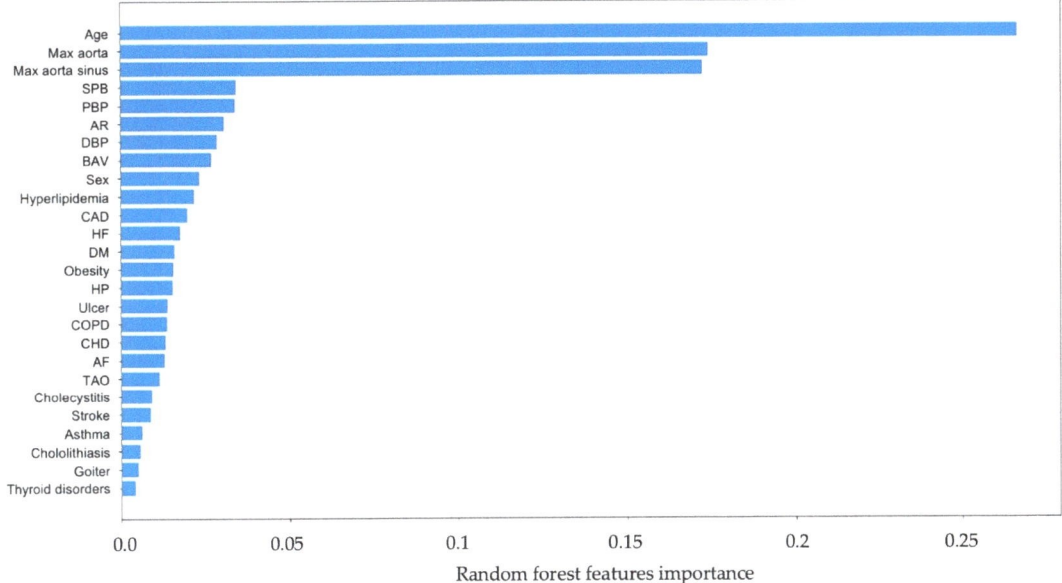

Figure 3. The results of the analysis of features important to the development of AS.

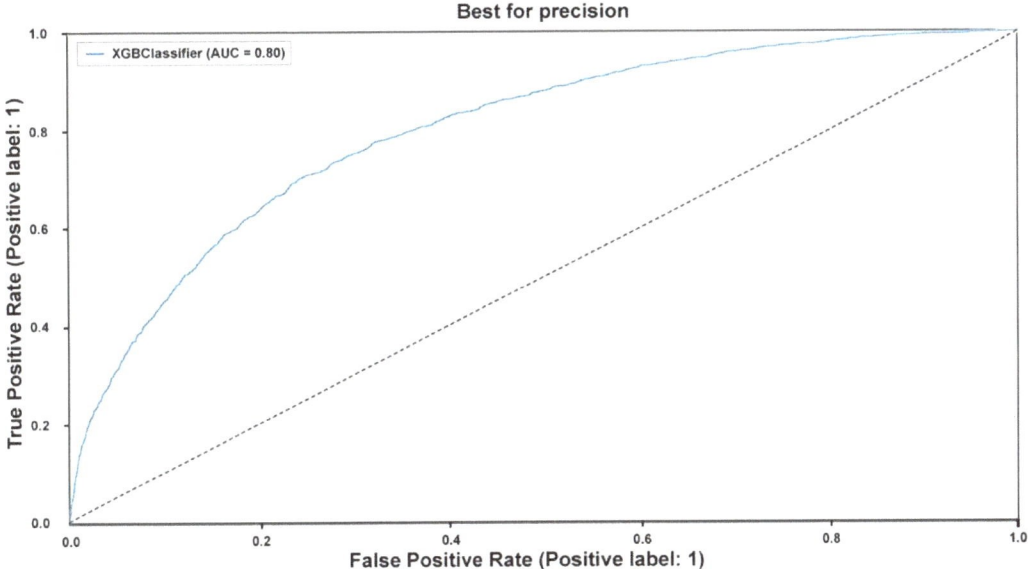

Figure 4. ROC for the classification model for the presence of AS.

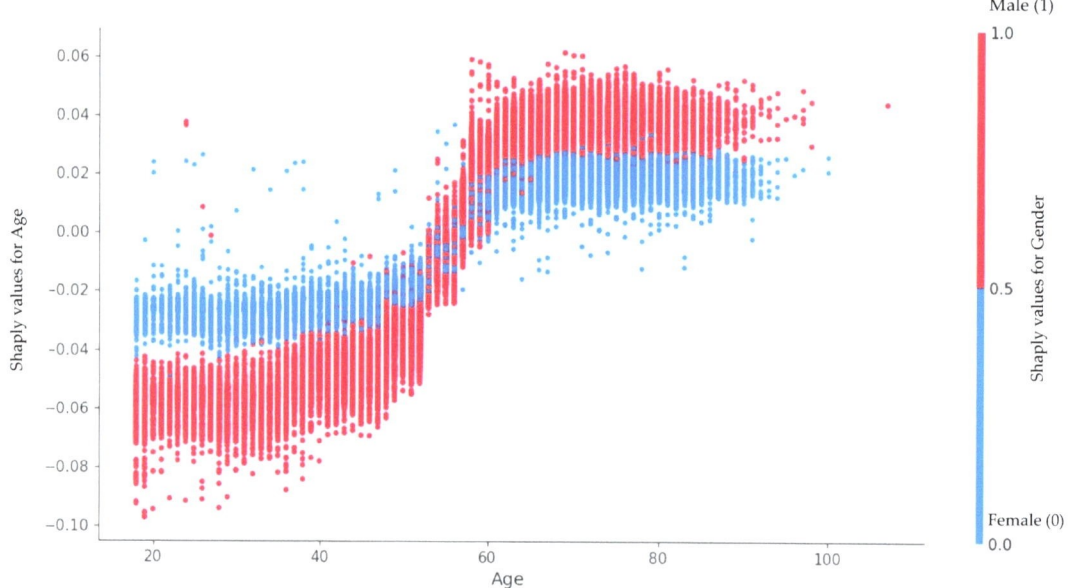

Figure 5. Influence of age in relation to gender on the formation of AS.

Figure 6 reveals an age-related difference in how Aortic Stenosis develops in men and women. It is clear that AS tends to appear at a younger age in women, while for men, it becomes significant at an older age. What is particularly interesting is that this shift occurs right around the age of 60, marking a turning point in the way age impacts AS formation in both genders.

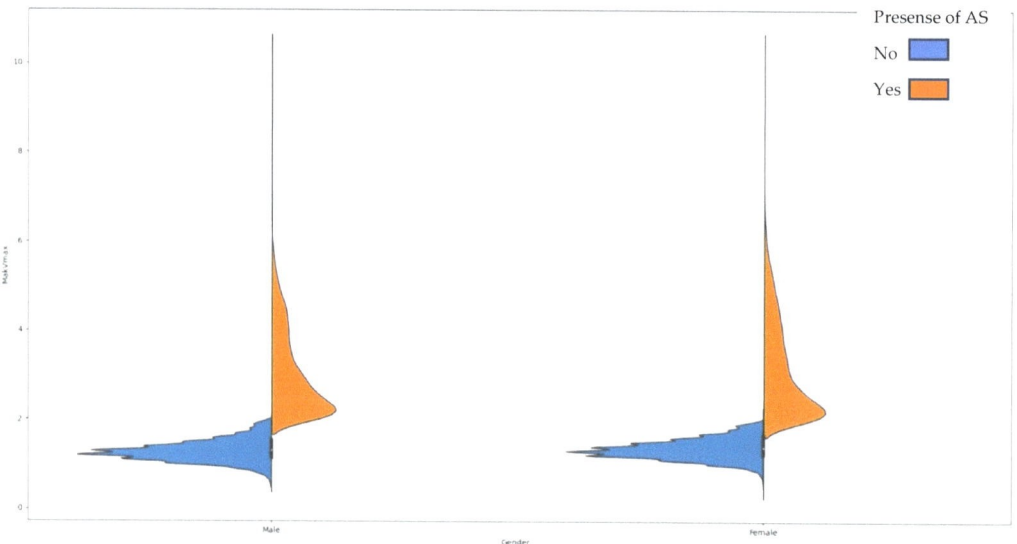

Figure 6. Distribution of the severity of AS depending on age and gender.

4. Discussion

The objective of our study was to conduct a comprehensive assessment of predictors and the prognostic significance of various factors on the prevalence of AS. As anticipated, age was identified as the primary factor associated with AS formation, aligning with previously reported findings. Additionally, aortic dilatation, hypertension, congenital heart defects, bicuspid aortic valve (BAV), and gender were also regarded as significant factors in our analysis.

4.1. Features Importance

We used a machine learning approach with Random Forest to determine the five most significant features for patients with AS. Two of them, namely older age and hypertension, are similar to the AscAD population in our previous publication [1]. The presence of BAV and dyslipidemia in AS patients was more significant than in AscAD patients. Moreover, important features of AS formation included an increase in the size of the ascending aorta. On the contrary, male sex was less important than in AscAD patients.

The best-performing model in the study was a Random Forest model. All feature importance measurements were made using this model. The application of Random Forest for this type of task can have the following benefits. Random Forest is less sensitive to outliers because it relies on the majority vote of multiple Decision Trees. Conventional statistical methods, like linear regression, can be heavily influenced by outliers. Random Forest provides a measure of feature importance, which can be valuable for variable selection and understanding which features contribute most to the prediction. Random Forest does not require assumptions about the distribution of the data, making them more versatile for analyzing various types of data, including both numerical and categorical variables. Random Forest can handle missing data without the need for imputation or specialized techniques.

In recent years, the differences in the course of AS depending on gender have been mentioned more and more often [11,26,27]. In our work, we also obtained significant differences between the groups, so in the following, we analyzed them separately.

Additionally, it was observed that women with AS (aortic stenosis) outnumbered men by more than 1000, despite the frequency of echoes being equal in both groups. Traditionally, AS has been believed to be 2–3 times more common in men [28]. However, recent research by Ana C. Iribarren et al. and Toyofuku Ms. et al. has challenged the notion of AS prevalence being dependent on gender. These studies showed that women with AS tend to be older and more common among patients over 75 years of age. We identified that gender changes its influence on AS at the age of 60. Women under 60 have a higher chance of developing AS than men of the same age. This changes after the crossover point at age 60 [12].

The hypothesis put forward was that women are more likely to seek medical care, including preventive care, which led to the assumption that women would have milder cases of AS. To investigate this hypothesis, additional analysis was conducted. Surprisingly, the results contradicted the hypothesis. The number of patients with mild and moderate stenosis did not differ significantly between men and women. However, a clear prevalence of women with severe stenosis was observed [29]. Ana C. Iribarren et al. demonstrated that due to physiological differences, severe AS is diagnosed later in women, resulting in delayed medical care-seeking [11,30]. The findings of this study suggested that men with severe AS may not seek medical care due to shorter life expectancy compared to women and other causes of death.

In our study, BAV was detected in 1544 patients, while TAV was detected in 83,316 patients. Patients with BAV were younger than TAV patients, as in the population. AS was diagnosed in 11,252 (13.26%) patients. AS was more frequent in the group of patients with BAV (58.77%) than in the group of TAV (12.4%).

The study included patients according to the ACC/AHA Guideline for the Management of Patients With Valvular Heart Disease [6], characterizing the presence of aortic stenosis (AS) when the aortic valve velocity was above 2 m/s. Out of 4432 patients, the median value of the ascending aorta diameter was 37 (33; 40) mm, and in the area of the sinuses of Valsalva, it was 36 (33; 39) mm. Aortic regurgitation of varying degrees of severity, predominantly mild, was observed in 17% of patients. Thus, we believe that normal aortic values and mild aortic regurgitation in the vast majority of included patients could not have influenced the aortic valve velocity measurements and the results of the analysis.

The findings from the study confirmed that age and bicuspid aortic valve are significant risk factors for AS. However, it was unexpected to discover that male sex was not among the top significant risk factors. Instead, aortic dilatation, aortic regurgitation (AR), and hypertension (HP) were found to be more prominent risk factors. This finding was consistent with the research of Shen M. et al. and Généreux P. et al., who demonstrated that the presence of AR, HP, and DM in patients with BAV and mild/moderate AS led to faster hemodynamic and anatomical progression of AS [31,32]. Upon analyzing clinical characteristics, it was observed that patients with BAV had AS recorded at an average age of around 50 years, whereas patients with Tricuspid Aortic Valve (TAV) were mostly diagnosed after the age of 60. Nevertheless, both groups of patients were notably older than those without AS, aligning with global data [33]. The study results showed that hypertension (HP) was present in 56% of patients with CHD:BAV and 71% of patients with TAV. According to the current analysis, the diameter of the ascending aorta was larger in the group of patients with AS and BAV compared to patients with normal valve morphology, which was in line with the results of other studies [34]. Additionally, aortic regurgitation (AR) was identified as a predictor of AS regardless of valve morphology, and varying degrees of AR was detected in one in four patients with BAV. Other studies have also reported the incidence of AR in patients with BAV to range from 13 to 65% [34,35]. Statistically, the median ejection fraction (EF) was within the normal range. However, it is worth mentioning that this median data were derived from a sample size of over 80,000 individuals. The quartiles indicate that EF levels below 55% were observed in all groups, and some patients were diagnosed with HF (heart failure) with preserved EF, considering the clinical context as well. To summarize, there were 35,192 patients diagnosed with HF, which is higher than the average frequency of occurrence. However, considering that it is a cardiology clinic with a specialized center for the treatment of HF, such a number of cases is expected [36].

Currently, echocardiography (ECHO) is recommended for patients with unexplained systolic noise on the aortic valve of the heart, second heart sound, a history of bicuspid aortic valve (BAV), or symptoms that could be attributed to AS [30]. However, this may not be sufficient considering the known information about delayed diagnosis of asymptomatic AS, including severe cases and instances of rapid AS progression, which are not uncommon [37]. In fact, AS has been accidentally diagnosed during examinations for other diseases, such as coronary artery disease (CAD), hypertension (HP), known valve heart disease (VHD), various arrhythmias, and other reasons. The optimal timing for follow-up examinations in cases of mild and moderate AS is still unknown [6], and the appropriate timing for the first ECHO in specific groups of asymptomatic individuals remains a question. We believe that men over the age of 60 should have a screening ECHO. These issues also pose logistical and economic challenges.

Therefore, it would be desirable to identify predictors of outcomes that enable risk assessment and more personalized management strategies.

Using the machine learning algorithm, we randomly identified significant features occurring in AS patients: age, HP, AR, AscAD, and BAV. Our findings could serve as additional indications for earlier observation and ECHO in specific patient groups. We think that it is necessary to perform ECHO more frequently to prevent the formation of AS and timely identify the indications for surgical treatment.

4.2. Study Limitations

The first limitation of this study is its retrospective nature and reliance on single-center data. Only one echocardiogram was analyzed in each case, so there was no assessment of AS progression within this population. The second limitation pertains to the referral nature of the center. The patients were not randomly selected from the general population but rather underwent examinations in a medical research center due to clinical indications and comorbidities. This fact may introduce some selection bias since this particular population of patients carries a higher risk.

In the confirmation of AS, we considered the mean aortic transvalvular pressure gradient and aortic valve area. However, it is important to note that these features were not present in all ECHO findings, which is a limitation of the current study. In addition to the ECHO features, we also used the ICD-10 codes I35.0, I35.1, I35.2, I35.8, and I35.9 for the confirmation of AS.

Machine learning analysis possesses inherent limitations associated with the availability and occupancy of the medical database. However, due to the utilization of a substantial dataset, these drawbacks are balanced out to a great extent.

Future research efforts should focus on early diagnostics and strategies to delay the progression of degenerative aortic valve disease by examining a more representative sample from the general population.

5. Conclusions

AS, one of the most common acquired valve heart diseases [2,3], was detected in 13.26% (11,252) of the population analyzed in this study. Therefore, the objective of our study was to identify significant factors and clinical conditions in patients with AS. Through the implementation of a machine learning algorithm, we randomly identified the following significant features in AS patients: age, hypertension (HP), aortic regurgitation (AR), ascending aortic dilatation (AscAD), and BAV. These findings highlight the main factors associated with AS. These findings could serve as additional indications for earlier observation and more frequent ECHO in specific patient groups for the earlier detection of developing AS.

Author Contributions: Conceptualization O.I.; methodology A.K.; validation V.U.; formal analysis M.G.; investigation G.K.; data curation O.M.; writing—original draft preparation O.I.; writing—review and editing M.B., E.S. and G.K.; visualization O.M.; supervision G.F.; project administration A.M. All authors have read and agreed to the published version of the manuscript.

Funding: This research was carried out with the financial support of the Ministry of Science and Higher Education of the Russian Federation (Agreement No. 075-15-2022-301).

Institutional Review Board Statement: The study was conducted in accordance with the Declaration of Helsinki, and approved by the Ethics Committee of Almazov National Research Center (protocol code 24 of 23.03.2020).

Informed Consent Statement: Informed consent was obtained from all subjects involved in the study.

Data Availability Statement: The datasets generated and analyzed for this study can be requested from the corresponding author.

Conflicts of Interest: The authors declare that the research was conducted in the absence of any commercial or financial relationships that could be construed as a potential conflict of interest.

References

1. Irtyuga, O.; Kopanitsa, G.; Kostareva, A.; Metsker, O.; Uspensky, V.; Mikhail, G.; Faggian, G.; Sefieva, G.; Derevitskii, I.; Malashicheva, A.; et al. Application of Machine Learning Methods to Analyze Occurrence and Clinical Features of Ascending Aortic Dilatation in Patients with and without Bicuspid Aortic Valve. *J. Pers. Med.* **2022**, *12*, 794. [CrossRef]
2. Nkomo, V.T.; Gardin, J.M.; Skelton, T.N.; Gottdiener, J.S.; Scott, C.G.; Enriquez-Sarano, M. Burden of valvular heart diseases: A population-based study. *Lancet* **2006**, *368*, 1005–1011. [CrossRef] [PubMed]

3. Vahanian, A.; Beyersdorf, F.; Praz, F.; Milojevic, M.; Baldus, S.; Bauersachs, J.; Capodanno, D.; Conradi, L.; De Bonis, M.; De Paulis, R.; et al. 2021 ESC/EACTS Guidelines for the management of valvular heart disease. *Eur. Heart J.* **2022**, *43*, 561–632. [CrossRef] [PubMed]
4. Yadgir, S.; Johnson, C.O.; Aboyans, V.; Adebayo, O.M.; Adedoyin, R.A.; Afarideh, M.; Alahdab, F.; Alashi, A.; Alipour, V.; Arabloo, J.; et al. Global, Regional, and National Burden of Calcific Aortic Valve and Degenerative Mitral Valve Diseases, 1990–2017. *Circulation* **2020**, *141*, 1670–1680. [CrossRef] [PubMed]
5. d'Arcy, J.L.; Coffey, S.; Loudon, M.A.; Kennedy, A.; Pearson-Stuttard, J.; Birks, J.; Frangou, E.; Farmer, A.J.; Mant, D.; Wilson, J.; et al. Large-scale community echocardiographic screening reveals a major burden of undiagnosed valvular heart disease in older people: The OxVALVE Population Cohort Study. *Eur. Heart J.* **2016**, *37*, 3515–3522. [CrossRef] [PubMed]
6. Writing Committee Members; Otto, C.M.; Nishimura, R.A.; Bonow, R.O.; Carabello, B.A.; Erwin, J.P., III; Gentile, F.; Jneid, H.; Krieger, E.V.; Mack, M.; et al. 2020 ACC/AHA Guideline for the Management of Patients With Valvular Heart Disease. *J. Am. Coll. Cardiol.* **2021**, *77*, e25–e197. [CrossRef]
7. Nightingale, A.K. Aortic sclerosis: Not an innocent murmur but a marker of increased cardiovascular risk. *Heart* **2005**, *91*, 1389–1393. [CrossRef]
8. Siu, S.C.; Silversides, C.K. Bicuspid Aortic Valve Disease. *J. Am. Coll. Cardiol.* **2010**, *55*, 2789–2800. [CrossRef]
9. Della Corte, A.; Bancone, C.; Quarto, C.; Dialetto, G.; Covino, F.E.; Scardone, M.; Caianiello, G.; Cotrufo, M. Predictors of ascending aortic dilatation with bicuspid aortic valve: A wide spectrum of disease expression. *Eur. J. Cardiothorac. Surg.* **2007**, *31*, 397–404. [CrossRef]
10. Agnese, V.; Pasta, S.; Michelena, H.I.; Minà, C.; Romano, G.M.; Carerj, S.; Zito, C.; Maalouf, J.F.; Foley, T.A.; Raffa, G.; et al. Patterns of ascending aortic dilatation and predictors of surgical replacement of the aorta: A comparison of bicuspid and tricuspid aortic valve patients over eight years of follow-up. *J. Mol. Cell Cardiol.* **2020**, *135*, 31–39; Erratum in *J. Mol. Cell. Cardiol.* **2020**, *143*, 159. [CrossRef]
11. Côté, N.; Clavel, M.A. Sex Differences in the Pathophysiology, Diagnosis, and Management of Aortic Stenosis. *Cardiol. Clin.* **2020**, *38*, 129–138. [CrossRef] [PubMed]
12. Iribarren, A.C.; AlBadri, A.; Wei, J.; Nelson, M.D.; Li, D.; Makkar, R.; Merz, C.N.B. Sex differences in aortic stenosis: Identification of knowledge gaps for sex-specific personalized medicine. *Am. Heart J. Plus Cardiol. Res. Pract.* **2022**, *21*, 100197. [CrossRef] [PubMed]
13. Tribouilloy, C.; Bohbot, Y.; Rusinaru, D.; Belkhir, K.; Diouf, M.; Altes, A.; Delpierre, Q.; Serbout, S.; Kubala, M.; Levy, F.; et al. Excess Mortality and Undertreatment of Women With Severe Aortic Stenosis. *J. Am. Heart Assoc.* **2021**, *10*, e018816. [CrossRef] [PubMed]
14. Banovic, M.; Putnik, S.; Penicka, M.; Doros, G.; Deja, M.A.; Kockova, R.; Kotrc, M.; Glaveckaite, S.; Gasparovic, H.; Pavlovic, N.; et al. Aortic Valve Replacement Versus Conservative Treatment in Asymptomatic Severe Aortic Stenosis: The AVATAR Trial. *Circulation* **2022**, *145*, 648–658. [CrossRef] [PubMed]
15. Rubin, J.; Aggarwal, S.R.; Swett, K.R.; Kirtane, A.J.; Kodali, S.K.; Nazif, T.M.; Pu, M.; Dadhania, R.; Kaplan, R.C.; Rodriguez, C.J. Burden of Valvular Heart Diseases in Hispanic/Latino Individuals in the United States: The Echocardiographic Study of Latinos. *Mayo Clin. Proc.* **2019**, *94*, 1488–1498. [CrossRef] [PubMed]
16. Kontogeorgos, S.; Thunström, E.; Basic, C.; Hansson, P.O.; Zhong, Y.; Ergatoudes, C.; Morales, D.; Mandalenakis, Z.; Rosengren, A.; Caidahl, K.; et al. Prevalence and risk factors of aortic stenosis and aortic sclerosis: A 21-year follow-up of middle-aged men. *Scand. Cardiovasc. J.* **2020**, *54*, 115–123. [CrossRef]
17. Rosenhek, R. Mild and moderate aortic stenosis Natural history and risk stratification by echocardiography. *Eur. Heart J.* **2004**, *25*, 199–205. [CrossRef]
18. Kopanitsa, G. Integration of Hospital Information and Clinical Decision Support Systems to Enable the Reuse of Electronic Health Record Data. *Methods Inf. Med.* **2017**, *56*, 238–247. [CrossRef]
19. Lang, R.M.; Badano, L.P.; Mor-Avi, V.; Afilalo, J.; Armstrong, A.; Ernande, L.; Flachskampf, F.A.; Foster, E.; Goldstein, S.A.; Kuznetsova, T.; et al. Recommendations for Cardiac Chamber Quantification by Echocardiography in Adults: An Update from the American Society of Echocardiography and the European Association of Cardiovascular Imaging. *J. Am. Soc. Echocardiogr.* **2015**, *28*, 1–39.e14. [CrossRef]
20. Pedregosa, F.; Varoquaux, G.; Gramfort, A.; Michel, V.; Thirion, B.; Grisel, O.; Blondel, M.; Müller, A.; Nothman, J.; Louppe, G.; et al. Scikit-learn: Machine Learning in Python. *J. Mach. Learn. Res.* **2011**, *12*, 2825–2830.
21. Prokhorenkova, L.; Gusev, G.; Vorobev, A.; Dorogush, A.V.; Gulin, A. CatBoost: Unbiased boosting with categorical features. In *Advances in Neural Information Processing Systems, Proceedings of the 32nd International Conference on Neural Information Processing Systems, Montréal, QC, Canada, 3–8 December 2017*; Curran Associates, Inc.: Red Hook, NY, USA, 2018; pp. 6639–6640.
22. Waskom, M. Seaborn: Statistical data visualization. *J. Open Source Softw.* **2021**, *6*, 3021. [CrossRef]
23. Hunter, J.D. Matplotlib: A 2D Graphics Environment. *Comput. Sci. Eng.* **2007**, *9*, 90–95. [CrossRef]
24. Chawla, N.V.; Bowyer, K.W.; Hall, L.O.; Kegelmeyer, W.P. SMOTE: Synthetic Minority Over-sampling Technique. *J. Artif. Intell. Res.* **2002**, *16*, 321–357. [CrossRef]
25. Lundberg, S.M.; Lee, S.I. A unified approach to interpreting model predictions. In *Advances in Neural Information Processing Systems, Proceedings of the 31st Annual Conference on Neural Information Processing Systems (NIPS 2017), Long Beach, CA, USA, 4–9 December 2017*; Curran Associates, Inc.: Red Hook, NY, USA, 2017; pp. 4768–4777.

26. Stewart, S.; Chan, Y.-K.; Playford, D.; Strange, G.A. Incident aortic stenosis in 49 449 men and 42 229 women investigated with routine echocardiography. *Heart* **2022**, *108*, 875–881. [CrossRef]
27. Büttner, P.; Feistner, L.; Lurz, P.; Thiele, H.; Hutcheson, J.D.; Schlotter, F. Dissecting Calcific Aortic Valve Disease—The Role, Etiology, and Drivers of Valvular Fibrosis. *Front. Cardiovasc. Med.* **2021**, *8*, 660797. [CrossRef] [PubMed]
28. Kong, W.K.; Regeer, M.V.; Ng, A.C.; McCormack, L.; Poh, K.K.; Yeo, T.C.; Shanks, M.; Parent, S.; Enache, R.; Popescu, B.A.; et al. Sex Differences in Phenotypes of Bicuspid Aortic Valve and Aortopathy: Insights From a Large Multicenter, International Registry. *Circ. Cardiovasc. Imaging* **2017**, *10*, e005155. [CrossRef]
29. Palacios-Fernandez, S.; Salcedo, M.; Belinchon-Romero, I.; Gonzalez-Alcaide, G.; Ramos-Rincón, J.M. Epidemiological and Clinical Features in Very Old Men and Women (≥80 Years) Hospitalized with Aortic Stenosis in Spain, 2016–2019: Results from the Spanish Hospital Discharge Database. *J. Clin. Med.* **2022**, *11*, 5588. [CrossRef]
30. Toyofuku, M.; Taniguchi, T.; Morimoto, T.; Yamaji, K.; Furukawa, Y.; Takahashi, K.; Tamura, T.; Shiomi, H.; Ando, K.; Kanamori, N.; et al. Sex Differences in Severe Aortic Stenosis-Clinical Presentation and Mortality. *Circ. J.* **2017**, *81*, 1213–1221. [CrossRef]
31. Evangelista, A. Aortic Stenosis in Bicuspid and Tricuspid Valves: A Different Spectrum of the Disease With Clinical Implications. *JACC Cardiovasc. Imaging* **2021**, *14*, 1127–1129. [CrossRef] [PubMed]
32. Généreux, P.; Pibarot, P.; Redfors, B.; Mack, M.J.; Makkar, R.R.; Jaber, W.A.; Svensson, L.G.; Kapadia, S.; Tuzcu, E.M.; Thourani, V.H.; et al. Staging classification of aortic stenosis based on the extent of cardiac damage. *Eur. Heart J.* **2017**, *38*, 3351–3358. [CrossRef]
33. Shen, M.; Tastet, L.; Capoulade, R.; Arsenault, M.; Bedard, E.; Clavel, M.A.; Pibarot, P. Effect of bicuspid aortic valve phenotype on progression of aortic stenosis. *Eur. Heart J. Cardiovasc. Imaging* **2020**, *21*, 727–734. [CrossRef] [PubMed]
34. Masri, A.; Svensson, L.G.; Griffin, B.P.; Desai, M.Y. Contemporary natural history of bicuspid aortic valve disease: A systematic review. *Heart* **2017**, *103*, 1323–1330. [CrossRef]
35. Butcher, S.C.; Fortuni, F.; Kong, W.; Vollema, E.M.; Prevedello, F.; Perry, R.; Ng, A.C.T.; Poh, K.K.; Almeida, A.G.; González-Gómez, A.; et al. Prognostic implications of left atrial dilation in aortic regurgitation due to bicuspid aortic valve. *Heart* **2022**, *108*, 137–144. [CrossRef] [PubMed]
36. Nagamine, T.; Gillette, B.; Pakhomov, A.; Kahoun, J.; Mayer, H.; Burghaus, R.; Lippert, J.; Saxena, M. Multiscale classification of heart failure phenotypes by unsupervised clustering of unstructured electronic medical record data. *Sci. Rep.* **2020**, *10*, 21340. [CrossRef]
37. Harris, A.W.; Pibarot, P.; Otto, C.M. Aortic Stenosis. *Cardiol. Clin.* **2020**, *38*, 55–63. [CrossRef] [PubMed]

Disclaimer/Publisher's Note: The statements, opinions and data contained in all publications are solely those of the individual author(s) and contributor(s) and not of MDPI and/or the editor(s). MDPI and/or the editor(s) disclaim responsibility for any injury to people or property resulting from any ideas, methods, instructions or products referred to in the content.

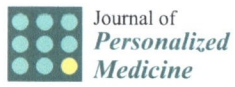

Review

Patient-Generated Health Data (PGHD): Understanding, Requirements, Challenges, and Existing Techniques for Data Security and Privacy

Pankaj Khatiwada [1,*], Bian Yang [1], Jia-Chun Lin [1] and Bernd Blobel [2]

1. Department of Information Security and Communication Technology (IIK), Norwegian University of Science and Technology (NTNU), 7034 Trondheim, Norway; bian.yang@ntnu.no (B.Y.); jia-chun.lin@ntnu.no (J.-C.L.)
2. Medical Faculty, University of Regensburg, 93053 Regensburg, Germany; bernd.blobel@klinik.uni-regensburg.de
* Correspondence: pankaj.khatiwada@ntnu.no

Citation: Khatiwada, P.; Yang, B.; Lin, J.-C.; Blobel, B. Patient-Generated Health Data (PGHD): Understanding, Requirements, Challenges, and Existing Techniques for Data Security and Privacy. *J. Pers. Med.* **2024**, *14*, 282.
https://doi.org/10.3390/jpm14030282

Academic Editor: Norman R. Williams

Received: 30 January 2024
Revised: 21 February 2024
Accepted: 28 February 2024
Published: 3 March 2024

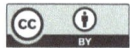

Copyright: © 2024 by the authors. Licensee MDPI, Basel, Switzerland. This article is an open access article distributed under the terms and conditions of the Creative Commons Attribution (CC BY) license (https://creativecommons.org/licenses/by/4.0/).

Abstract: The evolution of Patient-Generated Health Data (PGHD) represents a major shift in healthcare, fueled by technological progress. The advent of PGHD, with technologies such as wearable devices and home monitoring systems, extends data collection beyond clinical environments, enabling continuous monitoring and patient engagement in their health management. Despite the growing prevalence of PGHD, there is a lack of clear understanding among stakeholders about its meaning, along with concerns about data security, privacy, and accuracy. This article aims to thoroughly review and clarify PGHD by examining its origins, types, technological foundations, and the challenges it faces, especially in terms of privacy and security regulations. The review emphasizes the role of PGHD in transforming healthcare through patient-centric approaches, their understanding, and personalized care, while also exploring emerging technologies and addressing data privacy and security issues, offering a comprehensive perspective on the current state and future directions of PGHD. The methodology employed for this review followed the Preferred Reporting Items for Systematic Reviews and Meta-Analyses (PRISMA) guidelines and Rayyan, AI-Powered Tool for Systematic Literature Reviews. This approach ensures a systematic and comprehensive coverage of the available literature on PGHD, focusing on the various aspects outlined in the objective. The review encompassed 36 peer-reviewed articles from various esteemed publishers and databases, reflecting a diverse range of methodologies, including interviews, regular articles, review articles, and empirical studies to address three RQs exploratory, impact assessment, and solution-oriented questions related to PGHD. Additionally, to address the future-oriented fourth RQ for PGHD not covered in the above review, we have incorporated existing domain knowledge articles. This inclusion aims to provide answers encompassing both basic and advanced security measures for PGHD, thereby enhancing the depth and scope of our analysis.

Keywords: PGHD; health data; security; privacy; patient-generated health data

1. Introduction

This article is a completely revised and strongly extended version of our contribution to the pHealth 2022 Conference in Oslo [1]. In the predigital era, patient health data was mostly gathered during face-to-face consultation and manually recorded on paper. These records, mostly consisting of clinical observations, lab test data, physician notes, and imaging tests, were then archived as physical documents within healthcare facilities. The process had its shortcomings; not only was retrieving and disseminating these data cumbersome, but transferring such records between providers often meant mailing or faxing them, leading to potential delays or loss of vital information and security concerns. However, with technological advances in healthcare, there was a notable paradigm shift towards Electronic Health Records (EHRs) [2]. These digital systems streamlined the processes of storing, accessing, and sharing patient data. Concurrently, the healthcare sector has begun to employ standardized instruments and devices, allowing monitoring of specific health domains such as sleep or cardiac activity. This development is another key step towards the emergence of Patient-Generated Health Data (PGHD) [3]. With the advent of the digital era, patients have gained unprecedented access to an abundance of health information, leading to an increasing need for tools and platforms that enable monitoring of personal health metrics. The demand for better healthcare outcomes has been addressed by the advent of wearable devices and home-monitoring systems, which have provided valuable information outside the traditional boundaries of clinical settings [4]. Furthermore, the growing prevalence of digital platforms has improved the ease with which patients can record their daily experiences, including the onset of symptoms and the use of medications. The result of this is that doctors now have a more complete understanding of the health trajectory of their patients [5]. This transition has ramifications that extend beyond the scope of ordinary data collection. PGHD provides a holistic snapshot of a patient's health, highlighting details that are sometimes missed during occasional clinical visits. The continuous nature of this data collection ensures real-time monitoring, facilitating prompt interventions should anomalies arise. In a more significant manner, the utilization of PGHD has effectively encouraged patients to assume a major role in shaping their health narratives, thus promoting increased participation and compliance with medical treatment plans [6]. Fundamentally, the shift from physical paper records to digital systems and the development of PGHD represent an enormous transformation. It shifted the focus from provider-centric periodic care to ongoing patient-driven support. Due to this transformation, preventive medicine, individualized treatment, and patient participation are now front and center in the healthcare system [7].

PGHD can be understood and expressed in different ways by researchers, healthcare professionals, and industry stakeholders. Figure 1 presents a word cloud that illustrates the various terms associated with Patient-Generated Health Data (PGHD). These may encompass, but are not limited to: Patient-Generated Health Data (PGHD), Patient-Reported Outcome Measures (PROMs), Patient-Reported Outcomes (PROs), Self-Reported Health Data, Patient-Reported Data (PRD), Self-Monitored Health Data, Self-Recorded Health Data, Patient-Entered Health Data, Patient-Captured Health Data, Patient-Generated Data (PGD), Patient-Provided Health Data, Patient-Sourced Health Data, Patient Contributed Health Data, Patient-Recorded Information, Patient Derived Health Data, Personal Health Record (PHR), Electronic Personal Health Record (e-PHR), Personal Health Information (PHI), Health Diary, Health Journal, Health Log, Self-Tracking Data, Health Self-Monitoring, Digital Health Records (DHR), Personal Medical History, User-Generated Health Data (UGH Data), Self-Reported Medical Information, Self-Generated Health Information, Self-Documented Health Data, Self-Entered Health Data, Individual-Generated Health Data, Consumer Provided Health Data, User-Entered Health Information, Personal Health Data (PHD). Throughout this article, we consistently use the term PGHD (Patient-Generated Health Data) to refer to health data produced by patients. Whenever the term health data, patient data, or generated data appears, it should be understood as referring specifically to PGHD.

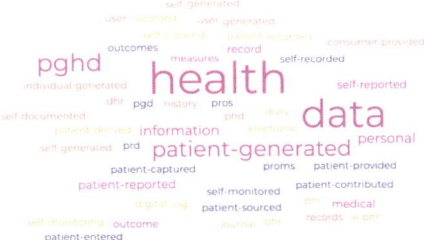

Figure 1. PGHD Related Word Cloud.

The article is structured into seven sections. Section 2 provides the main objective of the article. Here, we will introduce various research questions (RQs), mainly organized into four categories, Exploratory, Impact Assessment, Solution-Oriented, and Future-Oriented RQs. These questions will be discussed in detail in the subsequent section of the article. In Section 3, we will shift our focus to a concise overview of PGHD, covering its definition and types. This section also explores the growth of PGHD driven by technological advances, identifies its potential stakeholders, and discusses the challenges associated with it. Additionally, it examines the applications of PGHD, its global adoption trends, and anticipates its future developments. Section 4 outlines the methodology used for conducting the review, addressing the research questions (RQs) from three perspectives: Exploratory, Impact Assessment, and Solution-Oriented RQs. Section 5 is dedicated to addressing the Research Questions (RQs) highlighted in Section 3, as identified from the review article in Section 4. This section also tackles Future-Oriented RQs, which, although not part of the review, but answered separately and independently. In Section 6, we discuss the findings and results from Section 5, followed by the final conclusions presented in Section 7.

2. Objectives

The primary purpose of the article is to conduct a review and comprehensively explore and synthesize the current understanding of PGHD in terms of its origin, types, technological underpinnings, stakeholders involved, challenges (with a keen focus on privacy, security, and regulatory challenges), benefits for personalized care, global perspectives, and future prospects. The review seeks to elucidate the significance of PGHD in revolutionizing healthcare delivery, emphasizing its role in improving patient-centric approaches, enabling personalized interventions, and identifying emerging technologies and practices. A section of this article will also look at the privacy and security concerns associated with PGHD, highlighting the evolving regulatory landscape in different areas and its implications on the broader adoption and utilization of PGHD. This review would provide stakeholders from healthcare providers to technology developers and policymakers with a holistic view of the current landscape of PGHD, its implications, and its potential trajectory in the foreseeable future.

PGHD is where technology, healthcare and the power of patients come together. As we try to understand all of its different parts, some key questions arise. These questions help guide our research and what we want to learn from this review. Grouped by their type and what they aim to find, these questions help point us to the important information we need. We categorized them into four sections as follows:

(a) Exploratory Questions: (PGHD Understanding and Patient Perspective)
- RQE1: What are the primary sources of PGHD, and for what purpose are they being utilized in healthcare settings?
- RQE2: How do patients perceive the collection and utilization of their generated PGHD?

(b) Impact Assessment Questions:
- RQI1: What are the potential ramifications of data breaches pertaining to patient-generated health data on patient trust and healthcare outcomes?
- RQI2: What impact does the incorporation of patients and their PGHD have on healthcare decision-making

(c) Solution-Oriented Questions:
- RQS1: What are the recommended strategies for improving the security and privacy of PGHD?
- RQS2: In what ways may healthcare providers and technology developers engage in collaborative efforts to achieve an ideal equilibrium between the value of PGHD and the safeguarding of data privacy and security?

(d) Future-Oriented Questions:

- RQF1: How can PGHD prepare for the upcoming security and privacy problems brought on by the widespread adoption of AI and ML in healthcare?
- RQF2: How may the next decade's development of wearable technology and Internet of Medical Things devices affect the current state of PGHD security and privacy concerns?

Our approach will be to address the research questions from parts (a) Exploratory Questions (RQE1, RQE2), (b) Impact Assessment Questions (RQI1, RQI2), and (c) Solution-Oriented Questions (RQS1, RQS2) by leveraging the insights from the review conducted in Section 4. Regarding part (d) Future-oriented questions (RQF1, RQF2), due to the lack of extensive literature currently discussing these topics in PGHD, we will aim to provide answers by aligning them with the security of the Internet of Medical Things (IoMT) data and the security of health data, which are directly relatable to PGHD.

3. PGHD Understanding

This section focuses on providing the reader with a comprehensive overview of PGHD before discussing the RQs. It will differentiate PGHD from clinical data, discuss its various types, and explore its increasing prevalence. Additionally, it will identify key stakeholders involved, examine the challenges faced, and describe how PGHD is being used. The section will also dive into the adoption processes of PGHD and its ongoing advancements. As stated in the Introduction Section, PGHD refers to health-related data created, recorded, or gathered by or from patients (or family members or other caregivers) to address a health concern. This can include biometric data, symptoms, lifestyle choices, and other health-related information. PGHD is increasingly recognized for its potential to improve care and research, particularly in chronic disease management, mental health, and preventive care [2–20] [8]. Clinical data, on the other hand, refers to information collected by healthcare professionals in the course of providing care. This includes data from physical examinations, laboratory tests, imaging studies, and other diagnostic tools. Clinical data are typically considered more reliable because they are collected by professionals using standardized methods and equipment [9]. Below Table 1 provides the difference between the PGHD and clinical data:

Table 1. Difference between the Patient-Generated Health Data (PGHD) and Clinical data.

Factor	PGHD	Clinical Data
Source of Data	Generated by patients or caregivers using patients devices, apps, or self-reporting.	collected by healthcare professionals during visits, hospital stays, or by diagnostic procedures.
Accuracy and Reliability	Can vary; depends on the accuracy of the device and the patient's ability to accurately record data.	Generally high, collected through validated methods and equipment.
Scope and Context	Provides a broader view of the patient's health in daily life, including lifestyle and environmental factors.	Focuses on health status during clinical assessments; may miss daily life nuances.
Usage in Healthcare	Used for remote monitoring, chronic disease management, and patient participation in care.	Fundamental for diagnosis, treatment planning, and disease monitoring.
Integration Challenges	Integration with clinical workflows and EHRs can be challenging due to data variability.	Usually well-integrated, though interoperability between different EHR systems can be an issue.
Patient Engagement	Encourages active patient participation and self-management.	Typically, more passive, with healthcare professionals driving the process.

3.1. PGHD Type

As we already know, PGHD refers to health-related data created, recorded, or collected by or from patients (or family members or other caregivers) to help address a health concern. These data are often outside the traditional clinical setting and provide insights that can contribute to a more comprehensive view of a patient's health. The Figure 2 illustrates the different types of PGHD, with brief descriptions provided below.

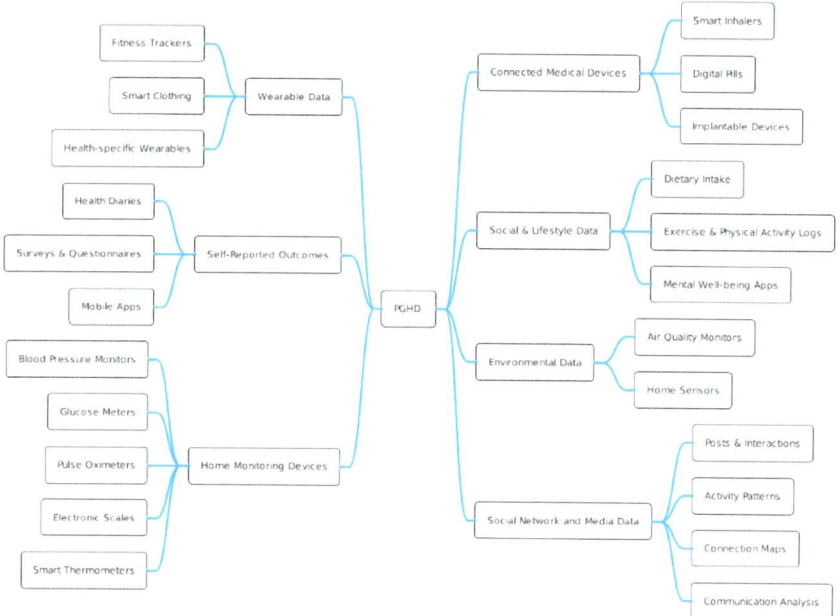

Figure 2. PGHD Types.

3.1.1. Wearable Data

- Fitness Trackers: Devices such as Fitbit, Garmin, or Apple Watch collect data on steps taken, heart rate, sleep patterns, calories burned, etc. [10].
- Health-specific Wearables: Devices that monitor specific health metrics, such as continuous glucose monitors for people with diabetes.
- Smart Clothing: Includes garments with embedded sensors that can monitor physiological markers such as heart rate, breathing rate, and muscle activity [11].

3.1.2. Self-Reported Outcomes [12]

- Health Diaries: Patients may keep a daily or weekly record of symptoms, diet, medication intake, and other health-related factors.
- Surveys & Questionnaires: Tools such as the Patient-Reported Outcomes Measurement Information System (PROMIS) offer standardized measures of physical, mental, and social well-being.
- Mobile Apps: Many health and wellness apps allow users to input data related to mood, nutrition, menstrual cycles, pain levels, etc.

3.1.3. Home Monitoring Devices [13]

- Blood Pressure Monitors: Devices that allow patients with hypertension or other conditions to monitor their blood pressure at home.
- Glucose Meters: Used by diabetics to regularly check blood sugar levels.
- Pulse Oximeters: Measure blood oxygen levels, which can be crucial for patients with respiratory conditions.
- Electronic Scales: For monitoring weight, especially useful for patients with heart failure or those undergoing certain treatments.
- Smart Thermometers: Digital devices that track and record temperature readings, often connecting to smartphone apps.

3.1.4. Connected Medical Devices [14]

- Smart Inhalers: Help patients with asthma or COPD track medication use and offer reminders.
- Digital Pills: Pills embedded with edible sensors that send signals to external devices upon ingestion, ensuring medication adherence.
- Implantable Devices: Some devices, such as certain cardiac monitors, can transmit data to external receivers.

3.1.5. Social & Lifestyle Data [15]

- Dietary Intake: Through apps or platforms where users input their daily meals and snacks.
- Exercise & Physical Activity Logs: Outside of wearables, users might manually record workouts or sports activities.
- Mental Well-being Apps: Tools like mood trackers or meditation apps can provide insight into mental health and stress levels.

3.1.6. Environmental Data [16]

- Air Quality Monitors: Devices that measure air quality within or outside the home, which can be valuable for patients with allergies or respiratory conditions.
- Home Sensors: Detect things like mold, pollen, or other environmental factors that might affect health.

3.1.7. Social Network and Media Data [17]

- Posts & Interactions: Analysis of posts, likes, comments, and shares on platforms like Facebook, Twitter, or Instagram can reveal emotional well-being, social support structures, and potential levels of stress or anxiety.
- Activity patterns: The time spent on social media platforms and the timing of activity can indicate sleep patterns and potentially correlate with mental health states.
- Connection Maps: Examination of the size and strength of a user's social network can provide insights into social isolation or social well-being.
- Communication Analysis: Studying the content and frequency of messages or posts exchanged can help gauge the quality of social interactions and its impact on health.

While PGHD offers rich insights and complements clinical data, integrating and interpreting these data in clinical practice presents challenges. Healthcare providers must ensure the accuracy and relevance of the data, and systems must be in place to protect patient privacy and data security. However, as technology and interoperability improve, PGHD will increasingly play a pivotal role in personalized healthcare and proactive patient management.

3.2. PGHD Technological Rise

Technological advancements, particularly in the realms of mobile apps and wearable devices, have significantly facilitated the rise and importance of Patient-Generated Health Data (PGHD). Here is how these technological breakthroughs have influenced the trajectory of PGHD as shown in Figure 3.

3.2.1. Ubiquity of Smartphones [18]

- Easy Data Entry: The widespread use of smartphones means that a large number of people have a powerful computer in their pocket, enabling them to easily input and track health data through specialized apps.
- Integration with Health Platforms: Operating systems like Apple's iOS have integrated health platforms (e.g., Apple Health) that aggregate data from various health and fitness apps, creating a comprehensive health profile.

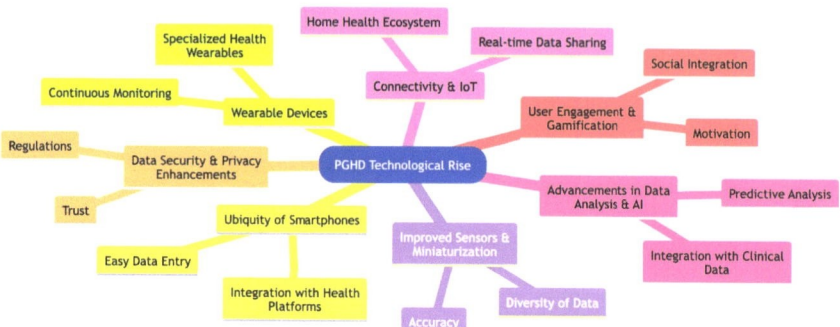

Figure 3. PGHD Technological Rise.

3.2.2. Wearable Devices [10,11]

- Continuous Monitoring: Wearable devices such as smartwatches and fitness trackers monitor users' health metrics continuously, capturing data such as heart rate, sleep patterns, and activity levels in real-time.
- Specialized Health Wearables: Beyond general fitness trackers, there are wearables tailored for specific conditions, such as continuous glucose monitors for diabetics, which offer real-time insights and alerts.

3.2.3. Improved Sensors & Miniaturization [19]

- Accuracy: Advancements in sensor technology mean that wearables and mobile devices can capture health data with increased accuracy, making the data more clinically relevant.
- Diversity of Data: From tracking UV exposure to measuring electrodermal activity (a potential stress indicator), technological progress has enabled a wider range of health metrics to be monitored.

3.2.4. Connectivity & IoT (Internet of Things) [20]

- Real-Time Data Sharing: Devices can instantly upload data to the cloud, allowing real-time sharing with healthcare providers or integration with electronic health records (EHRs).
- Home Health Ecosystem: Smart home devices, such as connected scales or blood pressure monitors, can now seamlessly integrate with other health devices and platforms.

3.2.5. Advancements in Data Analysis & AI [21]

- Predictive Analysis: With a large amount of PGHD being generated, advanced analytics and AI can identify patterns, predict potential health problems, and offer personalized health recommendations.
- Integration with Clinical Data: Advanced platforms can now integrate PGHD with traditional clinical data, offering healthcare providers a more holistic view of a patient's health.

3.2.6. User Engagement & Gamification [22]

- Motivation: Many health apps and wearables incorporate gamification elements, motivating users to achieve health goals, complete challenges, or maintain streaks, thus encouraging consistent data generation.
- Social Integration: Sharing achievements, joining fitness groups, or participating in community challenges can boost engagement and data generation.

3.2.7. Data Security & Privacy Enhancements [23]

- Trust: As technology companies prioritize data security and privacy, users are more inclined to share and store their health data.
- Regulations: Advances in technology have been complemented by regulations, ensuring that PGHD is handled with the same care and security as traditional health data.

In conclusion, the confluence of advances in mobile technology, wearables, connectivity, and data analysis has transformed PGHD from a niche concept to a central player in modern healthcare. The real-time, continuous, and diverse nature of the data captured has enormous potential to revolutionize patient care, drive proactive health management, and contribute to personalized medicine.

3.3. PGHD Stakeholders

PGHD has value for a wide range of stakeholders [7,24,25] within the healthcare ecosystem. Figure 4 represents a breakdown of some of the primary stakeholders and how they are impacted by or use PGHD.

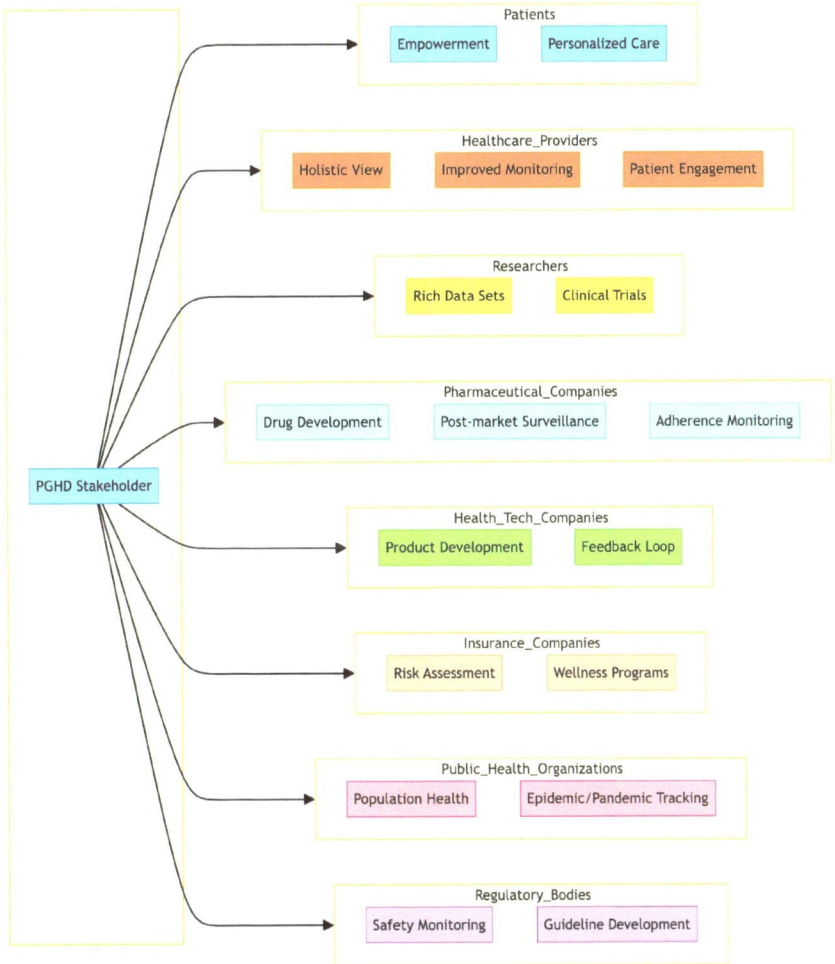

Figure 4. PGHD Stakeholders.

3.3.1. Patients

- Empowerment: PGHD allows patients to play a more active role in their health management, giving them insight into their health trends and patterns.
- Personalized care: With a more comprehensive data profile, patients can receive more personalized health advice and treatments.

3.3.2. Healthcare Providers

- Holistic View: PGHD complements clinical data, providing a more comprehensive picture of the health of the patient, including lifestyle and environmental factors.
- Improved monitoring: Especially for chronic conditions, PGHD enables providers to track patient health status in real time, allowing timely interventions.
- Patient Engagement: PGHD tools can foster better communication between patients and providers, improving adherence to care plans.

3.3.3. Researchers

- Rich Data Sets: With vast amounts of PGHD generated, researchers have access to diverse real-world data that can provide insight into health trends, disease patterns, and treatment outcomes.
- Clinical Trials: PGHD can be used to monitor participants in clinical trials, providing real-time data and potentially reducing costs.

3.3.4. Pharmaceutical Companies

- Drug Development: PGHD can provide information on how patients respond to medications in real-world settings, which can inform drug development and optimization.
- Post-market surveillance: After a drug is released, PGHD can help track its efficacy and any potential side effects in the broader population.
- Adherence Monitoring: Companies can understand how often patients take their medications and the factors that influence adherence.

3.3.5. Health Tech Companies

- Product Development: Companies can use PGHD to develop new devices, apps, and platforms tailored to user health needs.
- Feedback Loop: Continuous input from PGHD allows tech companies to refine and optimize their health tech offerings.

3.3.6. Insurance Companies

- Risk Assessment: PGHD can provide information on an individual's health habits, potentially influencing underwriting and policy pricing.
- Wellness Programs: Many insurers now offer wellness programs that leverage PGHD to incentivize healthy behaviors, potentially reducing claims in the long run.

3.3.7. Public Health Organizations

- Population Health: PGHD can offer information on health trends at the community or population level, helping to plan health campaigns and allocate resources.
- Epidemic/Pandemic Tracking: In situations such as the COVID-19 pandemic, PGHD from wearables or symptom-tracking apps can assist in early detection and monitoring of disease spread.

3.3.8. Regulatory Bodies

- Safety Monitoring: PGHD can be a source of data to monitor the safety and efficacy of medical devices or treatments in real world settings.
- Guideline development: Real-world data from PGHD can inform the development of health guidelines and standards.

As healthcare becomes more patient-centric and data-driven, the relevance of PGHD is set to grow. Each stakeholder in the healthcare ecosystem can harness the potential of PGHD to improve outcomes, optimize resources, and drive innovation. However, collaboration among these stakeholders is crucial to ensure that PGHD is used effectively and ethically.

3.4. PGHD Challenges

Certainly, while data security and privacy are the main concerns of PGHD, there are several other challenges associated with its use and implementation, as shown in Figure 5.

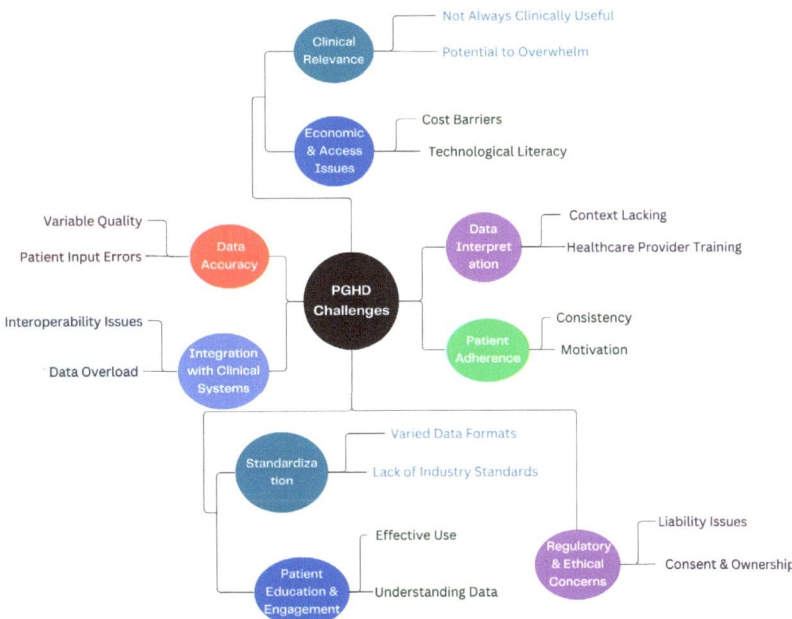

Figure 5. PGHD Challenges.

3.4.1. Data Accuracy [26]

- Variable Quality: Devices and apps vary in their accuracy and reliability. For instance, one fitness tracker might measure steps or heart rate differently from another.
- Patient Input Errors: Manual data entries by patients, such as symptom logs or dietary intakes, can be prone to inaccuracies or inconsistencies.

3.4.2. Integration with Clinical Systems [27]

- Interoperability Issues: Clinical systems like EHRs might not easily integrate with PGHD sources, leading to fragmented data.
- Data Overload: The sheer volume of PGHD can be overwhelming. Healthcare providers need efficient systems to sift through and extract relevant insights without being inundated.

3.4.3. Patient Adherence [28]

- Consistency: Patients might not consistently use wearables or input data into health apps, medication management leading to gaps in data.
- Motivation: Maintaining motivation to regularly input data or use health-tracking tools can wane over time, especially if patients do not see immediate benefits.

3.4.4. Data Interpretation [29]

- Context Lacking: Without proper context, PGHD can be misleading. For example, a spike in heart rate might be due to exercise, stress, or a health anomaly.
- Healthcare Provider Training: Not all providers may be trained or feel comfortable interpreting PGHD, especially given its diverse sources.

3.4.5. Standardization [29]

- Varied Data Formats: Data from different devices or apps might come in a variety of formats, making aggregation and analysis challenging.
- Lack of Industry Standards: Without universally accepted standards for the collection and interpretation of PGHD, its clinical utility can be limited.

3.4.6. Patient Education & Engagement [30]

- Effective Use: Patients need to be educated on how to effectively use devices or apps to ensure the data collected is of value.
- Understanding Data: Patients may misinterpret their data, leading to unnecessary anxiety or incorrect self-diagnosis.

3.4.7. Clinical Relevance

- Not Always Clinically Useful: Although PGHD can offer many insights, not all of it may be relevant for clinical decisions [31].
- Potential to Overwhelm: Excessive data can lead to "alert fatigue", in which healthcare providers become desensitized to numerous alerts or notifications, potentially overlooking important ones [32].

3.4.8. Economic & Access Issues [33]

- Cost Barriers: Not all patients can afford smart wearables or devices, potentially leading to disparities in who can benefit from PGHD.
- Technological literacy: Not everyone is tech-savvy, and some may find it challenging to navigate health apps or devices.

3.4.9. Regulatory & Ethical Concerns [34]

- Liability Issues: If a patient's PGHD indicates a health issue but is not acted on, it raises questions about liability.
- Consent & Ownership: Clear guidelines on who owns PGHD and how it can be used are essential to navigate potential ethical dilemmas. Ethical concerns in healthcare such as privacy, consent, and data security are increasingly significant. As a response, regulations are evolving to safeguard personal health data and mitigate associated risks. This evolution might lead to the development of new regulations encompassing a broader range of health data sources. Consequently, technology companies could face more stringent laws related to health data. Additionally, there need to be novel approaches introduced for individuals to consent to the use of their health data in research.

Addressing these challenges requires collaboration between technology developers, healthcare providers, regulators, and patients. As the field matures, solutions to many of these challenges are likely to emerge, paving the way for PGHD to realize its full potential in healthcare.

3.5. PGHD Health Use

PGHD stands as transformative data in the shift toward personalized medicine, fundamentally reshaping the patient-clinician relationship and the very nature of healthcare delivery. Figure 6 provides eight various uses of PGHD in promoting health and a more patient-centric approach, enabling personalized care.

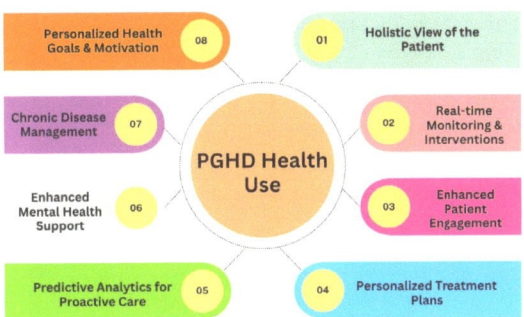

Figure 6. PGHD Health Use.

3.5.1. Holistic View of the Patient [7]

- Comprehensive Data: PGHD captures aspects of daily life, such as diet, exercise, stress levels, and sleep patterns. When combined with clinical data, providers get a fuller picture of a patient's health status and lifestyle.
- Environmental and Behavioral Context: Beyond just symptoms and clinical results, PGHD offers insights into the environments and behaviors affecting a patient's health.

3.5.2. Real-Time Monitoring & Interventions [29]

- Immediate Feedback: Devices that provide real-time data allow timely interventions. For example, a sudden drop in blood sugar levels captured by a continuous glucose monitor can trigger an immediate alert to a diabetic patient.
- Adjusting Treatment in Real-Time: Regular input of PGHD can help clinicians adjust medication dosages, exercise routines, or other treatment modalities based on current and actual data rather than waiting for periodic check-ups.

3.5.3. Enhanced Patient Engagement [35]

- Active Participation: By tracking and sharing their own data, patients become active participants in their care journey.
- Educated Decisions: Access to their data empowers patients with knowledge, enabling them to make informed decisions about their health and engage in meaningful discussions with healthcare providers.

3.5.4. Personalized Treatment Plans [36]

- Tailored Interventions: With PGHD insights, clinicians can develop care plans that are more aligned with a patient's unique circumstances, whether it is customizing a physical therapy routine or dietary recommendations.
- Drug Response Monitoring: By capturing how a patient feels or reacts after taking the medication, PGHD can help personalize drug regimens to maximize efficacy and minimize side effects.

3.5.5. Predictive Analytics for Proactive Care [37]

- Anticipating Health Issues: With the help of AI and machine learning, PGHD can be used to identify patterns and predict potential health problems before they become serious.
- Risk stratification: PGHD can aid in determining which patients are at higher risk for certain complications or conditions, enabling preemptive interventions.

3.5.6. Enhanced Mental Health Support [36]

- Emotional Well-being Tracking: Apps that track mood or mental well-being can inform interventions, helping providers understand triggers and patterns in mental health fluctuations.

- Personalized Therapeutic Interventions: Mental health practitioners can use PGHD to tailor therapeutic strategies, such as recommending specific stress reduction techniques based on tracked stressors.

3.5.7. Chronic Disease Management [38]

- Self-management: For chronic diseases such as diabetes or hypertension, PGHD allows patients to self-manage more effectively, adjusting behaviors in real time based on feedback from devices.
- Telehealth Integration: PGHD can be seamlessly integrated into telehealth platforms, allowing clinicians to provide remote care based on actual patient-generated metrics.

3.5.8. Personalized Health Goals & Motivation [39]

- Setting Achievable Targets: With the granularity of PGHD, patients can set and work toward specific, personalized health goals, whether it is achieving a certain activity level or maintaining a dietary regimen.
- Gamification and Incentives: Many health apps use gamification elements, providing rewards or achievements based on individual user data, thus motivating consistent healthy behaviors.

In summary, PGHD shifts the paradigm from a generalized, reactive healthcare model to a personalized, proactive one. With the individual at the center of the care model, interventions are expedited, treatments are more aligned with personal needs, and the entire healthcare experience is more collaborative and effective.

3.6. PGHD Adoption Worldwide

The adoption and utilization of PGHD vary significantly throughout the world, influenced by a combination of technological infrastructure, regulatory environments, cultural attitudes, and economic factors. Here is a brief look at the global perspective on PGHD:

3.6.1. North America (Primarily USA and Canada) [23,40,41]

- Advanced Adoption: The region has seen substantial growth in the adoption of wearable devices and health applications, supported by a robust technological infrastructure and a strong focus on healthcare innovation.
- Regulatory environment: Regulatory bodies like the FDA in the US provide guidelines for health applications and wearables, ensuring safety and efficacy.
- Challenges: Cost and insurance coverage can be barriers. Privacy concerns, especially in the US with regulations like HIPAA, also influence the utilization of PGHD.

3.6.2. Europe [23,42]

- Varied Adoption: Northern and Western European countries, such as the UK, Germany and Scandinavia, are at the forefront of PGHD adoption, with a strong emphasis on digital health and e-health strategies.
- Data Protection: The General Data Protection Regulation (GDPR) sets stringent standards for data privacy, affecting how PGHD is collected and used.
- Cultural Openness: In general, there is a positive attitude towards using technology to enhance healthcare, although individual perceptions can vary.

3.6.3. Asia [43–45]

- Rapid Growth: Countries such as Japan, South Korea, and Singapore are quickly adopting PGHD tools, driven by technological advancements and aging populations.
- Emerging markets: In India and China, the growth of the middle class and increasing tech-savviness are driving interest in personal health tracking, although full integration into healthcare systems is still in progress.
- Cultural Barriers: In certain areas, traditional beliefs about health can influence the acceptance and trust of digital health tools.

3.6.4. Australia & New Zealand [46]

- Positive Adoption: Both countries are progressively integrating PGHD into their healthcare systems, supported by national e-health strategies and initiatives.
- Challenges Geographic dispersion, especially in Australia, can pose challenges for consistent PGHD adoption across urban and rural areas.

3.6.5. Africa [47–49]

- Infrastructural Challenges: Limited technological infrastructure in many parts of the continent poses challenges to widespread adoption of PGHD.
- Innovative Solutions: Mobile phones are widely used in Africa, and there are health initiatives that leverage mobile technology for data collection, especially for community health.
- Cultural Differences Acceptance of PGHD varies, with some regions showing skepticism towards digital health interventions, while others are more receptive.

3.6.6. Latin America [50,51]

- Growing Interest: Urban centers in countries such as Brazil, Argentina, and Mexico are showing increasing interest in wearable devices and health apps.
- Infrastructural Limitations: Inconsistent access to the high-speed internet and advanced medical technology can limit the integration of PGHD.
- Cultural views: While there is general openness to PGHD in many areas, trust in technology and data privacy concerns can vary widely.

In conclusion, while the potential of PGHD is recognized globally, its actual adoption and utilization are heavily influenced by regional factors. Advanced technological infrastructure, supportive regulations, economic capabilities, and cultural beliefs all play a role in how different parts of the world approach and integrate PGHD into their healthcare systems.

3.7. PGHD Advancement

Certainly, the realm of PGHD is poised for continued growth and evolution. As technologies advance and healthcare evolves further towards patient-centric and preventive models, the role of PGHD will only become more central. Figure 7 provides the prospective future of the advancement of PGHD in healthcare.

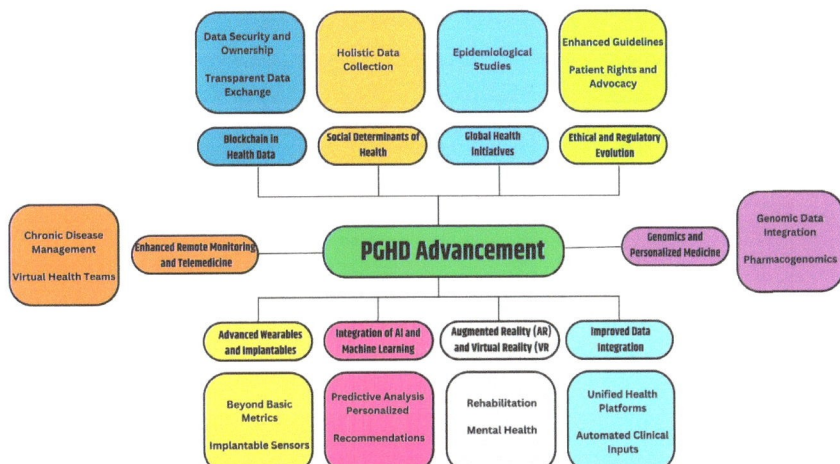

Figure 7. PGHD Advancement.

3.7.1. Advanced Wearables and Implantable [52]

- Beyond Basic Metrics: Future wearables will capture more than just heart rate or steps. They could monitor hydration levels, nutritional intake, stress biomarkers, or even blood oxygen levels in real-time.
- Implantable Sensors: Imagine tiny devices implanted under the skin or inside the body, continuously monitoring specific health parameters and sending alerts or recommendations when necessary.

3.7.2. Integration of AI and Machine Learning [53,54]

- Predictive Analysis: By analyzing vast amounts of PGHD, AI systems can identify patterns and predict health events or complications even before they manifest themselves overtly.
- Personalized recommendations: AI-driven apps could offer users daily health, diet, or exercise recommendations based on real-time data.

3.7.3. Augmented Reality (AR) and Virtual Reality (VR) [55,56]

- Rehabilitation: VR setups can be used for physical or cognitive therapy, with PGHD tracking progress and adjusting routines.
- Mental health: AR/VR environments can be therapeutic, especially when combined with real-time biofeedback.

3.7.4. Improved Data Integration [57,58]

- Unified Health Platforms: A consolidated platform where clinical data and PGHD converge, allowing seamless communication between healthcare providers and patients.
- Automated Clinical Inputs: Devices that not only collect data, but can also automatically input this into Electronic Health Records (EHRs) without manual intervention.

3.7.5. Genomics and Personalized Medicine [59,60]

- Genomic Data Integration: The decreasing cost of genome sequencing has facilitated the integration of genetic data with PGHD, allowing valuable insights into individual predispositions and the customization of preventive treatments.
- Pharmacogenomics: Personal drug regimens based on genetic makeup, lifestyle, and real-time health data.

3.7.6. Enhanced Remote Monitoring and Telemedicine [61]

- Chronic Disease Management: Real-time PGHD can be transmitted to healthcare providers, allowing them to monitor and manage chronic conditions from a distance.
- Virtual Health Teams: Based on PGHD inputs, virtual multidisciplinary teams can convene and make collaborative decisions.

3.7.7. Blockchain in Health Data [62]

- Data Security and Ownership: Blockchain can provide decentralized, immutable ledgers for health data, ensuring security and giving patients more control and ownership of their data.
- Transparent Data Exchange: Facilitating trust in the sharing of PGHD among patients, providers, and researchers.

3.7.8. Social Determinants of Health [63]

- Holistic Data Collection: Beyond biological parameters, future PGHD tools might capture data on social determinants such as environment, economic conditions, or social interactions, offering a comprehensive view of factors affecting health.

3.7.9. Global Health Initiatives [64]
- Epidemiological Studies: The large-scale collection of PGHD can help track disease outbreaks, understand public health trends, and shape health policies.

3.7.10. Ethical and Regulatory Evolution [23]
- Enhanced Guidelines: As PGHD becomes central to healthcare care, regulatory bodies will provide clearer guidelines to ensure data accuracy, privacy, and appropriate use.
- Patient Rights and Advocacy: Enhanced focus on patients' rights to their data, how it is used, and who has access.

In essence, the future of PGHD is a confluence of technology, personalized medicine, and patient empowerment. As innovations continue to emerge, the boundary between traditional healthcare settings and everyday life will blur, making health management an integrated aspect of our daily routines.

4. Methodology

The systematic review was carried out according to the Preferred Reporting Items for Systematic Reviews and Meta-Analyses (PRISMA) guidelines [65].

4.1. Search Strategy

To comprehensively review the existing literature on PGHD with a specific emphasis on its understanding, use, patient prospective, future trends and security and privacy, a systematic search strategy was formulated. The strategy was carefully tailored to each database, given its specificities and nuances.

Database Utilized
- PubMed
- Scopus
- IEEE Xplore
- Web of Science
- ACM Digital Library
- EBSCO host

4.2. Search Terms and Boolean Operators
- Patient Data Terms: Patient-Generated Health Data, PGHD, Patient-reported outcomes, Personal health records
- Security and Privacy Terms: security, privacy, encryption, health data security, health data privacy

The terms within each thematic group were combined using the "OR" Boolean operator, ensuring the breadth of the search within that theme. The two primary themes (Patient Data and Security & Privacy) were combined using the "AND" Boolean operator to ensure that the results pertain to both aspects.

Key Words Used: ("Patient-generated health data" OR "PGHD" OR "Patient-reported outcomes" OR "Personal health records" OR "PHR") AND ("security" OR "privacy" or "encryption" or "health data security" OR "health data privacy")

Search strategies for individual databases:

4.2.1. Pubmed

For the topic "patient-generated health data security and privacy" and focusing specifically on PubMed, it is recommend using a combination of MeSH (Medical Subject Headings) terms and free-text keywords. Search terms can be organized into thematic groups and combined using Boolean operators. ("Patient-generated health data" [MeSH] OR "PGHD" OR "Patient-reported outcomes" OR "Personal health records" OR "PHR") AND ("security" OR "privacy" or "encryption" or "health data security" OR "health data privacy").

4.2.2. Scopus

When designing a search strategy for Scopus, it is important to consider the database's specific syntax and features. Scopus does not use MeSH terms like PubMed; instead, you will focus on keyword and free-text searching.

TITLE-ABS-KEY ("Patient-generated health data" OR "PGHD" OR "Patient-reported outcomes" OR "Personal health records" OR "PHR") AND TITLE-ABS-KEY ("security" OR "privacy" OR "encryption" OR "health data security" OR "health data privacy")

In this query:

TITLE-ABS-KEY ensures that the search is focused on the titles, abstracts, and keywords of the documents, which are likely where the most relevant information will be.

We use parentheses to group related terms and use the Boolean operators AND and OR to specify our search requirements.

4.2.3. IEEE Xplore

IEEE Xplore is a platform that mainly contains literature in the fields of electronics, electrical engineering, and computer science. Thus, when designing a search strategy for IEEE Xplore, we should consider its audience and the likelihood that our terms will pull relevant results.

("Patient-generated health data" OR "PGHD" OR "Patient-reported outcomes" OR "Personal health records" OR "PHR") AND ("security" OR "privacy" or "encryption" or "health data security" OR "health data privacy")

Keep the following in mind when searching on IEEE Xplore:

Given the technical nature of the database, you are likely to encounter articles that deal with the technical aspects of PGHD security and privacy. This could be beneficial if you are interested in the technical solutions and challenges of PGHD.

It is crucial to review the results for relevance, as IEEE Xplore's focus on engineering and technology may yield some results that are tangential to the primary health-focused aspect of PGHD.

4.2.4. Web of Science

Web of Science (WoS) is a multidisciplinary database, which means that it is essential to have a well-structured search strategy to yield the most relevant results. Given your focus on "patient-generated health data" (PGHD) with an emphasis on security and privacy, here is a proposed search strategy for WoS:

TS = ("Patient-generated health data" OR "PGHD" OR "Patient-reported outcomes" OR "Personal health records" OR "PHR") AND TS = ("security" OR "privacy" OR "encryption" OR "health data security" OR "health data privacy")

In this search query:

TS = specifies that the search should look at topic, which includes title, abstract, author keywords, and Keywords Plus in WoS.

The terms within each group are combined using the OR operator to broaden the search within that theme.

The two main themes (PGHD and Security & Privacy concepts) are combined using the AND operator to ensure the results have elements of both.

4.2.5. ACM Library

When constructing a search strategy for the ACM Digital Library, remember that it mainly caters to the disciplines of computing and technology. Given your focus on "patient-generated health data" (PGHD) and its aspects of security and privacy, here is a possible search strategy for the ACM Digital Library:

[[All: "patient-generated health data"] OR [All: "pghd"] OR [All: "patient-reported outcomes"] OR [All: "personal health records"] OR [All: "phr"]] AND [[All: "security"] OR [All: "privacy" or "encryption" or] OR [All: "health data security"] OR [All: "health data privacy"]].

4.2.6. EBOSCO Host

EBSCOhost provides a variety of databases with a broad range of disciplines, so it is essential to ensure your search strategy is well-structured to yield relevant results.

("Patient-generated health data" OR "PGHD" OR "Patient-reported outcomes" OR "Personal health records" OR "PHR") AND ("security" OR "privacy" or "encryption" or "health data security" OR "health data privacy").

4.3. Inclusion and Exclusion Criteria for Studies

The inclusion and exclusion criteria are imperative to move through the results and ensure that the review captures the most relevant studies.

Inclusion Criteria:
- Articles that discuss or analyze patient-generated health data.
- Peer-reviewed articles, journal papers, conference papers, or books on PGHD.
- Articles published in English.
- Articles indexed in Google Scholar, SCOPUS, SCI, or SCIE.
- Both qualitative (primary and secondary research) and quantitative studies were included.
- Accessible through the university library and open access.
- Studies focusing on PGHD in the context of health data security.

Exclusion Criteria:
- Articles that only peripherally mention patient-generated health data without in-depth analysis or discussion.
- Articles not available in full text.
- Articles not in English or peer reviewed on PGHD.
- Poster, editorial and commentary papers excluded.
- Research mainly focused on extensive clinical data as opposed to PGHD.

4.4. Search Results

The search was conducted on 12 September 2023, and the initial results for each database were: Scopus = 1301, IEEE Xplore = 207, Web of Science = 703, PubMed. = 621, ACM Digital Library = 408, EBSCO Host = 242. Following the application of the inclusion and exclusion criteria, these numbers will be further refined to arrive at the final set of articles for review.

4.5. Study Selection and Screening Process

We used Rayyan, an online tool for systematic reviews, to collaboratively screen potential articles. First, Rayyan goes through the entries to eliminate duplicates. After that, the articles were shortlisted based on the review of their titles and abstracts. We then evaluated the full text of these articles using inclusion and exclusion criteria to determine their suitability for our systematic review. Any disagreements were addressed by team discussions until a mutual agreement was reached.

The Figure 8 shows a flow chart detailing the systematic review process for the selection of articles from various academic databases. It starts with the identification of studies, where a total of 3482 records were retrieved from databases such as Scopus (1301 records), IEEE Xplore (207 records), Web of Science (703 records), PubMed. (621 records), ACM Digital Library (408 records) and EBOSCO host (242 records). Before screening, duplicate records were removed, which amounted to 1492, narrowing the field to 1990 unique records that were screened for relevance using inclusion and exclusion criteria as explained above. From these, 245 reports were identified as potentially relevant and were retrieved for further assessment. Of these, a deeper evaluation was done on 52 reports to determine their eligibility based on predefined criteria relevant to the review's focus. This led to the exclusion of 20 reports that likely did not meet inclusion criteria such as study design, relevance to the research question, or quality thresholds. The final inclusion saw 32 studies that passed all previous filters and were deemed suitable for the review. These studies will be thoroughly reviewed and analyzed to answer the research question at hand. The flow chart provides a clear and structured outline of the literature selection process, ensuring a rigorous and transparent review method. This process is essential to minimize bias and ensure that the review is comprehensive and based on the best available evidence.

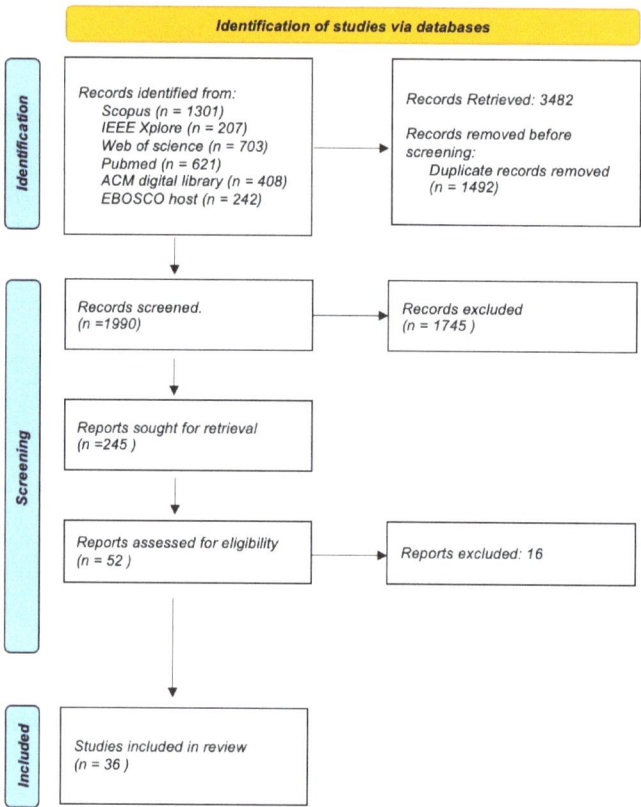

Figure 8. Selection Process.

4.6. Study Selection and Study Characteristics

The comprehensive review of the literature in this field yielded a total of 36 peer-reviewed articles eligible for citation, spanning several esteemed publishers and databases. These include 17 articles from PubMed, 5 from Scopus, 7 from Web of Science, 3 from IEEE Xplore, and 4 from ACM Library. The articles predominantly originated in the United States, with a considerable number also coming from various other countries throughout Europe, Asia, Australia, and North America. In terms of research type, the articles demonstrated a diverse range of methodologies: 15 were categorized as interviews, 16 as regular articles, 4 as review articles, and 1 as a comment paper. Furthermore, the research encompassed various study formats, including a survey, an empirical study, a Delphi study, and a unique blend of interviews and implementation. Geographically, the studies spanned multiple continents with the following detailed distribution: USA (n = 25), Australia (n = 3), UK (n = 2), Ireland (n = 1), Switzerland (n = 1), Canada (n = 1), Iraq (n = 1), India (n = 1), Slovenia (n = 1), Pakistan (n = 2), Sweden (n = 1), South Korea (n = 1), Netherlands (n = 1) and China (n = 1). This global representation highlights the widespread interest and applicability of the research topic.

The selected studies were categorized into various groups, providing insights into different aspects of the research topic. These categories included interviews (n = 15), regular articles (n = 16), review articles (n = 4), and other formats such as comment articles and empirical studies. This classification underscores the multifaceted nature of research and the diverse methodologies employed in exploring the field.

As mentioned previously, the first three research questions (RQs) (a) Exploratory Questions (RQE1, RQE2), (b) impact assessment questions (RQI1, RQI2) and (c) solution-oriented questions (RQS1, RQS2) are addressed by the articles in the review, as depicted in the Table 2.

Table 2. Articles included on PGHD Understsnding, Requirement, Challenges Review.

Category	Subcategory and References
PGHD	Research Question Exploratory
	RQE1 [6,26,33,58,65–67]
	RQE2 [3,7,68–71]
	Research Question Impact Assessment
	RQI1 [72]
	RQI2 [6,35,73–76]
	Research Question Solution-Oriented
	RQS1 [76–85]
	RQS2 [3,6,7,86–94]

Table 3 details the articles that contribute to the understanding of basic and advanced security measures in the PGHD domain, drawing on existing security techniques and protocols in related health sectors, such as medical device data security and health data security and privacy. These additional articles have been instrumental in addressing RQs (RQF1 and RQF2), compensating for the scarcity of literature specifically focused on the PGHD domain.

Table 3. Articles included on PGHD Basic and Advanced Security and Privacy Review.

Category	Subcategory and References
PGHD Security & Privacy	Research Question Future-Oriented
	RQF1: Basic Security Measure [3,23,24,77,84,85,95–101]
	RQF1: Advanced Security Measure [62,102–111]
	RQF2 [6,21,23–27,37,53,58,73,77–79,81,85,95,112]

5. Result

The findings related to the identified RQs are elaborated as follows.

5.1. RQE1: What Are the Primary Sources of PGHD, and for What Purpose Are They Being Utilized in Healthcare Settings?

Kawu et al. [27] identified the primary sources of PGHD used in healthcare settings as: Mobile health apps and wearable devices like fitness trackers, these collect various clinical measurements like heart rate, blood pressure, sleep data, etc. They are used for monitoring chronic conditions, weight management, fitness tracking, etc. Patient portals and personal health records (PHRs)—These allow patients to directly enter health data like symptoms, mood, food intake, pain levels, etc. Used for self-monitoring and sharing with providers. Social media posts—Posts describing health experiences, symptoms, etc. can provide insights especially for public health monitoring. Sensors and Internet-of-Things (IoT) devices—Various sensors and networked devices can transmit health data like ECG, glucose levels, etc. Used for remote monitoring. Interactive voice response systems—Allow patients to provide symptom or medication data via voice commands. Help track treatment progress. Virtual/mixed reality systems—Can be used for physical therapy, pain management, behavioral health, etc. The main purposes for using these sources of PGHD are: (1) To improve patient self-management of chronic conditions (2) Allow remote monitoring and care outside clinics (3) Provide a more holistic view of health by capturing patient experiences and lifestyle (4) Reduce burden on the healthcare system via automated data collection (5) Enable personalized care through additional patient context (6) Promote patient participation and empowerment in their own healthcare. However, the review mentions that more research is needed to incorporate emerging sources of PGHD like social networks, virtual reality, etc. into clinical workflows and health IT systems. Concerns around data privacy, quality, and interoperability also need to be addressed.

Petersen et al. [34] highlighted that PGHD encompasses a variety of sources that are increasingly being integrated into healthcare settings to improve patient care and outcomes. These sources include patient-reported outcomes (PRO), which assess how patients perceive their health status; patient-powered patient registries (PPR) that collect standardized information about specific patient groups; patient-powered research networks (PPRN) that consolidate multiple registries; and patient portals that offer web or mobile access to provider-created health information. In addition, remote sensors and smart wearable devices are becoming prevalent, transmitting personal data such as heart rate and activity levels for external analysis. The digital age has also seen the rise of social media platforms and mobile health (mHealth) apps as tools for patients to track, record, or share their health data. Integrating PGHD into healthcare care aims to improve care, facilitate research, assess treatment effectiveness, provide patients with access to their health information and foster better communication among patients, caregivers and healthcare providers. In essence, leveraging PGHD from a variety of sources provides a comprehensive view of patient experiences, making it possible to tailor care, expand research, and improve overall health outcomes.

Lai et al. [66] explain that PGHD comes from a variety of consumer health technologies including smartphones, wearable devices, sensors, patient portals, and personal health records. Patients can use these technologies to track health data such as vital signs, symptoms, lifestyle behaviors, and patient-reported outcomes. This data is being used in several ways. Patients are using PGHD for self-monitoring and self-management of health conditions, especially chronic diseases. PGHD also allows new methods to capture patient perspectives and outcomes in clinical research, such as clinical trials. In addition, PGHD is being integrated into electronic health records and provider workflows to inform clinical decision-making and care delivery, giving providers a more comprehensive view of patients. PGHD analysis from sources such as mobile health apps and online communities provides insights into patients' experiences, behaviors, and needs, guiding the design of better tools and interventions. In general, the main goal is to engage patients more actively in their health and care.

Lavallee et al. [7] describe several primary sources of PGHD that are being used in healthcare settings. Patients are generating PGHD through the use of wearable devices and mobile health apps that allow them to track metrics such as physical activity, heart rate, blood pressure, weight, sleep, and more. This type of data is often used by patients for their own health monitoring and management, or is shared with healthcare providers to facilitate data-driven care. Other sources of PGHD include patient portals and electronic health records, which allow patients to directly submit information like food/symptom logs, mood ratings, and customized health data to their providers. Validated clinical assessments and symptom trackers are also sources of PGHD that allow systematic tracking of patient-reported outcomes over time. Patients and caregivers are also using journals and diaries to capture highly customized PGHD that may not be easily recorded through devices and apps. On the provider side, healthcare systems are using PGHD for remote patient monitoring programs, particularly for chronic disease management. Telehealth technologies allow

PGHD to expand care access and oversight. Finally, both patients and providers described participating in clinical research efforts to collect PGHD, often with the goal of informing future clinical use cases and system-wide implementation. In summary, PGHD is generated from a diverse set of sources, including wearables, apps, portals, assessments, diaries, and research initiatives. Patients and providers are leveraging these sources of PGHD to enable data-driven care, patient engagement, population health, and care access improvements. However, fully integrating PGHD into clinical workflows and health IT systems remains an ongoing challenge.

Nittas et al. [67] state that PGHD originates primarily from health care consumers themselves, transforming their daily lives into a valuable source of health information. In healthcare settings, PGHD is increasingly used for a variety of purposes. The article highlights that a majority of studies integrate electronic PGHD with elements such as reflection, guidance, motivation, and education, which form a core part of digital prevention strategies. In particular, many of these interventions are fully automatized, demonstrating a shift towards resource-efficient care. These data not only strengthen proactive and person-centered healthcare approaches, but also play a pivotal role in disease prevention, health promotion, personalized counseling, and remote monitoring. The increasing reliance on PGHD underscores the evolving landscape of healthcare care, emphasizing digitalization and a more active role for consumers in their health management.

Austin et al. [95] examined various case studies of the use of PGHD in a healthcare system. They found that wearable devices and mobile/sensor technologies were the most common platforms for PGHD collection, used in 41% and 47% of case studies, respectively. These devices were used to collect data on physical activity, sleep, location, mood symptoms, and other metrics that reflect daily health and behaviors. The key goals cited for the use of PGHD were to improve the monitoring between clinical visits (8 case studies), personalize care plans (4 case studies) and assess outcomes (3 case studies). By capturing data on patient experiences and health patterns outside of clinical encounters, PGHD aimed to provide a more comprehensive view of health status to support care decisions. Overall, the use of wearables and mobile apps to collect patient-generated data allowed more continuous, personalized monitoring and care delivery in healthcare settings.

According to Bourke et al. [59] PGHD from sources such as smartphones, wearables, social media, and patient registries is emerging as a valuable complement to traditional healthcare data. Patients can actively contribute by recording symptoms, medication use, patient-reported outcomes on platforms such as apps and patient forums. Passive data collection via sensors in devices like smartwatches and ingestible pills also provides insights not typically captured in medical records, such as continuous physiologic parameters, detailed behaviors, and environmental exposures. The unique value of PGHD is that it offers the patient's perspective-experiences, attitudes, lifestyle factors, treatment adherence patterns, and more. While new methodological considerations exist, PGHD is being used to enable patient-centered research and care, capture data missing from routine clinical sources, study factors influencing health behaviors and outcomes, validate other data sources, and ultimately allow a more complete understanding of therapeutic interventions. Careful incorporation of this new patient-contributed data stream offers innovative opportunities for pharmacoepidemiology and improving health services.

Table 4 presents the insights and findings from the above discussion on primary source and utilization of PGHD in Healthcare Settings in a tabulated format.

Table 4. Primary Source and Utilization of PGHD in Healthcare Settings.

Article	Primary Sources	Purpose in Healthcare Settings
Bourke et al. [59]	Social media, Mobile apps, Online surveys, Speech recordings, Frequency of social communication	Gain person-centric insight not available in routine healthcare datasets, Enable better self-management and improve health outcomes, Support healthcare professionals in monitoring and managing patients, Improve relationships and communication with healthcare teams, Augment patient-driven quality of care assessment, Provide additional information to inform research in healthcare settings
Austin et al. [95]	Sensor devices, Mobile technologies	Enhance care delivery and outcomes, Support research and clinical practice, Improve health outcomes, Facilitate more "connected health" between patients and care teams
Nittas et al. [67]	Active data generation combined with Passive sensor-based trackers	Utilized for primary disease prevention and health promotion purposes, Used for exercise-based weight loss, well-being promotion, and healthy aging, Embedded in larger multicomponent preventive interventions, Combined with reflective, process guiding, motivational, and educational components
Lai et al. [66]	Mobile health technologies, Consumer-grade devices	Collecting and monitoring physiological signs of chronic conditions, Facilitating self-management of Inflammatory Bowel Disease (IBD), Monitoring patients in real-life settings through video surveillance, Integrating continuous glucose monitor data for Personal Health Record (PHR), Incorporating PGHD into clinical trials for more accurate patient information, Monitoring medication adherence and reminding patients to follow study protocols
Lavallee et al. [7]	Wearable devices, Mobile health apps, Geolocation technologies	To support care decisions and improve patient-provider communication and engagement, To expand care for individuals with limited access to healthcare, To improve care for those with acute or chronic conditions, To better engage patients in the use of patient portals and electronic health records, To ensure clinical data accurately reflects the health status of patients, To understand behaviors and health risks for better population health support
Petersen et al. [34]	Remote sensors, Smart wearable devices, Social media, Mobile health (mHealth) apps	Shift in medicine practice towards patient experience-based outcomes, Evaluation and choice of treatment options, Assessment of asthma control, Customized care plans and prediction of length of stay, Assessment of nutritional status
Kawu et al. [27]	mHealth apps, Wearables, Social media posts	Aid in decision-making and provision of personalized care, Provide additional information for healthcare professionals, Assist in the development of reimbursement structures, Facilitate the flow and use of PGHD by clinicians, Enable informed decisions about developing and sharing PGHD

5.2. RQE2: How Do Patients Perceive the Collection and Utilization of Their Generated PGHD?

Zhu et al. [68] in their interview study found that patients are motivated to collect PGHD to gain self-awareness and self-management skills, also tracking health data gives them insight into how their lifestyle and behaviors affect their health. They want to collect comprehensive PGHD to share with clinicians and collaborate on their healthcare and see it as a way of having informed discussions with clinicians. Some patients collect PGHD out of curiosity and seeing the effectiveness of treatments and collecting the data gives them hope and helps them feel that they are actively participating in their care. Patients want to use PGHD to alter treatment plans or medications also. They collect data to provide justification for changing medications or stopping medications. Sharing PGHD during clinical visits is perceived by some patients as burdensome. They have to select what is most relevant to share, given a limited visit time. Some patients perceive that their clinicians are not receptive to the PGHD they collect and initiate sharing on their own. This discourages them from collecting and sharing the data. Patients want clinicians to provide guidance on what PGHD is clinically relevant to collect. This would make the data more useful for clinicians to use. Patients want to be equal partners and collaborate with clinicians on their health care. Sharing PGHD is seen as a way to engage clinicians and alter treatment plans. In summary, patients are motivated to collect comprehensive PGHD to gain personal insight, share with clinicians, and collaborate on their care. But they need the guidance of clinicians on what is clinically relevant to collect. They perceive time constraints and clinician receptiveness as barriers to fully utilizing PGHD.

Lavallee et al. [7] interviews revealed that patients are intentional about when and what type of PGHD they share with providers. PGHD tracked solely for personal health goals or wellness purposes was typically not shared in formal healthcare settings. Patients decided to share PGHD with providers when they felt that it could support care decisions, improve communication about their health status and concerns, or provide data to inform treatment choices. Patients recognized that appointment time is limited, so sharing targeted PGHD is one way to maximize discussions and prepare in advance. However, if patients perceived that providers did not find the PGHD useful or relevant, they would be less likely to continue sharing it. Some patients even sought new providers who were more receptive to integrating PGHD into care. In general, patients were selective about sharing PGHD and considered factors such as perceived provider interest, relevance to care decisions, and visit time constraints when determining what data to bring to healthcare encounters.

Burns et al. [69] in an interview with the patient found that they perceive the collection and utilization of their generated PGHD as an overwhelmingly positive experience. Generating and using their own visual health data allows patients to feel more engaged, empowered, reassured, and in control when it comes to managing their health situations. The ability to visually track progress over time provides confidence that their conditions are improving. It aids comprehension and memory-making around their health journeys. Patients feel a greater sense of responsibility and control over their health outcomes by actively participating in monitoring and documentation. PGHD improves doctor-patient communication by providing visual evidence to accompany verbal descriptions of health problems. In general, patients find that collecting and using PGHD engages them more actively in their own care, improves doctor-patient relationships, and allows them to feel more empowered and confident through self-monitoring their conditions.

Adler-Milstei et al. [3] discuss that the patients' perceptions of the collection and utilization of their PGHD are multifaceted. They generally find that the types of data collected—health history, validated questionnaires and surveys, and biometric and health activity—align with their preferences and needs, with the notable exception of biometric and activity data collected by third parties, which raises privacy concerns. Patients are motivated to work with PGHD to achieve specific health goals, improve their understanding of their health, make office visits more efficient, and assist their providers in diagnosis and care management. They have reported positive results when PGHD was used effectively, such as achieving accurate diagnoses after previous errors. However, there are challenges in maintaining patient engagement with PGHD, including the manual effort and technical know-how required for data submission and the lack of clear communication from providers about the value and use of data. Patients do not expect immediate feedback on the PGHD they provide, but have noted problems with how these data are integrated into their interactions with healthcare providers. They also stress the importance of differentiating PGHD from data generated by clinicians within electronic health records. Furthermore, the communication between patients and providers is critical; patients are more likely to submit data if they understand its value to their care and if providers demonstrate how it informs clinical decisions. Policy-related challenges also emerge, particularly regarding the lack of reimbursement for PGHD and potential liability issues, which hinder the integration of PGHD into clinical workflows. Overall, while patients recognize the potential benefits of PGHD, their concerns about privacy, the submission process, and the clarity of its use in their healthcare are significant and need to be addressed to improve engagement and integration.

Kim et al. [70] found that patients have mixed perceptions regarding the collection and utilization of Patient-Generated Health Data (PGHD). On the one hand, they acknowledge that PGHD can improve transparency in the patient-provider relationship, potentially leading to better care. However, this transparency also raises concerns, as some patients may respond negatively by stopping collecting data, selectively sharing information or manipulating the data to appear compliant, driven by the desire to maintain a positive relationship with their healthcare providers. Clinicians recognize the value of PGHD despite possible inaccuracies and express concerns about the reliability of the data due to the reporting habits of patients. Older adults, in particular, find the monitoring aspect of PGHD intrusive and threatening their autonomy, leading to resistance. The need for education on how to collect and use PGHD is evident, but the responsibility to provide this education remains unclear, especially when the monitoring is initiated by patients themselves. There is also a noted uncertainty about how clinicians interpret PGHD and use it to benefit patient health. There is a mismatch between the available technology and the actual needs of patients and clinicians, with a preference for passively collected data due to its perceived accuracy. In general, while PGHD is seen as a tool that could potentially improve clinical care, it also presents challenges related to trust, privacy, and the balance between its benefits and its perceived intrusiveness.

Smith et al. [71] explore the perspectives of cancer survivors about providing patient-generated health data and patient-reported outcomes to central cancer registries. His study highlights significant insights into the perspectives of patients on the handling of their patient-generated health data (PGHD). Initially unfamiliar with the concept of cancer registry, patients became comfortable contributing diverse types of PGHD once they understood the objectives of the registry. Their motivation to share hinged on the altruistic potential to help fellow patients. Although some assumed that their information would remain private, others stipulated confidentiality as a prerequisite for sharing. They were prepared to provide data covering medical history, symptomatology, quality of life, functional ability, care experiences, lifestyle and economic factors. In particular, there was a prevalent demand for the inclusion of data on the enduring effects of cancer and the repercussions of treatments. Patients not only sought their data to enrich treatment options and facilitate their adaptation process but also to gain access to reciprocal information from the registries. This information ranged from side effects and survival rates to novel treatments and insights into quality of care. The preferred methods for submitting PGHD varied, including mail, phone, online surveys, and integration with patient portals. In essence, there is a strong willingness among patients to share their PGHD with registries in the hope of benefiting others, coupled with a clear expectation of privacy and the desire to receive valuable information in return.

Table 5 presents the insights and findings from the above discussion on patient perceptions and utilization of PGHD in a tabulated format.

Table 5. Patient Perceptions and Utilization of PGHD.

Article	Patient Perceptions	PGHD Utilization	Key Findings
Zhu et al. [68]	Positive: gain insights, participate in care, Negative: burdensome to share in visits	Self-management, Share with clinicians to inform treatment decisions	Patients motivated to collect PGHD for self-awareness, self-management, track effectiveness of treatments, Want to use PGHD to alter treatment plans and medications, Perceive sharing PGHD as burdensome due to time constraints, Want guidance from clinicians on relevant data to collect
Lavallee et al. [7]	Positive if providers find it useful/relevant, Negative if providers not receptive	Share targeted PGHD to inform treatment decisions, Discontinue sharing if provider not receptive	Selective in sharing PGHD based on perceived provider interest and relevance, Consider visit time constraints when deciding what PGHD to share, Less likely to continue sharing if providers don't find it useful

Table 5. *Cont.*

Article	Patient Perceptions	PGHD Utilization	Key Findings
Burns et al. [69]	Positive: engaging, empowering	Self-monitoring health conditions, Share with providers to improve communication	Collecting PGHD engages patients, enhances doctor-patient relationships, Allows patients to feel empowered, reassured, in control, Provides visual evidence to accompany descriptions of health issues
Adler-Milstei et al. [3]	Positive: enhances understanding, assist providers, Negative: privacy concerns, lack of communication on use	Achieve health goals, Diagnosis and care management	Aligns with patient preferences except 3rd party biometric data (privacy concerns), Motivated to achieve health goals, enhance understanding, assist providers, Concerns about manual effort required, lack of communication on value and use of data, Stress integrating PGHD into interactions with providers
Kim et al. [70]	Mixed: benefits but concerns on privacy, autonomy	Inform clinical care (but potential for manipulation)	Enhances transparency but also raises patient concerns about privacy, autonomy, Questions around reliability of data, need for education on collection and use, Mismatch between available technology and actual patient/provider needs
Smith et al. [71]	Positive: altruistic motivation, Expect privacy, reciprocity	Share with cancer registries to aid research	Motivated to share to aid other patients (altruistic), Want confidentiality, reciprocal information on treatments, side effects etc., Preferred methods: mail, phone, online surveys, patient portals

5.3. RQI1: What Are the Potential Ramifications of Data Breaches Pertaining to PGHD on Trust and Healthcare Outcomes?

Ostherr et al. [72] highlight key points emerge with respect to patient trust, data breaches, and health outcomes: Despite the high-profile data breaches, patients expressed little concern about sharing their health data with corporations. Some felt that the transactional nature of consenting to the terms of service overrode privacy concerns. However, when approached for research purposes and informed about the risks of data privacy, the patients became more wary. This suggests an asymmetry in which companies face less scrutiny than researchers for the handling of health data. Many patients felt that sharing data in general could improve health outcomes more than lab research alone. However, recruiting participants was still difficult when privacy risks were highlighted. There is a disconnect between attitudes on corporate data sharing versus research/clinical data sharing. The public discourse on data privacy threats also contrasts with lax reading of terms of service.

The regulatory environment lags behind real-world data sharing practices and attitudes. More public dialogue on the benefits/harms of health data is needed. In summary, the conclusion focuses on how patient trust differs based on context, the need to update regulations, and the complex relationship between data sharing and perceived health outcomes. Although patients tolerate corporate data practices, highlighting risks reduces trust, signaling a need for greater transparency.

However, some potential ramifications of data breaches of PGHD on patient trust and healthcare outcomes include the following:

- Loss of trust in companies and technologies collecting patient health data. The article mentions users' comfort in sharing health data with corporations, despite the potential for exploitation. Data breaches could erode this trust and make patients more cautious about using health apps and devices.

- Unwillingness to share health data. The article notes that researchers already face challenges in getting people to share health data for studies due to privacy concerns. Data breaches could exacerbate this and inhibit research using patient-generated data.
- Negative impacts on care. The article suggests that patient-generated data could improve outcomes by providing information on health / illness. If data breaches discourage patients from sharing data, it could hinder these potential health benefits.
- Reluctance to disclose sensitive information. Patients may be less forthcoming with potentially relevant health details during clinical encounters if concerned about data privacy and breaches. This could negatively impact care.
- Increased stress/anxiety. Data breaches involving sensitive health information could lead to emotional distress for patients whose data is exposed. This psychological impact could also take a toll on wellbeing.

In summary, by undermining patient trust and inhibiting data sharing, health data breaches could limit the progress and benefits expected from access to patient-generated data, leading to detrimental impacts on care, health research, and patient well-being. Maintaining rigorous data privacy and security is critical to realizing the potential of PGHD.

5.4. RQI2: What Impact Does the Incorporation of Patients and Their PGHD Have on Healthcare Decision-Making?

According to Jim et al. [73] PGHD can have several important impacts on healthcare decision making:

- Improving symptom monitoring and management: PGHD, such as patient-reported outcomes (PROs), allow for more comprehensive and real-time assessment of patient symptoms and side effects. This enables earlier detection and treatment of issues that can impact quality of life or clinical outcomes.
- Informing treatment choices: PGHD provides additional information on patient experiences that can better inform shared decision-making about treatment options. For example, PRO data on side effect profiles can help patients and physicians select the optimal treatment regimen.
- Predicting health events: The longitudinal analysis of PGHD can uncover patterns predictive of disease progression, treatment complications, or health emergencies. This can allow for preventive interventions. For example, a rapid decline in activity monitoring data could indicate an upcoming need for hospitalization.
- Population health management: PGHD aggregates can help identify trends, disparities, and opportunities to improve care delivery across patient populations. This is useful for quality improvement initiatives.
- Clinical trial outcomes: Incorporating PGHD as secondary endpoints in the trials provides a more comprehensive view of treatment effects on quality of life and symptomatic adverse events from the perspective of the patient.
- Regulatory decisions: Drug and device approvals are increasingly informed by patient experience data from PGHD. This ensures that the patient's voice is represented in the benefit-risk determinations.
- Remote patient monitoring: PGHD enables care outside traditional settings through telehealth, reducing hospital visits. During the COVID-19 pandemic, remote monitoring using PGHD became especially important.

In summary, PGHD allows care to be tailored to patients' unique needs and preferences, predict risks, and improve health outcomes across entire populations. Its integration into decision-making processes can improve patient-centeredness, quality of care, and value.

Singh et al. [74] elaborate the impact of incorporating PGHD on healthcare decision-making are:

- PGHD from mobile apps and wearables provides additional and more up-to-date information about the patient compared to only relying on healthcare professional-generated data (HPGD) from EHRs. This can lead to faster and improved healthcare decision making.

- PGHD allows continuous monitoring of patient health parameters such as adherence to medications, exercise, sleep, etc. These real-time data can enable timely interventions and personalized care that lead to better health outcomes.
- Integration of PGHD and HPGD provides a more holistic view of the patient's health. Decisions can be based on both historical clinical data as well as current lifestyle and health indicators tracked by the patient.
- Patient participation and empowerment increase with PGHD as they take greater ownership over monitoring and managing their health. This can improve their adherence to care plans.
- Quality of decision-making can potentially be improved by speeding up decision time, reducing errors, improving patient outcomes, and reducing healthcare costs. Metrics to quantify improvements need further research.
- Challenges like data integration, privacy/security, regulatory issues, impact on provider workload need to be addressed for effective utilization of PGHD in decision making.

In summary, incorporating patient-generated data facilitates patient-centered care by engaging patients in their own health management. This, together with the integration with clinical data, provides a foundation for more informed and timely shared decision-making between providers and patients.

Petersen et al. [35] discuss the significant role of PGHD in the medical decision-making process. It highlights that patients are actively involved in collecting and sharing their health data in order to improve their treatment outcomes. Such proactive sharing facilitates more productive and informed consultations with healthcare providers. Furthermore, PGHD contributes to greater patient participation and equips physicians with valuable information about the health of their patients beyond the clinical environment, thereby improving the decision-making process. When PGHD is reviewed collectively, it not only promotes better health results, but also encourages patients to participate more in activities beneficial to their health. Transparent exchange of PGHD also encourages honesty in patient-provider interactions, leading to decisions grounded in accurate information. Despite these benefits, the lack of standardized protocols for PGHD is a significant obstacle to its full integration into clinical practice. In conclusion, the inclusion of PGHD enriches the clinician-patient dynamic, improves collaborative decisions, and promotes improved health outcomes, although standardization and effective integration into healthcare systems remain areas for development.

Cohen et al. [6] examine the impact of incorporating PGHD in clinical decision-making and care. The authors interviewed clinicians and researchers involved in five studies testing PGHD collection tools. They found that PGHD provides valuable insights between visits and reveals patient problems that may be missed during appointments. Incorporating PGHD into healthcare care provides clinicians with a comprehensive view of a patient's health over time, allowing for better disease management and more personalized care. PGHD offers detailed information that may be missed in routine visits, helping to adjust care plans more effectively and potentially reducing unnecessary clinic visits. However, it requires the development of specific protocols for data collection, integration into EHR and response to data, while also considering the privacy and security of the stored information. Moreover, PGHD empowers patients by giving them control over their health data, fostering greater autonomy, and transforming the patient-clinician dynamic.

Wood et al. [75] explains that the incorporation of PGHD into healthcare decision making can improve treatment efficacy, identify patients at risk of treatment toxicity, and inform personalized treatment plans. PGHD allows for a better understanding of the long-term impacts of treatments on quality of life, informs the conduct of clinical trials, and provides prognostic value in clinical outcomes. In addition, PGHD can contribute to the evaluation of new therapeutics and potentially influence regulatory decisions. By tracking metrics such as symptoms, medication adherence, and lifestyle factors, PGHD can also play a role in clinical research to improve patient well-being. In general, PGHD promotes more personalized and informed healthcare decisions that benefit patient experiences and outcomes, while also advancing clinical research.

Petersen et al. [76] discusses policy recommendations to facilitate the use of PGHD from apps, wearables, etc. in shared decision making between patients and clinicians. Incorporating PGHD makes care more patient-centric by bringing in the patient perspective. Accessing their own data also allows patients to take an active role in managing their health. For clinicians, PGHD provides a more holistic view of patients for tailored care plans and allows tracking of health status over time. At the population level, aggregated PGHD can reveal health trends to guide public health efforts. However, concerns such as privacy risks, ensuring accuracy, building clinician trust in PGHD, and avoiding marginalization need to be addressed. The authors suggest policy changes such as stronger data protections and consent processes so patients can trust that their data are safe. Patients should be able to easily access their PGHD. The collection and use of PGHD should be transparent and ethical. While PGHD holds promise in healthcare decision-making, policies must balance maximizing its benefits with minimizing potential harms, especially for vulnerable groups. If implemented effectively, PGHD can make care more collaborative and empower the patient.

Table 6 presents the insights and findings from the above discussion on impact on incorporation of patients and their PGHD in healthcare decision-making in a tabulated format.

Table 6. Impact on incorporation of patients and their PGHD in healthcare decision-making.

Article	Patient Incorporation	PGHD Incorporation
Jim et al. [73]	Allow care to be tailored to patient's unique needs and preferences; Inform treatment choices; Predicts health events; Population health management; Clinical trial outcomes; Regulatory decisions; Remote patient monitoring	Improves symptom monitoring and management; Provides additional and more up-to-date information about the patient; Allows continuous monitoring of health parameters like medication adherence, exercise, sleep, etc.; Integrates PGHD and HPGD for a more holistic view of the patient's health; Increases patient engagement and empowerment; Potentially improves quality of decision-making; Addresses challenges like data integration, privacy/security, regulatory issues
Singh et al. [74]	Facilitates patient-centered care; Enhances shared decision-making	Provides additional and more up-to-date information about the patient; Allows continuous monitoring of health parameters such as medication adherence, exercise, sleep, etc.; Integrates PGHD and HPGD for a more holistic view of the patient's health; Increases patient engagement and empowerment; Potentially improves quality of decision-making; Addresses challenges such as data integration, privacy/security, regulatory issues
Petersen et al. [35]	Actively involved in collecting and sharing health data; Facilitates productive, informed consultations with healthcare providers; Contributes to greater engagement from patients; Encourages honesty in patient-provider interactions	Provides valuable insights between visits and reveals patient issues that may be missed during appointments; Provides comprehensive view of patient's health over time; Empowers patients by giving them control over their health data; Enhances patient autonomy and transforms patient-clinician dynamic; Necessitates development of specific protocols for data collection and integration into EHR; Addresses privacy and security concerns
Wood et al. [75]	-	Enhances treatment efficacy; Identifies patients at risk of treatment toxicity; Informs personalized treatment plans; Contributes to evaluation of novel therapeutics; Tracks metrics to improve patient well-being
Petersen et al. [76]	Brings in the patient perspective; Empowers patients to take an active role in managing their health	Provides a more holistic view of patients for tailored care plans; Enables tracking of health status over time; Reveals health trends at the population level; Addresses issues like privacy risks, ensuring accuracy, and building clinician trust in PGHD; Suggests policy changes for transparent and ethical collection and use of PGHD

5.5. RQS1: What Are the Recommended Strategies for Improving the Security and Privacy of PGHD?

Improving the security and privacy of PGHD involves several strategies:

(a) Restrict Access to Data and Applications: Limiting who can access PGHD can help prevent unauthorized use. To ensure the security and privacy of patient information inside healthcare systems, many main tactics are employed. These include the implementation of multifactor authentication (MFA) [77], the use of role-based access control (RBAC) [78], the adherence to the principle of least privilege, conducting frequent audits, and the deployment of firewalls and virtual private networks (VPNs) [79]. Multifactor authentication (MFA) improves security by necessitating the provision of two or more distinct forms of proof by users as a prerequisite for access, such as a password and a fingerprint. Role-Based Access Control (RBAC) is a security mechanism that allocates user roles and permissions according to the specific requirements of their job responsibilities. This approach guarantees that users are granted access only to the data that are essential for the execution of their designated duties. The idea of least privilege enhances control measures by restricting user access to only the essential level required to perform their responsibilities. Implementing routine audits plays a critical role in the identification of security vulnerabilities and the enforcement of approved access protocols. Firewalls serve as protective measures against illegal network invasions, whilst Virtual Private Networks (VPNs) provide the security of remote access. In conclusion, maintaining regular software updates, encompassing both security and medical applications, is vital to protect against any vulnerabilities that might be exploited. These techniques together strive to ensure the security of patient data, allowing access exclusively to individuals who have been authorized for legal purposes.

(b) Implement Data Usage Controls: The implementation of data usage controls in the healthcare sector is of utmost importance, also in order to protect PGHD and ensure that its utilization is in accordance with patient permission and legal obligations. This involves the implementation of robust access controls to restrict data visibility only to authorized individuals, the use of encryption techniques to safeguard data integrity, and the establishment of audit trails to ensure accountability. Strict adherence to regulatory frameworks, such as the Health Insurance Portability and Accountability Act (HIPAA) in the United States and the General Data Protection Regulation (GDPR) in Europe, is imperative and leaves little room for negotiation. Consequently, it is essential to establish and maintain robust systems to ensure compliance with these requirements. It is imperative for healthcare companies to establish and maintain explicit policies and procedures that undergo continuous updates in order to align with the ever-changing legal and ethical norms. It is important to provide training to healthcare personnel about data privacy and security protocols, while also ensuring that patients are adequately informed about their rights and the extent of their control over their personal data. The involvement of stakeholders in the process of policy creation and the establishment of effective communication channels are crucial in ensuring that regulations on data usage are well-informed and comprehensive. Continuous monitoring, frequent audits, and feedback loops play a crucial role in facilitating continual progress, while being abreast of technology changes can further bolster endeavors aimed at safeguarding data. Collectively, these steps establish a safe milieu for the management of PGHD, cultivating confidence among individuals and guaranteeing the responsible and efficient utilization of their data for healthcare provision.

Petersen et al. [76] underscores the importance of enhancing the security and privacy of PGHD by recommending several key strategies. Policymakers are called upon to fortify privacy and security protections for PGHD, bridging gaps in existing laws and ensuring strict enforcement. It advocates for individual access to PGHD in real-time and electronically, reinforcing transparency and personal data control. The need to clarify informed consent processes is emphasized, ensuring individuals are well-informed about how their data is managed and shared, with the flexibility to revise their consent. The use of PGHD should be ethically bound, with a prohibition on potentially harmful non-health applications. Additionally, the article suggests individuals should have the option to securely share their PGHD for research purposes, with privacy intact. Regular review processes for PGHD analytics, updated HIPAA regulations to reflect current practices, and clear, enforceable penalties for data misuse are also recommended. Collectively, these measures aim to establish robust policy changes, augmenting privacy, security, and ethical use of PGHD while giving individuals enhanced control over their data.

(c) Logs and Monitor Use: Keeping track of who is accessing PGHD and when can help identify any potential security breaches. Prosper et al. [80] emphasize the increases in healthcare data breaches and highlight the need for analyzing security practices like access logs in EHR systems which could also relate to PGHD. The paper simulates EHR logs data since real logs are highly confidential. The simulated logs have normal accesses and some anomalous accesses imitating attackers. For role classification, Decision Tree and Random Forest perform best with 0.89 accuracy. For anomaly detection, all methods have high recall but low precision. Soft classification works better than hard classification. Bernoulli Naive Bayes on non-normalized data performs best with F1-score of 0.893 for anomaly detection. The high recall means the methods can help narrow down data for further investigation of anomalies by hospital IT staff. Future work is needed to better distinguish between anomalies and true malicious events. More comparisons on real data could also help. The paper proposes an anomaly detection method to detect potentially illegitimate access to patient records in electronic health records (EHR) systems. The method uses machine learning algorithms to classify user activities into roles. It then detects anomalies by comparing a user's daily activity to the expected activity for their role. Several machine learning algorithms are evaluated including Naive Bayes, SVM, Neural Networks, KNN, Logistic Regression, Random Forest, and Decision Trees.

(d) Encrypt Data at Rest and in Transit: Encryption can protect PGHD from being intercepted or accessed by unauthorized individuals. Shaik et al. [81] presents a novel cryptographic algorithm designed to secure unencrypted non-data database files both at rest and in transit. Recognizing the vulnerability of non-data files, which are often overlooked by standard encryption methods like Transparent Data Encryption (TDE), the authors propose a two-level encryption logic that incorporates a passcode lock, ensuring that file owners maintain complete control over their encryption. This approach addresses the security and compliance shortcomings of third-party encryption tools by providing a robust, in-house solution for protecting sensitive database information from unauthorized access. The practical application of this algorithm is validated with real-world results, showcasing its effectiveness in enhancing the security of database files beyond the capabilities of existing methods.

(e) Secure Mobile Devices: Many healthcare providers use mobile devices in their work, and also the patient uses the mobile devices to collect PGHD these can be a potential security risk if not properly secured. Vrhovec et al. [82] examines the proliferation of mobile devices in healthcare and the consequent security risks, noting that 44% of data breaches in healthcare are linked to mobile device use. It highlights the benefits of mobile devices, such as improved healthcare worker coordination and reduced data redundancy, while also addressing the significant security challenges posed by rapid technology adoption, including device theft, insecure applications, and inadequate security management. To mitigate these risks, the paper recommends establishing comprehensive security management practices, including administrative measures, physical security, secure data exchange, continuous adaptation to technological changes, and particularly emphasizes the importance of training and raising awareness among healthcare workers about the secure use of mobile devices.

(f) Mitigate Connected Device Risks: Devices that are connected to the internet can be vulnerable to hacking, so steps should be taken to mitigate these risks. To mitigate the risks associated with connected medical devices Yaqoob et al. [83] explain a multifaceted approach is essential. This includes understanding and addressing programming issues in legacy devices, adhering to FDA regulations by reviewing pre-market submissions for safety and security, and implementing robust access control mechanisms. Additionally, the development of lightweight secure algorithms is crucial for resource-constrained implantable and wearable devices to prevent attacks that compromise confidentiality, integrity, and availability. Attestation-based architectures are also recommended to protect against run-time attacks that exploit programming vulnerabilities. Furthermore, ongoing research and development are imperative to analyze and improve upon current countermeasures, ensuring the security of these critical devices in the face of sophisticated cyber threats. Communication technologies and standards must be scrutinized for security features, with a focus on both wireless and wired technologies used by these medical devices.

(g) Conduct Regular Risk Assessments: Regular assessments can help identify any potential weaknesses or vulnerabilities in the system. Yaqoob et al. [84] implementation of the Integrated Security, Safety, and Privacy (ISSP) Risk Assessment Framework for medical devices involves a systematic approach that includes identifying security vulnerabilities and safety-related bugs, considering past issues, and predicting future ones. The framework uses FDA recalls considering past software/electrical/mechanical (SW/EM/UI) issues and predicts their impact on patient safety. It also incorporates the Common Vulnerability Scoring System (CVSS) to assess security vulnerabilities and FDA recalls evaluating SW/EM/UI failures. The framework calculates the ISSP risk of medical devices by considering the unified impact of safety, security, and privacy risks on patient well-being. It suggests appropriate security controls with respect to the device's classification, addressing vulnerabilities that could affect patient privacy and health. The framework is compared against NIST best practices, ISO standards, and FDA guidance documents, demonstrating its systematic approach to determining security, privacy, and safety risks and suggesting security controls relative to the device's class. For further details on the implementation steps, the document outlines the important steps of the ISSP framework, which are exhibited in a figure within the document and discussed in subsequent sections. This includes the identification of events that trigger hazards and threats, analysis of available controls required by regulatory bodies for device approval, and the emphasis on the criticality and sensitivity of data and information. The framework is validated using a case scenario of an infusion pump and is evaluated by comparing it to current practices, showing that it provides a unified approach to considering different types of risks associated with medical devices.

(h) Educate Healthcare Staff: The human element remains one of the biggest threats to security across all industries, this is also case in the healthcare field. Nifakos et al. [85] outlines the importance of educating healthcare staff to reduce security threats through a combination of strategies. It emphasizes the need for collaborative and standardized training programs and awareness campaigns that inform on the nature and types of cyber threats. Emphasis is placed on maintaining cyber hygiene and information governance through mandatory training, which is crucial for understanding risks, particularly regarding information leakage on social media. The document also highlights the effectiveness of tailored training programs and simulation exercises for management executives to underscore the often-overlooked importance of cybersecurity compared to other emergencies. Best practices recommended by healthcare experts should be widely promoted among all healthcare stakeholders, and there is a call for the development of formal training and educational standards to address human factors in cybersecurity. Additionally, it is suggested that IT systems should be adept at detecting social engineering attacks, while healthcare professionals should be equipped with the knowledge to recognize such threats. The document concludes that there is a critical need for a systematic methodology to harmonize research findings for objective evaluation by cybersecurity experts in the healthcare industry.

In addition to these, it's important to consider the integration of PGHD into electronic health records (EHRs).This process is still in its early stages, and efforts are needed to understand how to optimize PGHD integration into EHRs considering resources, standards for EHR delivery, and clinical workflows.It's also crucial to develop a secure architecture compatible with the EHR vendor proprietary non-FHIR web services.

5.6. RQS2: In What Ways May Healthcare Providers and Technology Developers Engage in Collaborative Efforts to Achieve an Ideal Equilibrium between the Value of PGHD and the Safeguarding of Data Privacy and Security?

The research suggests various ways in which healthcare providers and technology developers can collaborate to balance the value of PGHD with data privacy and security:

(a) Integration of PGHD into Clinical Care: PGHD collected through technical applications can provide deeper insight into a patient's condition and health between clinic visits, which can lead to more accurate patient information and revised care plans for improved health goal achievement. This can also reduce unnecessary clinic visits [6].

(b) Overcoming Barriers: While wearable devices and mobile health apps allow individuals to collect PGHD outside of healthcare encounters, which can improve patient-provider communication and engagement, significant barriers include data validity, actionability, and the burden of integrating PGHD into existing care processes [7].

(c) Data Sharing and Anonymity: Healthcare organizations can collaborate to disclose significant quantities of personal biomedical data without violating anonymity, which suggests that data privacy can be maintained while sharing valuable health data [86].

(d) Privacy and Public Benefits: Analysis of real-world data can offer stakeholders practical protocols/guidelines for publicizing patient information and design implications for future systems, such as automatic privacy sensitivity checking, to strike a balance between privacy and public benefits [87].

(e) Patient Concerns and Health System Challenges: Health systems face challenges related to lack of reimbursement, data quality, and clinical usefulness of PGHD. Patients have concerns about data security and the value of reporting, which must be addressed [3].

(f) Governance Framework: To strengthen the social license for data sharing, conditions such as value, privacy, risk minimization, data security, transparency, control, information, trust, responsibility, and accountability must be operationalized in a governance framework [88].

(g) Routine Data Sharing: Doctors routinely share health data electronically under HIPAA, and sharing with patients and patients' third-party health apps should be just as routine, provided it is consistent with privacy regulations [89].

(h) Privacy-Preserving Data Aggregation: A privacy-preserving health data aggregation scheme can securely collect health data from multiple sources and guarantee fair incentives for contributing patients [90].

(i) Ethics and Privacy Framework: An integrated approach to ethics and privacy can help achieve consensus on privacy and ethics principles, which could accelerate health data access in data-driven research projects [91].

(j) Research Directions for Privacy Concerns: There is a need for research directions for techniques and mechanisms to address patient's data privacy concerns in cloud-assisted healthcare systems [92].

(k) EHR Integration Efforts: Mobile health app developers should examine PGHD information needs to inform Electronic Health Record (EHR) integration efforts [93].

(l) Policy Considerations for Interoperability: Policy considerations for improving specific aspects of health information's interoperability while preserving patient data privacy and security are necessary [94].

These findings indicate that a multi-faceted approach involving technical, ethical, legal, and policy considerations is essential for the successful integration of PGHD while ensuring data privacy and security.

5.7. RQF1: How Can PGHD Prepare for the Upcoming Security and Privacy Problems Brought on by the Widespread Adoption of AI and ML in Healthcare?

Below the Table 7 includes more detailed descriptions focusing specifically on PGHD and security measures for AI and ML applications in healthcare:

Table 7. Basic Security Measures for PGHD.

Security Measure	Detailed Description
Data Collection Policies [95]	Establish comprehensive policies that govern the collection of PGHD, ensuring that all data types, collection methods, and data flows are well-defined and documented. These policies should also dictate the lifecycle of the data from collection to deletion, including use cases for AI and ML applications.
Consent and Transparency [23]	Implement mechanisms to obtain explicit patient consent for the use of their PGHD in AI and ML applications, providing transparency regarding the purpose of data collection, processing, and sharing. This involves clear communication with patients about their data rights and the measures in place to protect their privacy.
Secure Data Transmission [96]	Utilize end-to-end encryption methods to secure the transmission of PGHD from patients' devices to healthcare systems. This ensures that data remains confidential and is protected against interception or unauthorized access during transmission.
Robust Authentication [77]	Apply strong authentication measures to verify the identity of patients and healthcare providers accessing PGHD. This might include the use of multi-factor authentication (MFA), biometric verification, or unique patient identifiers.
Data Minimization [3]	Collect only the PGHD that is necessary for specific AI and ML healthcare applications. This approach minimizes the volume of sensitive data that could be compromised in a breach and limits exposure to only essential elements.
Data Storage Security [97]	Secure the storage of PGHD with encryption and other protective measures. Ensure that databases and storage environments adhere to health industry security standards and best practices, such as using encrypted databases and secure cloud services with health data compliance certifications.
Endpoint Security [98]	Strengthen the security of patient-owned devices that generate PGHD, including mobile phones, wearables, and home monitoring devices. This may involve the deployment of security software, regular security updates, and secure configuration guides for patients.
Network Security [99]	Deploy comprehensive network security solutions, including firewalls, intrusion detection/prevention systems, and secure Wi-Fi protocols, to protect the networks over which PGHD is transmitted. Regularly monitor network traffic for anomalies and conduct penetration tests to detect vulnerabilities.
Data Anonymization [100]	When using PGHD for AI and ML training, apply data anonymization techniques to remove or obfuscate personal identifiers, reducing the risk of patient re-identification. This can involve techniques such as differential privacy, where "noise" is added to the data to prevent individual identification while still maintaining the data's utility for analysis and model training.
Regular Security Audits [84]	Perform periodic security audits and risk assessments on systems handling PGHD to ensure compliance with policies and to identify any new threats or vulnerabilities. This can help in proactively addressing security gaps and updating defenses accordingly.
Data Integrity Checks [24]	Implement checksums, digital signatures, and other data validation methods to ensure the integrity of PGHD throughout its lifecycle. This helps in detecting any unauthorized alterations or corruption of data, which is crucial for the accuracy and reliability of AI and ML outputs.
Secure Application Development [101]	Adhere to secure software development life cycle (SDLC) practices when developing AI and ML applications that process PGHD. This includes regular code reviews, security testing, and the incorporation of security by design principles to minimize vulnerabilities in applications that will handle sensitive health data.

Table 7. *Cont.*

Security Measure	Detailed Description
Disaster Recovery and Business Continuity [84]	Develop and maintain comprehensive disaster recovery and business continuity plans to ensure the resilience of systems managing PGHD. These plans should provide for the rapid restoration of data and services in the event of an incident, with minimal disruption to healthcare services and patient care.
Legal and Regulatory Compliance [23]	Stay informed and compliant with all relevant legislation and regulations concerning PGHD, such as HIPAA, HITECH, GDPR, and other regional data protection and privacy laws. Compliance should be continuously monitored and updated in response to legislative changes, especially those related to the use of PGHD in AI and ML applications.
Training and Awareness [85]	Regularly conduct comprehensive training programs for all stakeholders involved in the collection and processing of PGHD, including healthcare professionals, IT staff, and patients. This training should focus on the importance of data security, privacy best practices, and the proper use of AI and ML applications in healthcare.

These detailed measures provide a framework for securing PGHD in the context of AI and ML in healthcare, ensuring that as technology advances, patient privacy and data integrity remain at the forefront of healthcare initiatives.

Also, we include more of those advanced security measures in the context of securing PGHD for AI and ML applications in healthcare in the Table 8 below:

Table 8. Advanced Security Measures for PGHD.

Security Measure	Detailed Description
Federated Learning [102]	Implement federated learning to train AI models on decentralized data. In this approach, the data remains on the patient's device or local server, and only model updates are shared to a central server for aggregation. This reduces the amount of PGHD transferred and stored centrally, thus minimizing exposure and enhancing privacy.
Blockchain Technology [62]	Utilize blockchain technology to create a secure, immutable ledger of transactions related to PGHD. This can be used to manage consent, track data access, and ensure data integrity. Since blockchain records are tamper-evident and decentralized, they provide a robust framework to audit and verify the provenance and handling of PGHD, ensuring transparency and trust in the system.
Homomorphic Encryption [103,104]	Apply homomorphic encryption to allow computation on encrypted PGHD, enabling AI and ML analysis without decrypting sensitive data. This type of encryption allows data to remain encrypted even during the analysis process, greatly reducing the risk of data exposure. AI models can be trained and refined using encrypted data, thus preserving patient privacy throughout the AI lifecycle.
Secure Multi-party Computation [105]	Engage in secure multi-party computation (SMPC) protocols to enable a group of parties to jointly compute a function over their inputs while keeping those inputs private. This could allow for collaborative AI model training or data analysis on PGHD without exposing individual patient data to any of the involved parties, including the model trainer.
Differential Privacy [106]	Incorporate differential privacy techniques in the data analysis and AI training processes to add statistical noise to PGHD. This approach ensures that the output of the analysis or the behavior of the trained model does not reveal sensitive information about any individual, thereby providing a quantifiable level of privacy.
Zero-Knowledge Proofs [107]	Integrate zero-knowledge proof systems to enable the verification of data integrity and authenticity without revealing the underlying data. This can be particularly useful in verifying patient identities and the authenticity of PGHD without exposing the actual data, ensuring that only necessary data is processed and reducing the risk of privacy breaches.
Advanced Persistent Threat (APT) Protection [108]	Adopt APT protection strategies to defend against sophisticated, prolonged cyber-attacks aimed at stealing data. This involves a combination of advanced security technologies and practices such as network segmentation, behavioral analytics, threat intelligence, and proactive hunting for threats to protect PGHD and the systems that process it.

Table 8. *Cont.*

Security Measure	Detailed Description
AI Security Audits [109]	Conduct specialized security audits focusing on the AI components involved in processing PGHD, examining the model's robustness against adversarial attacks, data poisoning, and other AI-specific threats. This also includes ensuring the AI system's transparency and explainability, which is vital for trust and compliance in healthcare applications.
Decentralized Identity Management [110]	Deploy decentralized identity management systems that give patients control over their digital identities and the sharing of their PGHD. Such systems can employ blockchain technology and support selective disclosure, allowing patients to prove certain aspects of their identity or health data without revealing more information than necessary.
Continuous Security Monitoring [111]	Establish continuous security monitoring practices, using advanced security information and event management (SIEM) systems, to detect and respond to anomalies in real time. This is crucial to protect the integrity of PGHD during collection, storage, and processing for AI and ML applications.

5.8. RQF2: How May the Next Decade's Development of Wearable Technology and Internet of Medical Things Devices Affect the Current State of PGHD Security and Privacy Concerns?

The development of wearable technology and Internet of Medical Things (IoMT) devices over the next decade is likely to have a significant impact on PGHD security and privacy concerns in several ways:

(a) Increased Data Volume [26]: As wearable technology becomes more prevalent, the volume of PGHD will increase exponentially. This will pose greater challenges in securing the data against unauthorized access and ensuring privacy, as there will be more data points and potentially more sensitive information available.

(b) Advanced Data Analytics [21,37]: With more data, there will be a push for advanced analytics to make sense of the information. This could lead to the development of more sophisticated algorithms for data processing, which could either strengthen data security (by identifying and mitigating breaches more quickly) or create new vulnerabilities (if the algorithms themselves are not secure).

(c) Improved Security Measures [77–79,81]: The rise in security threats could drive innovation in security technologies. We might see the development of more robust encryption methods, secure data transmission protocols, and advanced user authentication processes specifically designed for wearable and IoMT devices.

(d) Regulatory Evolution [23]: As technology advances, regulations and standards will need to keep pace. This could mean new or updated legislation around data protection specific to health data generated by wearables and IoMT devices, which could help address privacy concerns.

(e) Public Awareness and Education [85]: With the proliferation of these devices, consumers may become more aware of the potential risks to their data. This could lead to increased public demand for better security and privacy protections, which in turn could pressure manufacturers and service providers to prioritize these concerns.

(f) Integration Challenges [24,25,27,53,58]: As wearables and IoMT devices become more integrated with other healthcare systems, the complexity of ensuring end-to-end security and privacy protections increases. There will be a need for standardized protocols and interoperability frameworks that can maintain security and privacy across different platforms and devices.

(g) Ethical and Legal Implications [6,23]: The next decade may also bring to the forefront ethical questions about data ownership, consent for data use, and the balance between individual privacy and public health benefits. This could reshape the landscape of PGHD security and privacy concerns, leading to new legal precedents and ethical guidelines.

(h) Market-Driven Solutions [95]: As competition in the wearable technology and IoMT space intensifies, companies may differentiate themselves through superior privacy and security features. This could lead to market-driven improvements in PGHD security and privacy.

(i) Personalization of Security [112]: There may be a trend towards personalized security settings, where users can set their own preferences for data sharing and privacy, giving them more control over their PGHD.

(j) Global Disparities [73]: The impact on PGHD security and privacy concerns will likely be uneven across the globe, with disparities in technological advancement, regulatory environments, and public awareness affecting how these issues are addressed.

It's important to note that these are projections, and the actual impact will depend on a variety of factors, including technological breakthroughs, market dynamics, regulatory changes, and shifts in consumer behavior.

6. Discussion

Research Questions Discussion

RQE1 [7,27,34,59,66,67,95] helps to identify the major sources of PGHD include mobile health applications, wearable devices, patient portals and personal health records, remote monitoring sensors/IOM devices, virtual/mixed reality systems, social media platforms, validated assessments, and patient diaries. Patients are using these technologies to collect, track and share various health metrics with providers, spanning symptoms, lifestyle behaviors, physiological data, and customized patient-reported outcomes. Healthcare systems are increasingly using PGHD to enable patient self-monitoring/management, facilitate continuous care between visits, capture patient perspectives to personalize treatment plans, support clinical decision making with more comprehensive data, assessing outcomes, informing system design, promoting patient engagement, and advance clinical research including treatment effectiveness and precision medicine efforts. While PGHD integration offers innovations in research and care delivery, open questions remain around ensuring data quality, system interoperability, and appropriate use regulations.

RQE2 [3,7,68–71] focuses on exploring how patients view the collection and use of their PGHD. Insights from interviews conducted by various researchers reveal that patient perspectives encompass multiple aspects, which include:

- Motivation and Barriers: Patients collect PGHD to improve self-awareness, manage their health, assess treatment effectiveness, provide reasons for changes in medications, and collaborate with healthcare professionals. However, they face challenges in discerning clinically relevant data and dealing with obstacles such as short appointment durations and varying levels of clinician engagement.
- Selective Sharing: When deciding to share PGHD, patients weigh factors such as the healthcare provider's interest, the relevance to care, and time constraints during appointments. If they perceive a lack of receptiveness from providers, patients may withhold information or seek alternative healthcare professionals.
- Impact on Patient Engagement: Using PGHD can make patients feel more involved, empowered and reassured about their health management. It also improves their understanding, memory, communication with physicians, and responsibility for health outcomes.
- Perceptions and Concerns: Patients acknowledge the benefits of PGHD but also express significant worries about privacy, the process of data submission, understanding of PGHD use, and the trade-off between benefits and intrusiveness. Addressing these concerns is crucial for enhancing patient engagement.
- Familiarity and Willingness to Share: Initially, patients may be unfamiliar with the uses of PGHD but tend to become more open to sharing it once they comprehend its objectives, especially when motivated by the potential to aid others. Confidentiality is a key concern, and patients often expect reciprocal access to information.

In conclusion, while patients recognize the potential advantages of PGHD, they also identify significant challenges related to the process, privacy, communication, and mutual benefits. These issues must be resolved to foster more effective and sustained patient engagement and use of PGHD.

RQI2 [6,35,73–76] emphasize the incorporation of PGHD and its understanding from sources like mobile apps and wearables has wide-ranging impacts on healthcare decision-making. PGHD provides more comprehensive, real-time data about patients' health and experiences, enabling more informed, personalized, and timely treatment decisions. It also facilitates continuous remote monitoring, allowing earlier interventions for better outcomes. While promising, utilizing PGHD poses some challenges regarding privacy, accuracy, integration into clinical workflows, and avoiding marginalization of disadvantaged groups. However, overall PGHD is transforming decision-making to be more patient-centered and collaborative. Through participatory tracking and data sharing, patients are empowered in managing their health. Meanwhile clinicians gain fuller understanding of patients for tailored care plans. Effective policies must balance maximizing PGHD's benefits for decision quality while minimizing potential harms.

RQS1 [76–85] explores several important strategies that can help safeguard the security and privacy of PGHD. These include restricting data access to authorized personnel only, implementing robust data usage controls, maintaining audit trails to monitor data access, encrypting data at rest and in transit, securing mobile devices used to collect PGHD, mitigating risks associated with connected devices, conducting regular risk assessments to identify vulnerabilities, educating healthcare staff about security protocols, and carefully considering how to integrate PGHD into electronic medical record systems. Employing a multilayered approach that encompasses technological solutions, strong policies, and human accountability can help provide comprehensive protection for sensitive patient information.

RQS2 [3,6,7,86–94] investigates how healthcare providers and technology developers can collaborate effectively to balance the value of PGHD with the safeguarding of data privacy and security. The research identifies multiple approaches for this: integrating PGHD into clinical care for more accurate patient information and improved health goals; addressing barriers like data validity and integration challenges; maintaining data privacy while sharing valuable health data; developing practical protocols for balancing privacy with public benefits; addressing patient concerns and health system challenges regarding data security and the usefulness of PGHD; creating a governance framework that operationalizes value, privacy, and risk minimization; making routine data sharing with patients and their apps as common as current health data exchanges; implementing privacy-preserving data aggregation schemes; adopting an integrated approach to ethics and privacy in health data; researching techniques to address privacy concerns in cloud-assisted healthcare; focusing on PGHD integration in Electronic Health Records (EHRs); and considering policies for improving health information interoperability. This multi-faceted approach requires technical, ethical, legal, and policy considerations for successful PGHD integration while ensuring data privacy and security.

RQF1 distinctly highlights the security measure that could arise from the extensive use of AI and ML in healthcare. In this context, we have pinpointed a range of security measures, varying from basic [3,23,24,77,84,85,95–101] to advanced [62,102–111], which can be effectively implemented to ensure the secure usage and management of PGHD. RQF2 [6,21,23–27,37,53,58,73,77–79,81,85,95,112] suggests that the development of wearable devices and internet-connected medical devices over the next decade will profoundly impact PGHD security and privacy. Key influences include a massive increase in PGHD volume, advanced data analytics, improved security measures, new regulations, greater public awareness, systems integration challenges, ethical implications, market-driven solutions, personalized security settings, and global disparities. While projections are uncertain, it is likely the confluence of technological, regulatory, and societal changes will reshape how PGHD security and privacy concerns are addressed. Companies and policymakers should proactively develop robust, flexible frameworks to keep pace with these expected changes.

7. Conclusions

In conclusion, the evolving landscape of PGHD that ranges from social media data to physiological data presents both transformative opportunities and significant challenges in the realm of healthcare. The substantial increase in the variety and interconnectedness of the patient-generated data, which are seen as PGHD, improves the ability to predict individual behaviors, health conditions, and diseases. But in many countries, laws particularly safeguard health-related data, recognizing its sensitivity. The current extensive integration of diverse data sets, which can include a wide range of data landscapes, has the potential to reclassify data not traditionally viewed as health-related into sensitive health information [113]. The integration of PGHD into healthcare models also offers profound benefits, including enhanced patient engagement, improved accuracy of health records, and more personalized care. However, this integration is not without its complexities, particularly with regard to the security and privacy of sensitive health data. The key challenges identified include ensuring the authenticity and accuracy of PGHD, seamlessly integrating these data into existing healthcare systems, and addressing the substantial privacy and security concerns associated with digital health data. The article underscores the critical need for robust security measures, including end-to-end encryption, secure data transmission protocols, and stringent access controls, to safeguard against unauthorized access and cyber threats. Furthermore, the article highlights the importance of developing comprehensive privacy frameworks and governance models that prioritize patient consent and transparency. This includes the need for continuous adaptation to emerging technologies like AI and machine learning, which require novel approaches to data security and privacy. To optimize the value of PGHD while protecting patient privacy and data integrity, a collaborative effort is required among stakeholders, including healthcare providers, technology developers, policy makers and patients themselves. This involves not only technological solutions but also ethical, legal, and policy considerations. The dynamic nature of PGHD, coupled with the rapid advancement of technology, requires ongoing research and development in this field. Future directions should focus on developing innovative security techniques, exploring new models for effective data integration, and continuously updating regulatory frameworks to keep pace with technological advancements. In essence, the successful and secure integration of PGHD into healthcare models hinges on a multifaceted approach that combines technological innovation with strong policy frameworks, ethical considerations, and active stakeholder engagement. This approach will be crucial to realize the full potential of PGHD in enhancing healthcare delivery and patient outcomes while maintaining the highest standards of data privacy and security.

Author Contributions: Conceptualization and Writing—original draft by P.K., Writing—review & editing by B.Y., J.-C.L. and B.B. All authors have read and agreed to the published version of the manuscript.

Funding: This work has been carried out in the context of the research project Digi Remote and Health Democratization, funded by the Research Council of Norway in the IKTPLUSS program, grant number 310137 and 288856.

Institutional Review Board Statement: Not Applicable. The current study did not involve humans or animals.

Informed Consent Statement: Not applicable. The current study did not involve humans.

Data Availability Statement: Data not available. The current study did not generate any new data.

Acknowledgments: We utilize writing tools such as Grammarly and Writefull to refine our writing, grammar check, and strengthen our English language for this article, striving to improve proficiency and accuracy.

Conflicts of Interest: The authors declare no conflict of interest.

References

1. Khatiwada, P.; Yang, B. *An Overview on Security and Privacy of Data in IoMT Devices: Performance Metrics, Merits, Demerits, and Challenges*; pHealth: Oslo, Norway, 2022; pp. 126–136.
2. Hunt, L.M.; Bell, H.S.; Baker, A.M.; Howard, H.A. Electronic health records and the disappearing patient. *Med. Anthropol. Q.* **2017**, *31*, 403–421. [CrossRef]
3. Adler-Milstein, J.; Nong, P. Early experiences with patient-generated health data: Health system and patient perspectives. *J. Am. Med. Inform. Assoc.* **2019**, *26*, 952–959. [CrossRef] [PubMed]
4. Korjian, S.; Gibson, C.M. Digital technologies and the democratization of clinical research: Social media, wearables, and artificial intelligence. *Contemp. Clin. Trials* **2022**, *117*, 106767. [CrossRef] [PubMed]
5. Medina, S.G.; Isomursu, M. The Use of Patient-Generated Health Data From Consumer-Grade Mobile Devices in Clinical Workflows: Protocol for a Systematic Review. *JMIR Res. Protoc.* **2023**, *12*, e39389. [CrossRef] [PubMed]
6. Cohen, D.J.; Keller, S.R.; Hayes, G.R.; Dorr, D.A.; Ash, J.S.; Sittig, D.F. Integrating patient-generated health data into clinical care settings or clinical decision-making: Lessons learned from project healthdesign. *JMIR Hum. Factors* **2016**, *3*, e5919. [CrossRef] [PubMed]
7. Lavallee, D.C.; Lee, J.R.; Austin, E.; Bloch, R.; Lawrence, S.O.; McCall, D.; Munson, S.A.; Nery-Hurwit, M.B.; Amtmann, D. mHealth and patient-generated health data: Stakeholder perspectives on opportunities and barriers for transforming healthcare. *Mhealth* **2020**, *6*, 8. [CrossRef] [PubMed]
8. US Health and Human Services. Consumer eHealth: Patient-Generated Health Data. Available online: https://www.healthit.gov/topic/scientific-initiatives/pcor/patient-generated-health-data-pghd (accessed on 9 October 2023).
9. McGinnis, J.M.; Olsen, L.A.; Goolsby, W.A.; Grossmann, C. *Clinical Data as the Basic Staple of Health Learning: Creating and Protecting a Public Good: Workshop Summary*; National Academies Press: Washington, DC, USA, 2011.
10. Zeng, N.; Gao, Z. Health wearable devices and physical activity promotion. In *Technology in Physical Activity and Health Promotion*; Taylor & Francis: London, UK, 2017; pp. 148–164.
11. Muhammad Sayem, A.S.; Hon Teay, S.; Shahariar, H.; Luise Fink, P.; Albarbar, A. Review on smart electro-clothing systems (SeCSs). *Sensors* **2020**, *20*, 587. [CrossRef]
12. Martin, R.L.; Irrgang, J.J. A survey of self-reported outcome instruments for the foot and ankle. *J. Orthop. Sport. Phys. Ther.* **2007**, *37*, 72–84. [CrossRef]
13. Liu, L.; Stroulia, E.; Nikolaidis, I.; Miguel-Cruz, A.; Rincon, A.R. Smart homes and home health monitoring technologies for older adults: A systematic review. *Int. J. Med. Inform.* **2016**, *91*, 44–59. [CrossRef]
14. El Amrani, L.; Engberink, A.O.; Ninot, G.; Hayot, M.; Carbonnel, F. Connected health devices for health care in French general medicine practice: Cross-sectional study. *JMIR MHealth UHealth* **2017**, *5*, e7427. [CrossRef]
15. Brown, R.; Coventry, L.; Sillence, E.; Blythe, J.; Stumpf, S.; Bird, J.; Durrant, A.C. Collecting and sharing self-generated health and lifestyle data: Understanding barriers for people living with long-term health conditions—A survey study. *Digit. Health* **2022**, *8*, 20552076221084458. [CrossRef] [PubMed]
16. Rahi, P.; Sood, S.P.; Bajaj, R.; Kumar, Y. Air quality monitoring for Smart eHealth system using firefly optimization and support vector machine. *Int. J. Inf. Technol.* **2021**, *13*, 1847–1859. [CrossRef]
17. Alshaikh, F.; Ramzan, F.; Rawaf, S.; Majeed, A. Social network sites as a mode to collect health data: A systematic review. *J. Med. Internet Res.* **2014**, *16*, e171. [CrossRef] [PubMed]
18. Trifan, A.; Oliveira, M.; Oliveira, J.L. Passive sensing of health outcomes through smartphones: Systematic review of current solutions and possible limitations. *JMIR MHealth UHealth* **2019**, *7*, e12649. [CrossRef]
19. Tricoli, A.; Nasiri, N.; De, S. Wearable and miniaturized sensor technologies for personalized and preventive medicine. *Adv. Funct. Mater.* **2017**, *27*, 1605271. [CrossRef]
20. Kashani, M.H.; Madanipour, M.; Nikravan, M.; Asghari, P.; Mahdipour, E. A systematic review of IoT in healthcare: Applications, techniques, and trends. *J. Netw. Comput. Appl.* **2021**, *192*, 103164. [CrossRef]
21. Wang, C.; He, T.; Zhou, H.; Zhang, Z.; Lee, C. Artificial intelligence enhanced sensors-enabling technologies to next-generation healthcare and biomedical platform. *Bioelectron. Med.* **2023**, *9*, 17. [CrossRef]
22. Ilhan, A.; Fietkiewicz, K.J. Learning for a healthier lifestyle through gamification: A case study of fitness tracker applications. In *Perspectives on Wearable Enhanced Learning (WELL) Current Trends, Research, and Practice*; Springer: Cham, Switzerland, 2019; pp. 333–364.
23. Winter, J.S.; Davidson, E. Harmonizing regulatory regimes for the governance of patient-generated health data. *Telecommun. Policy* **2022**, *46*, 102285. [CrossRef]
24. Webber, C.M.; Riberdy Hammer, A.; Saha, A.; Marinac-Dabic, D.; Caños, D.A.; Tarver, M.E. Integrating Patient-Generated Health Data Throughout the Total Product Life Cycle of Medical Devices. *Ther. Innov. Regul. Sci.* **2023**, *57*, 952–956. [CrossRef]
25. Blondon, K.; Ehrler, F. Integrating patient-generated health data in an electronic medical record: Stakeholders' perspectives. In *Integrated Citizen Centered Digital Health and Social Care*; IOS Press: Amsterdam, The Netherlands, 2020; pp. 12–16.
26. Codella, J.; Partovian, C.; Chang, H.Y.; Chen, C.H. Data quality challenges for person-generated health and wellness data. *IBM J. Res. Dev.* **2018**, *62*, 3:1–3:8. [CrossRef]
27. Kawu, A.A.; Hederman, L.; O'Sullivan, D.; Doyle, J. Patient-generated health data and electronic health record integration, governance and socio-technical issues: A narrative review. *Inform. Med. Unlocked* **2022**, *37*, 101153. [CrossRef]

28. Huang, Y.; Upadhyay, U.; Dhar, E.; Kuo, L.J.; Syed-Abdul, S. A Scoping Review to Assess Adherence to and Clinical Outcomes of Wearable Devices in the Cancer Population. *Cancers* **2022**, *14*, 4371. [CrossRef] [PubMed]
29. Abdolkhani, R.; Gray, K.; Borda, A.; DeSouza, R. Patient-generated health data management and quality challenges in remote patient monitoring. *JAMIA Open* **2019**, *2*, 471–478. [CrossRef] [PubMed]
30. Krist, A.H.; Tong, S.T.; Aycock, R.A.; Longo, D.R. Engaging patients in decision-making and behavior change to promote prevention. *Inf. Serv. Use* **2017**, *37*, 105–122. [CrossRef]
31. Omoloja, A.; Vundavalli, S. Patient-generated health data: Benefits and challenges. *Curr. Probl. Pediatr. Adolesc. Health Care* **2021**, *51*, 101103. [CrossRef]
32. Blondon, K.; Ehrler, F. Design Considerations for the Use of Patient-Generated Health Data in the Electronic Medical Records. In *Challenges of Trustable AI and Added-Value on Health*; IOS Press: Amsterdam, The Netherlands, 2022; p. 229.
33. Wilson, J.; Heinsch, M.; Betts, D.; Booth, D.; Kay-Lambkin, F. Barriers and facilitators to the use of e-health by older adults: A scoping review. *BMC Public Health* **2021**, *21*, 1–12. [CrossRef]
34. Petersen, C.; DeMuro, P. Legal and regulatory considerations associated with use of patient-generated health data from social media and mobile health (mHealth) devices. *Appl. Clin. Inform.* **2015**, *6*, 16–26.
35. Petersen, C. Use of patient-generated health data for shared decision-making in the clinical environment: Ready for prime time. *Mhealth* **2021**, *7*, 39. [CrossRef]
36. Wu, D.T.; Xin, C.; Bindhu, S.; Xu, C.; Sachdeva, J.; Brown, J.L.; Jung, H. Clinician perspectives and design implications in using patient-generated health data to improve mental health practices: Mixed methods study. *JMIR Form. Res.* **2020**, *4*, e18123. [CrossRef]
37. Nagpal, M.S.; Barbaric, A.; Sherifali, D.; Morita, P.P.; Cafazzo, J.A. Patient-Generated Data Analytics of Health Behaviors of People Living With Type 2 Diabetes: Scoping Review. *JMIR Diabetes* **2021**, *6*, e29027. [CrossRef]
38. Park, Y.R.; Lee, Y.; Kim, J.Y.; Kim, J.; Kim, H.R.; Kim, Y.H.; Kim, W.S.; Lee, J.H. Managing patient-generated health data through mobile personal health records: Analysis of usage data. *JMIR MHealth UHealth* **2018**, *6*, e9620. [CrossRef] [PubMed]
39. Kim, K.K.; Jalil, S.; Ngo, V. Improving self-management and care coordination with person-generated health data and mobile health. In *Consumer Informatics and Digital Health: Solutions for Health and Health Care*; Springer: Cham, Switzerland, 2019; pp. 221–243.
40. International Association of Privacy Professionals. Wearables: Where Do They Fall within the Regulatory Landscape? Available online: https://iapp.org/news/a/wearables-where-do-they-fall-within-the-regulatory-landscape/ (accessed on 13 November 2023).
41. Insights, D. Wearable Technology in Healthcare. Available online: https://www2.deloitte.com/us/en/insights/industry/technology/wearable-technology-healthcare-data.html (accessed on 13 November 2023).
42. EU Data Europa. Patient-Generated Health Data. Available online: https://data.europa.eu/en/news-events/news/patient-generated-health-data (accessed on 13 November 2023).
43. Raghavan, A.; Demircioglu, M.A.; Taeihagh, A. Public health innovation through cloud adoption: A comparative analysis of drivers and barriers in Japan, South Korea, and Singapore. *Int. J. Environ. Res. Public Health* **2021**, *18*, 334. [CrossRef] [PubMed]
44. Nakashima, N.; Hu, Y.; Maruf, R.I.; Ahmed, A. Personal health record in Japan, China, and Bangladesh. In *Mobile Technologies for Delivering Healthcare in Remote, Rural or Developing Regions*; Institution of Engineering and Technology: Fukuoka, Japan, 2020; pp. 165–177.
45. Seldon, H.; Moghaddasi, H.; Seo, W.J.; JoNah, S.W. Personal Health Records in SE Asia Part 2-A Digital Portable Health Record. *Electron. J. Health Inform.* **2014**, *8*, e2.
46. Group, B.C. Australia and New Zealand Digital Health Strategy. Available online: https://www.bcg.com/publications/2023/australia-and-new-zealand-digital-health-strategy (accessed on 4 January 2024).
47. Hampshire, K.; Mwase-Vuma, T.; Alemu, K.; Abane, A.; Munthali, A.; Awoke, T.; Mariwah, S.; Chamdimba, E.; Owusu, S.A.; Robson, E.; et al. Informal mhealth at scale in Africa: Opportunities and challenges. *World Dev.* **2021**, *140*, 105257. [CrossRef] [PubMed]
48. Foundation, C. Mobile Health: How Phones Are Reshaping Healthcare in Africa. Available online: https://www.cdcfoundation.org/content/mobile-health-how-phones-are-reshaping-healthcare-africa (accessed on 14 November 2023).
49. Chukwuneke, F.; Ezeonu, C.; Onyire, B.; Ezeonu, P. Culture and biomedical care in Africa: The influence of culture on biomedical care in a traditional African society, Nigeria, West Africa. *Niger. J. Med.* **2012**, *21*, 331–333. [PubMed]
50. Forecast, M.D. Latin America Smart Wearables Market. Available online: https://www.marketdataforecast.com/market-reports/latin-america-smart-wearables-market (accessed on 14 November 2023).
51. Guanais, F.; Doubova, S.V.; Leslie, H.H.; Perez-Cuevas, R.; Garcia-Elorrio, E.; Kruk, M.E. Patient-centered primary care and self-rated health in 6 Latin American and Caribbean countries: Analysis of a public opinion cross-sectional survey. *PLoS Med.* **2018**, *15*, e1002673. [CrossRef] [PubMed]
52. Shi, Q.; Yang, Y.; Sun, Z.; Lee, C. Progress of advanced devices and internet of things systems as enabling technologies for smart homes and health care. *ACS Mater. Au* **2022**, *2*, 394–435. [CrossRef]
53. Hu, V.; Chen, E.; Bridgeman, M.; Jariwala, S. Utility of Patient-Generated Health Data and Artificial Intelligence in the Prediction of Asthma Exacerbations. *J. Allergy Clin. Immunol.* **2022**, *149*, AB185. [CrossRef]

54. Melstrom, L.G.; Rodin, A.S.; Rossi, L.A.; Fu, P., Jr.; Fong, Y.; Sun, V. Patient-generated health data and electronic health record integration in oncologic surgery: A call for artificial intelligence and machine learning. *J. Surg. Oncol.* **2021**, *123*, 52–60. [CrossRef]
55. Goharinejad, S.; Goharinejad, S.; Hajesmaeel-Gohari, S.; Bahaadinbeigy, K. The usefulness of virtual, augmented, and mixed reality technologies in the diagnosis and treatment of attention deficit hyperactivity disorder in children: An overview of relevant studies. *BMC Psychiatry* **2022**, *22*, 1–13. [CrossRef]
56. Carroll, J.; Hopper, L.; Farrelly, A.M.; Lombard-Vance, R.; Bamidis, P.D.; Konstantinidis, E.I. A scoping review of augmented/virtual reality health and wellbeing interventions for older adults: Redefining immersive virtual reality. *Front. Virtual Real.* **2021**, *2*, 655338. [CrossRef]
57. Tiase, V.L.; Hull, W.; McFarland, M.M.; Sward, K.A.; Del Fiol, G.; Staes, C.; Weir, C.; Cummins, M.R. Patient-generated health data and electronic health record integration: A scoping review. *JAMIA Open* **2020**, *3*, 619–627. [CrossRef]
58. Dinh-Le, C.; Chuang, R.; Chokshi, S.; Mann, D. Wearable health technology and electronic health record integration: Scoping review and future directions. *JMIR MHealth UHealth* **2019**, *7*, e12861. [CrossRef] [PubMed]
59. Bourke, A.; Dixon, W.G.; Roddam, A.; Lin, K.J.; Hall, G.C.; Curtis, J.R.; van der Veer, S.N.; Soriano-Gabarró, M.; Mills, J.K.; Major, J.M.; et al. Incorporating patient-generated health data into pharmacoepidemiological research. *Pharmacoepidemiol. Drug Saf.* **2020**, *29*, 1540–1549. [CrossRef] [PubMed]
60. Hull, S. Patient-generated health data foundation for personalized collaborative care. *CIN Comput. Inform. Nurs.* **2015**, *33*, 177–180. [CrossRef]
61. Foster, C.; Schinasi, D.; Kan, K.; Macy, M.; Wheeler, D.; Curfman, A. Remote monitoring of patient-and family-generated health data in pediatrics. *Pediatrics* **2022**, *149*, e2021054137. [CrossRef] [PubMed]
62. Subramanian, H. A Decentralized Marketplace for Patient-Generated Health Data: Design Science Approach. *J. Med. Internet Res.* **2023**, *25*, e42743. [CrossRef]
63. Magnan, S. Social determinants of health 201 for health care: Plan, do, study, act. *NAM Perspect.* **2021**, *2021*. [CrossRef]
64. Choo, H.; Kim, M.; Choi, J.; Shin, J.; Shin, S.Y. Influenza screening via deep learning using a combination of epidemiological and patient-generated health data: Development and validation study. *J. Med. Internet Res.* **2020**, *22*, e21369. [CrossRef]
65. Moher, D.; Liberati, A.; Tetzlaff, J.; Altman, D.G.; Group PRISMA. Preferred reporting items for systematic reviews and meta-analyses: The PRISMA statement. *Int. J. Surg.* **2010**, *8*, 336–341. [CrossRef]
66. Lai, A.M.; Hsueh, P.Y.; Choi, Y.K.; Austin, R.R. Present and future trends in consumer health informatics and patient-generated health data. *Yearb. Med. Inform.* **2017**, *26*, 152–159. [CrossRef] [PubMed]
67. Nittas, V.; Lun, P.; Ehrler, F.; Puhan, M.A.; Mütsch, M. Electronic patient-generated health data to facilitate disease prevention and health promotion: Scoping review. *J. Med. Internet Res.* **2019**, *21*, e13320. [CrossRef] [PubMed]
68. Zhu, H.; Colgan, J.; Reddy, M.; Choe, E.K. Sharing patient-generated data in clinical practices: An interview study. *AMIA Annu Symp Proc.* **2016**, *2016*, 1303–1312. [PubMed]
69. Burns, K.; McBride, C.A.; Patel, B.; FitzGerald, G.; Mathews, S.; Drennan, J. Creating consumer-generated health data: Interviews and a pilot trial exploring how and why patients engage. *J. Med. Internet Res.* **2019**, *21*, e12367. [CrossRef] [PubMed]
70. Kim, B.; Ghasemi, P.; Stolee, P.; Lee, J. Clinicians and Older Adults' Perceptions of the Utility of Patient-Generated Health Data in Caring for Older Adults: Exploratory Mixed Methods Study. *JMIR Aging* **2021**, *4*, e29788. [CrossRef] [PubMed]
71. Smith, T.; Dunn, M.; Levin, K.; Tsakraklides, S.; Mitchell, S.; van de Poll-Franse, L.; Ward, K.; Wiggins, C.; Wu, X.; Hurlbert, M.; et al. Cancer survivor perspectives on sharing patient-generated health data with central cancer registries. *Qual. Life Res.* **2019**, *28*, 2957–2967. [CrossRef] [PubMed]
72. Ostherr, K.; Borodina, S.; Bracken, R.C.; Lotterman, C.; Storer, E.; Williams, B. Trust and privacy in the context of user-generated health data. *Big Data Soc.* **2017**, *4*, 2053951717704673. [CrossRef]
73. Jim, H.S.; Hoogland, A.I.; Brownstein, N.C.; Barata, A.; Dicker, A.P.; Knoop, H.; Gonzalez, B.D.; Perkins, R.; Rollison, D.; Gilbert, S.M.; et al. Innovations in research and clinical care using patient-generated health data. *CA Cancer J. Clin.* **2020**, *70*, 182–199. [CrossRef]
74. Singh, N.; Varshney, U.; Sarkar, S. Patient-Generated Health Data: Framework for Decision Making. In Proceedings of the 55th Hawaii International Conference on System Sciences, Honolulu, HI, USA, 4–7 January 2022.
75. Wood, W.A.; Bennett, A.V.; Basch, E. Emerging uses of patient-generated health data in clinical research. *Mol. Oncol.* **2015**, *9*, 1018–1024. [CrossRef]
76. Petersen, C.; Edmunds, M.; McGraw, D.; Priest, E.L.; Smith, J.R.; Kemp, E.; Campos, H. A Policy Framework to Support Shared Decision-Making through the Use of Person-Generated Health Data. *ACI Open* **2021**, *5*, e104–e115. [CrossRef]
77. Suleski, T.; Ahmed, M.; Yang, W.; Wang, E. A review of multi-factor authentication in the Internet of Healthcare Things. *Digit. Health* **2023**, *9*, 20552076231177144. [CrossRef]
78. Fareed, M.; Yassin, A.A. Privacy-preserving multi-factor authentication and role-based access control scheme for the E-healthcare system. *Bull. Electr. Eng. Inform.* **2022**, *11*, 2131–2141. [CrossRef]
79. Santhosh, B. Internet of Medical Things in Secure Assistive Technologies. In *AI-Based Digital Health Communication for Securing Assistive Systems*; IGI Global: Pennsylvania, PA, USA, 2023; pp. 244–270.
80. Yeng, P.K.; Fauzi, M.A.; Yang, B. Comparative analysis of machine learning methods for analyzing security practice in electronic health records' logs. In Proceedings of the 2020 IEEE International Conference on Big Data (Big Data), Atlanta, GA, USA, 10–13 December 2020; pp. 3856–3866.

81. Shaik, V.; Natarajan, K. Flexible and cost-effective cryptographic encryption algorithm for securing unencrypted database files at rest and in transit. *Methodsx* **2022**, *9*, 101924. [CrossRef] [PubMed]
82. Vrhovec, S.L. Challenges of mobile device use in healthcare. In Proceedings of the 2016 39th International Convention on Information and Communication Technology, Electronics and Microelectronics (MIPRO), Opatija, Croatia, 30 May–3 June 2016; pp. 1393–1396.
83. Yaqoob, T.; Abbas, H.; Atiquzzaman, M. Security vulnerabilities, attacks, countermeasures, and regulations of networked medical devices—A review. *IEEE Commun. Surv. Tutor.* **2019**, *21*, 3723–3768. [CrossRef]
84. Yaqoob, T.; Abbas, H.; Shafqat, N. Integrated security, safety, and privacy risk assessment framework for medical devices. *IEEE J. Biomed. Health Inform.* **2019**, *24*, 1752–1761. [CrossRef] [PubMed]
85. Nifakos, S.; Chandramouli, K.; Nikolaou, C.K.; Papachristou, P.; Koch, S.; Panaousis, E.; Bonacina, S. Influence of human factors on cyber security within healthcare organisations: A systematic review. *Sensors* **2021**, *21*, 5119. [CrossRef]
86. Malin, B. Secure construction of k-unlinkable patient records from distributed providers. *Artif. Intell. Med.* **2010**, *48*, 29–41. [CrossRef]
87. Jung, G.; Lee, H.; Kim, A.; Lee, U. Too much information: Assessing privacy risks of contact trace data disclosure on people with COVID-19 in South Korea. *Front. Public Health* **2020**, *8*, 305. [CrossRef]
88. Kalkman, S.; van Delden, J.; Banerjee, A.; Tyl, B.; Mostert, M.; van Thiel, G. Patients' and public views and attitudes towards the sharing of health data for research: A narrative review of the empirical evidence. *J. Med. Ethics* **2022**, *48*, 3–13. [CrossRef]
89. Savage, M.; Savage, L.C. Doctors routinely share health data electronically under HIPAA, and sharing with patients and patients' third-party health apps is consistent: Interoperability and privacy analysis. *J. Med. Internet Res.* **2020**, *22*, e19818. [CrossRef]
90. Tang, W.; Ren, J.; Deng, K.; Zhang, Y. Secure data aggregation of lightweight E-healthcare IoT devices with fair incentives. *IEEE Internet Things J.* **2019**, *6*, 8714–8726. [CrossRef]
91. Liyanage, H.; Liaw, S.T.; Di Iorio, C.; Kuziemsky, C.; Schreiber, R.; Terry, A.; de Lusignan, S. Building a privacy, ethics, and data access framework for real world computerised medical record system data: A Delphi study. *Yearb. Med. Inform.* **2016**, *25*, 138–145. [CrossRef] [PubMed]
92. Sajid, A.; Abbas, H. Data privacy in cloud-assisted healthcare systems: State of the art and future challenges. *J. Med. Syst.* **2016**, *40*, 155. [CrossRef]
93. Tiase, V.L.; Sward, K.A.; Del Fiol, G.; Staes, C.; Weir, C.; Cummins, M.R. Patient-generated health data in pediatric asthma: Exploratory study of providers' information needs. *JMIR Pediatr. Parent.* **2021**, *4*, e25413. [CrossRef] [PubMed]
94. Shrivastava, U.; Song, J.; Han, B.T.; Dietzman, D. Do data security measures, privacy regulations, and communication standards impact the interoperability of patient health information? A cross-country investigation. *Int. J. Med. Inform.* **2021**, *148*, 104401. [CrossRef] [PubMed]
95. Austin, E.; Lee, J.R.; Amtmann, D.; Bloch, R.; Lawrence, S.O.; McCall, D.; Munson, S.; Lavallee, D.C. Use of patient-generated health data across healthcare settings: Implications for health systems. *JAMIA Open* **2020**, *3*, 70–76. [CrossRef] [PubMed]
96. Kruse, C.S.; Smith, B.; Vanderlinden, H.; Nealand, A. Security techniques for the electronic health records. *J. Med. Syst.* **2017**, *41*, 1–9. [CrossRef]
97. Ghubaish, A.; Salman, T.; Zolanvari, M.; Unal, D.; Al-Ali, A.; Jain, R. Recent advances in the internet-of-medical-things (IoMT) systems security. *IEEE Internet Things J.* **2020**, *8*, 8707–8718. [CrossRef]
98. Rohloff, K.; Polyakov, Y. An end-to-end security architecture to collect, process and share wearable medical device data. In Proceedings of the 2015 17th International Conference on E-health Networking, Application & Services (HealthCom), Boston, MA, USA, 14–17 October 2015; pp. 615–620.
99. Koutras, D.; Stergiopoulos, G.; Dasaklis, T.; Kotzanikolaou, P.; Glynos, D.; Douligeris, C. Security in IoMT communications: A survey. *Sensors* **2020**, *20*, 4828. [CrossRef]
100. Nair, A.K.; Sahoo, J.; Raj, E.D. Privacy preserving Federated Learning framework for IoMT based big data analysis using edge computing. *Comput. Stand. Interfaces* **2023**, *86*, 103720. [CrossRef]
101. Asha, N.; Krishnan, S.R.; Gitanjali, J. Integration of artificial intelligence in software development process for implementing a secure healthcare system—A review. *Int. J. Med. Eng. Inform.* **2023**, *15*, 293–310. [CrossRef]
102. Patel, V.A.; Bhattacharya, P.; Tanwar, S.; Gupta, R.; Sharma, G.; Bokoro, P.N.; Sharma, R. Adoption of federated learning for healthcare informatics: Emerging applications and future directions. *IEEE Access* **2022**, *10*, 90792–90826. [CrossRef]
103. Basilakis, J.; Javadi, B.; Maeder, A. The potential for machine learning analysis over encrypted data in cloud-based clinical decision support—Background and review. *Health Inform. Knowl. Manag. (HIKM'15)* **2015**, *164*, 3–13.
104. Lin, C.P.; Wu, Z.Y.; Liu, C.H. Privacy Protection Scheme for Personal Health Record System Using Blockchain Based on Homomorphic Encryption. In Proceedings of the 2023 IEEE 6th Eurasian Conference on Educational Innovation (ECEI), Singapore, 3–5 February 2023; pp. 212–215.
105. Melanson, D.; Maia, R.; Kim, H.S.; Nascimento, A.; De Cock, M. Secure Multi-Party Computation for Personalized Human Activity Recognition. *Neural Process. Lett.* **2023**, *55*, 2127–2153. [CrossRef]
106. Li, Z.; Wang, B.; Li, J.; Hua, Y.; Zhang, S. Local differential privacy protection for wearable device data. *PLoS ONE* **2022**, *17*, e0272766. [CrossRef] [PubMed]
107. Tomaz, A.E.B.; Do Nascimento, J.C.; Hafid, A.S.; De Souza, J.N. Preserving privacy in mobile health systems using non-interactive zero-knowledge proof and blockchain. *IEEE Access* **2020**, *8*, 204441–204458. [CrossRef]

108. Kolokotronis, N.; Dareioti, M.; Shiaeles, S.; Bellini, E. An intelligent platform for threat assessment and cyber-attack mitigation in IoMT ecosystems. In Proceedings of the 2022 IEEE Globecom Workshops (GC Wkshps), Rio de Janeiro, Brazil, 4–8 December 2022; pp. 541–546.
109. Falco, G.; Shneiderman, B.; Badger, J.; Carrier, R.; Dahbura, A.; Danks, D.; Eling, M.; Goodloe, A.; Gupta, J.; Hart, C.; et al. Governing AI safety through independent audits. *Nat. Mach. Intell.* **2021**, *3*, 566–571. [CrossRef]
110. Javed, I.T.; Alharbi, F.; Bellaj, B.; Margaria, T.; Crespi, N.; Qureshi, K.N. Health-ID: A blockchain-based decentralized identity management for remote healthcare. *Healthcare* **2021**, *9*, 712. [CrossRef]
111. Coppolino, L.; D'Antonio, S.; Romano, L.; Sgaglione, L.; Staffa, M. Addressing security issues in the eheatlh domain relying on SIEM solutions. In Proceedings of the 2017 IEEE 41st Annual Computer Software and Applications Conference (COMPSAC), Turin, Italy, 4–8 July 2017; Volume 2, pp. 510–515.
112. Lafky, D.B.; Horan, T.A. Personal health records: Consumer attitudes toward privacy and security of their personal health information. *Health Inform. J.* **2011**, *17*, 63–71. [CrossRef]
113. Schneble, C.O.; Elger, B.S.; Shaw, D.M. All our data will be health data one day: The need for universal data protection and comprehensive consent. *J. Med. Internet Res.* **2020**, *22*, e16879. [CrossRef]

Disclaimer/Publisher's Note: The statements, opinions and data contained in all publications are solely those of the individual author(s) and contributor(s) and not of MDPI and/or the editor(s). MDPI and/or the editor(s) disclaim responsibility for any injury to people or property resulting from any ideas, methods, instructions or products referred to in the content.

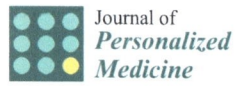

Article

Future pHealth Ecosystem-Holistic View on Privacy and Trust

Pekka Ruotsalainen [1,*] and Bernd Blobel [2]

[1] Faculty of Information Technology and Communication Sciences (ITC), Tampere University, 33100 Tampere, Finland
[2] Medical Faculty, University of Regensburg, 93053 Regensburg, Germany; bernd.blobel@klink.uni-regensburg.de
* Correspondence: pekka.ruotsalainen@tuni.fi

Abstract: Modern pHealth is an emerging approach to collecting and using personal health information (PHI) for personalized healthcare and personalized health management. For its products and services, it deploys advanced technologies such as sensors, actuators, computers, mobile phones, etc. Researchers have shown that today's networked information systems, such as pHealth ecosystems, miss appropriate privacy solutions, and trust is only an illusion. In the future, the situation will be even more challenging because pHealth ecosystems will be highly distributed, dynamic, increasingly autonomous, and multi-stakeholder, with the ability to monitor the person's regular life, movements, emotions, and health-related behavior in real time. In this paper, the authors demonstrate that privacy and trust in ecosystems are system-level problems that need a holistic, system-focused solution. To make future pHealth ethically acceptable, privacy-enabled, and trustworthy, the authors have developed a conceptual five-level privacy and trust model as well as a formula that describes the impact of privacy and trust factors on the level of privacy and trust. Furthermore, the authors have analyzed privacy and trust challenges and possible solutions at each level of the model. Based on the analysis performed, a proposal for future ethically acceptable, trustworthy, and privacy-enabled pHealth is developed. The solution combines privacy as personal property and trust as legally binding fiducial duty approaches and uses a blockchain-based smart contract agreement to store people's privacy and trust requirements and service providers' promises.

Keywords: privacy; trust; holistic view; fiducial duty; privacy law; smart contract

Citation: Ruotsalainen, P.; Blobel, B. Future pHealth Ecosystem-Holistic View on Privacy and Trust. *J. Pers. Med.* **2023**, *13*, 1048. https://doi.org/10.3390/jpm13071048

Academic Editor: Yi Guo

Received: 10 May 2023
Revised: 18 June 2023
Accepted: 21 June 2023
Published: 26 June 2023

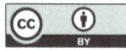

Copyright: © 2023 by the authors. Licensee MDPI, Basel, Switzerland. This article is an open access article distributed under the terms and conditions of the Creative Commons Attribution (CC BY) license (https://creativecommons.org/licenses/by/4.0/).

1. Introduction

Nowadays, we live in almost borderless digital environments where products are increasingly interchangeable with intellectual and informational goods and services [1]. They also require the availability of "Big Data" related to human's experiences, relationships, behaviors, and environments. Novel health service models such as tele-health, mHealth, pHealth, eHealth, and digital health are examples of those services. pHealth focuses on personal/personalized health and health care services, and it presents a horizontal view of health care, eHealth, and mHealth [2]. Modern pHealth services are data-driven and vary in focus and size. The pHealth service can be a sensor system that is focused on a dedicated personal health or wellness problem, or it can be a personal health recommender system using a holistic view of a person's health [3]. Nowadays, pHealth services are increasingly part of a dynamic, multi-stakeholder, cross-organizational, cross-border, and cross-jurisdictional ecosystem. In pHealth, technological innovations have always been adapted on the front lines. Currently, the deployment of smart sensors, mobile devices, wireless networks, web technologies, digitalized services, Cloud platforms, algorithms, artificial intelligence (AI), machine learning (ML), and blockchains for online personalized health services is common. Ongoing paradigm shifts in health care from organization-centered and reactive healthcare to person-centered preventive and predictive care are well adapted in pHealth [4].

Today's information technology enables Web sites, computer applications, and networks to routinely collect, use, store, and share all kinds of personally identifiable information (PII) about a person's health problems, including health-related information about the person's life. Modern sensors, wearables, and smart wrists have the ability to measure a person's physical activity, blood pressure, heart rate, quality of sleep, social activities, stress, emotions, and mood [5]. Furthermore, behavioral activities are invisibly tracked online when using computers, mobile phones, and health services via networks [6,7]. According to Zuboff, almost unlimited data collection and surveillance are daily practices in the digital age [8]. Video surveillance systems in public spaces can monitor our social and health-related behaviors. Data analytics companies both sell our raw data and use our PII in the form of behavioral profiles and predictive products [9].

The Internet of Things (IoT) and artificial intelligence of things interfaces (AIoT) are new emerging technologies that enable real-time data collection. According to Ziegeldorf et Al., the IoT moves the collection of personal data and behaviors from the internet and public spaces to homes and working places [10]. The novel neurotechnology has the ability to go even further. According to Berger et al., it can impact technology indirectly through wearable devices that read data from the head and also write data using neuromodulation. According to Berger et al., in the future, neurotechnology may have the ability to influence people's behavior, emotions, values, and thoughts [11].

During the last few years, both the public sector and private organizations have shown increasing interest in the collection and use of personal health data for innovations, new products, and services, and they have built technology environments such as ecosystems where services offered are dependent on the collection of PHI, users' behaviors, and interactions [12]. This development has raised the question of the ownership of PHI and whether or not health data should be understood as a public good (a commodity produced without profit for all) or personal property [13]. Currently, there is no unanimous answer to this question. According to Piasecki et al., the ownership concept cannot solve problems associated with the sharing of PHI [14]. In a workshop report, Crossmann et al. summarize that health care data should be established as a public good [15]. Taylor sees that nowadays, data as a public good model fits best with corporate reality and existing models for data sharing [16]. On the other side, propertization of personal information, according to Schwarz, responds best to people's concerns about privacy [17]. The new European Health Data Space proposal goes even further by considering health data according to the common good model. In this proposal, health data is understood to include not only EHR and clinical trials but also the content of PHR and personal wellness data [18].

These days, the Internet brokers and data giants have well understood the commercial value of health data and the potential of AI and have adapted and established the business model of data collection and commercialization [19]. Increasing commercialization of PHI is a big problem for human rights, and it raises the danger that, in the future, expected economic benefits will override people's needs for privacy and autonomy. It is notable that the United Nations has confirmed that privacy remains a human right even in the digital age, and "sharing health data as a public good requires making data available with the right degree of openness or restriction to achieve maximum benefit, while reducing any potential for harms" [20]. It is evident that privacy is a big problem in real-life networks and ecosystems [21]. Therefore, information privacy is inevitable in the digital age [22]. Researchers have shown that traditional security-based privacy protection solutions cannot guarantee privacy, and a person cannot control the collection, use, and sharing of his or her personal information (PII) in today's networked information systems [2].

Building trust in a dynamic ecosystem is a big challenge for the service user. In today's information systems, it is widely expected that people blindly trust organizations' and service providers' promises that they process PII fairly. In other words, it is expected that a service user believes without any proof that structures such as guarantees, regulations, promises, legal recourse, and procedures are in place (i.e., structural assurance) and that the environment is in proper order (i.e., situational normality) [23]. Unfortunately, researchers have shown that in real life, this is far from true. And in dynamic multi-stakeholder ecosystems, it is almost impossible to know who and why to trust [24]. Furthermore, researchers have observed that digital information systems are seldom designed with privacy in mind, i.e., in today's digital information systems, trust is only an illusion [25,26]. As pHealth services are built over the same general ITC technology used in commercial information systems and platforms, they share the same privacy and trust concerns [26–29]. It is a specific feature of pHealth ecosystems that some of the stakeholders can be non-regulated health care providers or private organizations. This means that parts of personal health information (PHI) collected and used are not regulated by health care-specific laws. Together with the sensitivity of PHI collected and used, this raises additional privacy concerns, especially because the content and implementation of privacy laws vary in different countries [30].

The future of pHealth has the potential to offer personalized, preventive, and predictive services to its service users. However, for it to be successful, it needs a huge amount of PHI and health-related personal behavioral data covering a person's regular life, social relations, economic activities, and psychological status [2]. This data (i.e., personal big health data) can be used for different analyses, to calculate detailed personal health profiles, to detect changes in personal health and disease, and to develop new applications such as personal health recommendation services [3]. According to researchers, future pHealth will rely on Internet of Things (IoT)-based data collection and advanced computer methods such as machine learning (ML), artificial intelligence (AI), and deep learning (DL) [27,29,30]. It is evident that in the future, pHealth privacy and trust challenges will be much bigger than they are today. To realize even a part of the promises of data-driven pHealth (e.g., innovations, new products, better health, and economic growth) and to prevent short- and long-term negative consequences for human values such as privacy, dignity, integrity, and autonomy, it is necessary to find new solutions for privacy, trust, and ownership of PHI.

This paper is an extension of the work originally presented to the pHealth 2022 Conference [2]. In that paper, the authors have studied methods and solutions that have the ability to prevent the situation where PHI can be invisible collected, shared, and misused, where there is no information privacy, and where predefined trust in technology and service providers' fairness is just expected [22,27]. As healthcare-specific laws and general privacy regulations grant several rights to the data subject (e.g., access to their own health data, rectification, objection, data portability, and the right to block data sharing), this paper is focused on the collection, processing, storage, and sharing of PHI that takes place outside the health care domain and medical research [31]. The authors' starting point is that future pHealth should be ethically acceptable, trustworthy, and empower the service user or data subject (DS) to maintain information privacy by expressing their own privacy needs and expectations. For future pHealth, potential ICT solutions and their weaknesses are discussed, and the authors also propose a holistic set of principles and solutions that, when used together, have the power to make future pHealth ethically acceptable and trustworthy.

The rest of the article is organized as follows: Chapter 2 briefly summarizes the main features of widely used privacy and trust models and the principles of information ethics. In chapter 3, the authors define how the pHealth ecosystem is understood in this paper and present a user's view of it. In Chapter 4, privacy and trust challenges existing in current pHealth ecosystems are discussed. Then (Chapter 5), features of new privacy and trust approaches developed by researchers are analyzed. In chapter 6, a five-level holistic model and a formula describing factors that influence the level of privacy and trust in an ecosystem are presented. In Chapter 7, the authors propose a holistic solution for a trustworthy, privacy-enabled, and ethically acceptable pHealth ecosystem. Chapter 8 covers the limitations of this paper and outlines the necessary future steps needed to reach the authors' goal.

2. Privacy, Trust and Information Ethics

Privacy and trust are vague, dynamic, situational, and context-dependent concepts with many definitions [2,27,32]. Almost all cultures value privacy, but they differ in how they obtain it [33]. It is widely accepted that privacy is a human and constitutional right [34]. Information privacy is a subset of the concept of privacy [35]. According to Floridi, two theories of information privacy are popular: the reductionist interpretation and the ownership-based interpretation. The first theory looks for undesirable consequences caused by the misuse of data, and the second theory defines that a person owns his or her information (privacy is defined in terms of intellectual property) [36]. According to Smith et al., the person who owns PII can also trade privacy for other goods or services [37]. For Decew, privacy is a common value because all individuals value some amount of privacy [33].

At a general level, privacy addresses the question "what would we like others to know about us". In western countries, privacy is widely based on concepts of autonomy and informational self-determination, which refer to a person's right and expected ability to control the flow of his/her own personal information. This implies that a person has the right to control when, by whom, and why personal information is collected and shared, and to protect himself/herself against surveillance, unnecessary data collection and processing, dissemination, unauthorized use, and harm caused by the unfair use of PII [38–40].

Other widely used privacy models are privacy as a concern, legal construct, risk-based concept, behavioural concept, and social good [27,41,42]. The concept of privacy as a commodity understands privacy as an economic good that can be traded. The privacy as a concern approach refers to individuals' anxiety regarding the collection, processing, and unfair use and sharing of data. Privacy as a regulative (legal) construct tries to regulate the way data is collected, used, and shared [43]. The risk-based approach to privacy focuses on risks such as harm caused by unnecessary data collection, misuse, disclosure, surveillance, and behavioral manipulation [44,45].

In real life, the nature of privacy and the lack of availability of reliable privacy related information make the measurement of the actual (objective) level of privacy challenging [45]. Furthermore, researchers have found that privacy preferences vary drastically from individual to individual. They can change over time and are context-dependent [46]. Furthermore, in many countries, privacy is not an absolute right. Instead, it can be balanced with, or overridden by, others' concerns and priorities, including business needs, public safety, and national security. According to Friedewald, the right to privacy requires a forward-looking privacy framework that positively outlines the parameters of privacy in order to prevent intrusions [22]. A meaningful challenge is that, while technical solutions provide some protection against data misuse, the existence of such protection does not necessarily mean that users will disclose more information [47].

Some researchers have pointed out that current privacy models do not work in distributed and digital information systems, and there is a need to redefine how we understand privacy [21,48]. Furthermore, Friedewald has proposed that in the digital age, the concept of privacy should be expanded to include the following aspects: privacy of the person, privacy of personal behavior and actions, privacy of personal communication, privacy of data and images, privacy of thoughts and feelings, privacy of location and space, and privacy of association (including group privacy) [22].

According to Sætra, an individualistic model of privacy is insufficient, and privacy should be understood as a public good, i.e., everyone in a society should have the right to enjoy privacy [49]. DaCosta has proposed a novel privacy-as-property approach. Its fundamental idea is that "you have the right to control yourself, and this property interest in oneself extends to the external objects you own, including your data" [50]. Acquisti et al. have proposed that in the digital age, privacy should include not only personal data but also behaviors and actions, personal communication, thoughts and feelings, and associations [51].

Traditionally, trust is understood to exist between persons; however, researchers agree that trust is also needed between a person and an organization (organizational trust) and between a person and technology (trust in technology) [29]. Trust is needed in situations where the trustor has insufficient information about the features and behavior of the trustee [52]. Therefore, to build a relationship of trust, there must be confidence that the other partner will act in a predictable manner [39]. Trust can also be defined as a personal expectation of other partners' future behavior [53]. Trust is widely understood as a disposition, attitude, belief, feeling, expectancy, psychological state, personal trait, social norm, subjective feature, willingness to be vulnerable, and perception based on one's own previous experiences or others' recommendations. Trust has been understood as the willingness to depend on other parties expected or unexpected actions without the ability to monitor or control them [54]. Perceived trust is a personal opinion based on information gleaned from one's own senses or from others. Computational trust is an algorithmic imitation of human-based measured features of the trustor and the used information system. Thus, trust is often based on emotions or feelings, which also include cognition. According to Ikeda, trust can be based on justifiable reasons such as laws and science [55]. That kind of trust, aka "rational trust" is based on rational arguments [56]. In the case of rational trust, the trustor should have facts on which the trust is based [57].

In digital information systems, people should increasingly trust technology. According to Mc Knight, trust in technology is often a belief that the technology used is reliable, secure, and protects information privacy, and that appropriate governance is established and enforced [58]. Furthermore, the level of trust depends on the understanding of the system and its behavior, i.e., the system's willingness and ability to correctly perform [59].

Ethics is a set of principles and concepts that judge whether a behavior is right or wrong. The basic principles of general ethics are autonomy, justice, non-maleficence, privacy, and solidarity. Normative theories of ethics include consequence-based theories, duty-based theories, rights-based theories, and virtue-based theories to guide how to interact properly with others [60]. Information ethics (which is closely related to computer ethics) is an applied ethics that focuses on the relationship between the creation, organization, dissemination, and use of information and the ethical standards and moral codes governing human conduct in society [61]. Information ethics intertwines with other areas of applied ethics such as computer ethics, data ethics, internet ethics, engineering ethics, and business ethics. In this paper, the authors emphasize that information ethics covers not only humans but also any actor in the ecosystem, such as applications and technologies, including implantable and wearable devices. As today's networked information systems, or more generally, ecosystems, impact human values such as life, health, happiness, freedom, knowledge, resources, power, and opportunity in many ways, researchers have highlighted that information systems should function in an ethically acceptable way [62]. The European Union has proposed the following ethical principles for information systems using AI: The system must not negatively affect human autonomy, violate the right to privacy, or directly or indirectly cause social or environmental harm to an individual. Instead, the system should support freedom and dignity. Furthermore, the AI system should be accountable and transparent to its stakeholders and end-users [63]. The authors state the above-discussed ethical principles as mandatory for all information systems processing PHI.

3. User View on Privacy and Trust in pHealth Ecosystems

The concept "ecosystem" was originally developed in the fields of ecology and biology [64]. Today, it is transferred to many other contexts and widely used in the field of information science to describe networked communities consisting of interconnected and interrelated technical and non-tangible elements [54]. Typical non-tangible elements are data, digital services, and stakeholders. Technical elements include networks, platforms, programs, and communication lines. Architecture presents its structure, function, and relations [64]. The goal of the ecosystem is to create value for all stakeholders [64]. A pHealth ecosystem is typically a socio-technical system that is characterized by its stakeholders' business models, roles, and relations, its services and products, information flows, the information itself, and the underlying infrastructure [65]. Nowadays, pHealth ecosystems are increasingly platform ecosystems. In the pHealth ecosystem, there can be conflicting objectives; e.g., stakeholders want to maximize their profit by collecting and using a maximal amount of PHI, and users try to minimize short- and long-term harms through disclosed data while at the same time getting benefits from services. In pHealth ecosystems, a service user typically has a direct connection to one service provider. On the other hand, other parts of the ecosystem, including its other stakeholders, architecture, deployed privacy technology, regulations, business goals, and relations, are usually invisible to the service user, i.e., the ecosystem looks at the service user as a black box (Figure 1).

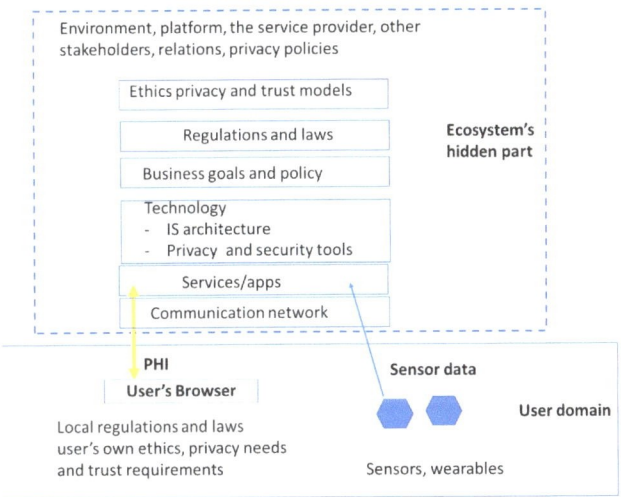

Figure 1. Users' view on pHealth ecosystem.

This means that the service user is strongly dependent on the service provider's willingness to use and share the service user's PHI ethically and fairly. The service user cannot build trust in the pHealth ecosystem and make privacy-based decisions without sufficient information about the ecosystem's invisible features, which the service provider should make available. According to Dobkin, service providers who collect and utilize user data are fiduciaries to customers [66], and the information fiduciary duty of service providers could ensure that they use data only in ways that are consistent with users' expectations [67]. This implies that there exists a specific informational and fiducial relationship between the service user and service provider in pHealth ecosystems. Thereby, the service provider has an obligation to act in the best interests of the service user.

4. Privacy and Trust Challenges in pHealth Ecosystems

When we currently use information systems, we leave trails that expose our interests and traits that expose our actions, beliefs, intentions, and targets of interests to commercial entities and also to our governments [51]. On the Web, there are tens of thousands of health apps collecting and using PHI [32]. In today's information systems, a person's behavioral health data is systematically and secretly collected by Web service providers, health apps, and Web platforms. According to Dobkin et al., at least 77.4% of Websites globally track visitors' data and people's behavior [66]. Zuboff has noted that behavioral tracking is not only used to measure body signals but also our physical and social behaviors and how we use information systems [8]. Therefore, persons do not have sufficient knowledge of what information other people, organizations, and firms have about them, by whom and how that information is used, and what the consequences are for the data subject (DS). This situation is often described by decision-makers and firms as a win-win situation, i.e., people, organizations, firms, and society benefit from data sharing. Unfortunately, in real life, benefits to a person are often only promises or beliefs, and invisible data collection and sharing not only breaches trust and privacy, but it can also generate harm to the person.

Researchers have shown that traditional privacy solutions such as notification and choice (consent) as well as fair information processing principles have failed to guarantee privacy in today's networked environment. Although the new privacy regulations, such as the EU-GDPR, oblige companies to specify how the collected data is used, in real life, organizations' privacy policies (if available) are written in a legalistic and confusing manner and are difficult to understand and use [68]. For the same reasons, transparency in the form of an organization's privacy policy does not work well. Furthermore, many big Web actors and service providers simply do not care about privacy laws [45,69]. Finally, the service user's privacy decision takes place in a complex, multidimensional situation, and his or her bounded rationality makes rational privacy choices difficult [70].

Currently, most Web services are free of charge for the consumer, but in real life, people are paying for the use of services through disclosed PII (i.e., PII is traded and monetarized). The option of buying an application with the option of not disclosing personal information to the company, which may subsequently sell that data, does not exist [68]. Service providers and platform managers often expect that they can freely use and sell disclosed data [2]. Service providers are also prioritizing their business needs and benefits over service users privacy needs. There is also a tension between public and commercial interests in collecting and using PII on the one hand and people's needs for privacy on the other. Industry widely sees personal information as raw material for products and services and society as a public good. This makes it challenging to balance a person's individual need for privacy on the one hand and the use of PII for meaningful public benefits or for making profit on the other [27].

The unlimited collection of a person's behavioral data is a big problem in today's digital information systems. Behavioral data talks about our routines, habits, and medical conditions. Behavioral data can also be used to uniquely identify individuals [71] and web-browsing behavior [72]. Another problem is that in ecosystems, the DS cannot know how data will be used in the future, what its potential uses are, or whether other people's PHI will be linked to it [73].

Lack of trust is also a meaningful problem in ecosystems, where the user has to trust not only the service provider but also other frequently unknown stakeholders and surrounding information technology. In ecosystems, the service user does not have reasonable knowledge of stakeholders' trust features and relations and has no power to negotiate privacy rules and safeguards or force the service provider or platform manager to take personal privacy and trust needs into account [2]. Instead, the service user is typically forced to accept a service provider's privacy promises (policy) and trust manifesto in the form of a take-it-or-leave-it approach [66]. Unfortunately, commercial service providers often have low incentives to enforce strong privacy policies, and they often do not keep the privacy promises expressed in their policy documents [73,74]. This all indicates that policy-makers and technology firms fail to provide the user with reasons to trust, and codes of conduct and privacy policies will not provide sufficient reasons to trust [75].

As discussed earlier, the vagueness of privacy and trust concepts makes it difficult to conceptualize and measure them and to make them understandable for computer programs. To solve this problem, different proxies such as service level agreements, external third-party seals, service provider's privacy policy documents, reputation, direct observations, and degree of compliance with laws or standards have been used instead [27]. Preserving behavioral privacy requires more sophisticated approaches than just removing direct identifiers (IP address, social security number (SSN), blurring a face) or intuitive quasi-identifiers (gender, age, ethnicity) from databases [72].

Consequently, a person today has just a few or no possibilities to maintain privacy in networked information systems, and therefore just a few reasons to trust. According to Goldberg, the service user can only use feelings or personal opinions as measures of the level of privacy and trust [39], reject the use of the service, filter the amount of PII he or she is willing to disclose, or add noise to data before disclosure [76]. This all indicates that the current situation is unsatisfactory.

5. Novel Approaches for Privacy and Trust

As discussed earlier, current privacy and trust models and solutions are insufficient to provide an acceptable level of privacy in networked and highly distributed information systems. Furthermore, a service user has few or no reasons to trust the service provider or the ecosystem as a whole. To solve these problems, researchers have created different privacy and trust approaches and solutions. Most of them focus on reducing the negative consequences of the use and sharing of personal information by offering more control and the possibility of using computer-understandable policies. There are also solutions, providing insight that the control model and the use of consent are inadequate and that a more radical solution is needed (Table 1).

Table 1. Examples of new privacy and trust approaches and solutions.

Approach	Examples of Solutions
More personal control Transparency	Privacy nudges User tailored privacy Personalized privacy Person/Patient controlled or PHR Personal privacy policies Explainable trust
Ownership model	Privacy as intellectual property
Duty based model	Informational duties Trust as duty
Regulatory model	Trust as legal binding duty Accountability Privacy risk analysis
Computational models	Calculated level of privacy Calculated trust
Contractual models	Privacy negotiation Smart contract
Cryptographic based models	Blockchain Differential privacy Homomorphic encryption
Obfuscation methods Disclosure limitation	Data hiding by masking Adding noise or laying
Architectural solutions	Edge/Fog computing Federated learning
Ethics based approaches	Ethical design Ethical agents
Distributed trust approaches	Blockchain

The aim of the privacy as control approach is to give the DS or service users more control over what data they wish to share with whom and how and for what purposes the data can be used. Privacy nudges offer the person a ready-made template to make personal choices. On the other side, it is only a normative "one-size-fits-all" solution to make normative assumptions about the value of privacy [77]. User-tailored privacy solutions offer the user more flexibility by automatically tailoring IS's privacy settings to fit the user's privacy preferences [78]. As AI applications have the ability to predict a user's privacy preferences by determining privacy needs based on the user's previous data sharing history, AI can be used to contextually tailor a user's privacy needs.

The person-controlled EHR (Electronic Health Record)/PHR (Personal Health Record) approach gives a person full control over his/her own PHI (e.g., the person grants or rejects granular access to the stored PHI in a context). Typically, rules that are expressed in the form of personal policies and data encryption methods are used together. The encrypted data can be stored on a blockchain [79]. Yue et al. have proposed a person-controlled blockchain solution that enables the patient to own, control, and share their own data securely without violating privacy [71].

Computational privacy models use mathematical methods to calculate the level of privacy using measured attributes and mathematical methods. According to Ruotsalainen et al., computational privacy offers a better approximation for the actual level of privacy than risk probabilities and privacy perceptions [48]. A contractual agreement, such as a legally binding service level agreement (SLA), is widely used between organizations. Ruotsalainen et al. have proposed the use of legally binding digital (Smart) contracts between the pHealth customer and service provider [27,80]. A smart contract is a set of rules that can be executed in a network of mutually distrusted nodes without the need for a centralized, trusted authority [81]. To guarantee the integrity, availability, and non-repudiation of the contract, it can be stored on a Blockchain. In a smart contract, the service user's personal privacy policy is part of the contract between the person and the pHealth service provider. The personal policy can regulate not only how the service provider uses PHI but also the sharing and secondary use of PHI in the ecosystem [54].

New cryptographic solutions such as encryption, differential privacy, k-anonymity, and homomorphic encryption offer ways to maintain privacy. Homomorphic encryption allows some calculations with the data without decryption [82]. Architectural solutions such as edge-and-fog computing can also support privacy. The edge consists of human-controlled devices, such as PCs, smart phones, IoT devices, personal health devices, and local routers [83]. In edge computing, the processing of sensitive data takes place at the local level, and the Edge router controls the data flow between the edge domain and other worlds [84].

Some researchers have stated that the current privacy and trust models are unsatisfactory and that a radical (paradigmatic) change is necessary [54]. According to Ritter, today's highly distributed information systems, such as ecosystems and the Internet of Things (IoT), have raised legal questions such as who is the owner of PHI and behavioral personal data by defining a new class of property by legislation [85]. He also noted that today's defensive privacy laws should be expanded to support new contractual models such as smart contracts, and the consumer should have a veto right concerning privacy [85]. Another radical solution is to make the person the legal owner of his or her PHI. This informational property rights model gives the person the power and ability to define how and by whom PHI is used. According to Samuelson, the informational property rights model empowers individuals to negotiate with organizations and firms about how data is used [86]. Koos has proposed a variant of this model where the PHI can be licensed by the customer [87]. Ruotsalainen et al. have proposed PHI as a personal property model, where a person defines policies for the use and sharing of PHI in the ecosystem [27]. To be effective, the property model requires legal support [85]. The property model can also be expanded to cover a person's behavioral data.

Trust creation by information and explanations regarding how information systems function seems to make information systems more trustworthy [88]. Challenges in this transparency model are the lack of reliable information about system trust features and the fact that explanations and increased information overload the user in a situation. To outweigh this, Ruotsalainen et al. have proposed for pHealth the use of a computational trust model that is based on information about the ecosystem's measured/published features. In this solution, a Fuzzy Linguistic method is used to calculate the merit of service (fuzzy attractiveness rating) for the whole ecosystem [48]. Depending on the quality of the available attributes (i.e., attributes should be measurable if possible), this model can support the idea of building rational trust.

A radical approach is the use of the concept of informational duties instead of privacy. Information duties imply that individuals and institutions acting as data controllers or processors have specific information duties towards data subjects [89,90]. For privacy, Balkin has proposed the deployment of the concept of information fiduciary as a specific duty [67]. Fiduciaries must act in the interests of another person, i.e., a fiduciary has a responsibility to accept and act based on privacy needs expressed by a person. Fiduciaries also have obligations of loyalty and care toward another person and the responsibility not to do harm [67]. Therefore, according to Barret, the information fiduciary model has the power to strengthen equality and autonomy in the digital society and to offer better privacy protection [91]. According to Dobkin, the principle of the information fiduciary should be legally imposed as a duty in digital information systems [66].

The fiduciary relationship, as a legal duty, can also be used as a trust builder. According to Mayer, trust in fiduciary relationships is based on the professional's competence and integrity [92]. Waldman sees that privacy in an information-sharing context is a social construct based on trust. He has proposed for privacy the privacy as trust model. According to Waldman, privacy as trust creates a fiduciary relationship between data subjects and users. In this approach, a private context is also a trusted context [38].

Blockchain technology can be used as a trust builder because it offers decentralized trust. In blockchain, people do not need interpersonal trust, but users must trust mathematics, algorithms, and indirectly, the creators of the blockchain system [93].

In an ecosystem, a single privacy or trust solution alone is hardly a silver bullet, and the combination of different methods shown in Table 1 offers a better solution. Ruotsalainen et al. have developed a solution that combines privacy as a personal property model, trust as a fiducial duty, a legally binding smart contract, and blockchain-based repositories for pHealth [27]. Thereby, the smart contract is a digital SLA agreement the service provider has a legal duty to follow.

As already mentioned, the information processing in the pHealth ecosystem should be ethically acceptable. Therefore, pHealth information systems should be compliant with the principles of information ethics (non-maleficence, beneficence, justice, and respect for autonomy). Hand has proposed a solution for an ethical information system that is based on the following ethical principles: integrity, honesty, objectivity, responsibility, trustworthiness, impartiality, nondiscrimination, transparency, accountability, and fairness [94].

6. A Holistic View to Privacy and Trust in pHealth Ecosystems

As discussed in earlier chapters, the authors expect that future pHealth will be part of a highly distributed and dynamic multi-stakeholder ecosystem, i.e., an information system that collects and shares all kinds of PHI and intensively uses AI, ML, and DL for detailed personal health analysis. In an ecosystem, some stakeholders can be virtual; PHI and results are shared not only between the user and the service provider but increasingly with other stakeholders across contexts and jurisdictions [2]. Furthermore, stakeholders in the pHealth ecosystem often have different business and privacy policies as well as trust features. To dare to use offered services, the user needs to know the aggregated level of privacy and reasons to trust not only a service provider but the ecosystem as a whole. In this chapter, the authors create a holistic solution to this challenge.

According to Holt et al., in modern highly distributed ecosystems, infrastructure, policies, citizen rights, national and international regulations and laws, as well as cultural preferences and corporate policies, make the maintenance of privacy and trust an extremely complex task [95]. Elrik has noted that ecosystem interrelations between members define how the ecosystem works, and a holistic approach to privacy is needed [96]. The authors state that in future pHealth ecosystems, privacy and trust cannot be built using a single method or solution. Instead, a holistic, systemic view is needed. Furthermore, for privacy and trust, a user-centric approach should be used [47].

For the future pHealth ecosystem, the authors have created a holistic, six-level, user-centric conceptual model (Figure 2). This model also supports the idea of explainability, i.e., that service users of the ecosystem should understand how their PHI is processed and used and how their privacy and trust needs are implemented by different stakeholders. The authors also expect that explainability fosters trust in the ecosystem [97].

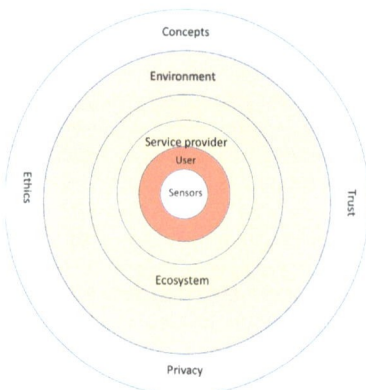

Figure 2. User centric five-level conceptual model for future pHealth ecosystem.

For each level of the conceptual model, the authors have analysed from the user's point of view the privacy and trust challenges and their possible solutions. The content of Table 2 creates a holistic view of privacy and trust in a future pHealth ecosystem.

Using the "Conceptual Model of Everyday Privacy in Ubicompo" developed by Lederer et al. [98], as a starting point, the authors have conceptualized the influence of privacy and trust factors discussed in Table 2 and developed the following formula:

$$\text{Level of privacy and trust} = f\ (M, E, Te, IA, SR, SP, KN, USPr, USPt, DS) \qquad (1)$$

where
  M = Models for ethics, privacy, and trust
  E = Environment (e.g., Laws, regulations, standards) [98]
  Te = technology (e.g., safeguards, encryption) [99]
  IA = Information architecture [98,100]
  SR = stakeholders' privacy and trust features and their relations [48]
  SP = service provider's privacy and trust features (attributes) [48]
  KN = knowledge [101]
  USPr = service user's privacy needs
  USPt = service users trust requirements and trust threshold
  DS = sensitivity of data [98].

Using the analysis made in the previous chapter and the content of Table 2, the authors have also developed a proposal for an ethically acceptable, trustworthy, and privacy-enabled pHealth ecosystem. Concerning the ethical model, the authors state that consequentialism (i.e., consequences to a person caused by the collection, use, and disclosure of PHI) alone is insufficient for future pHealth. Instead, the authors propose that a combination of consequentialism, duty ethics, and utilitarianism (i.e., the use of PHI should be available to improve the population's health) should be used in the environment. Furthermore, the privacy as personal property model is proposed to be used. This implies that the DS or service user has legal ownership of their own PHI, including personal health behaviors.

Table 2. Holistic view to privacy and trust in a future pHealth ecosystem.

Levels	Content	Possible Solutions	Challenges
Concepts and models	Ethical model, principles and values	Consequentialism Utility or duty ethics.	Stakeholders' ethical models, values and principles are seldom known
	Trust model	Trust as informational duty Computational trust	Stakeholders' privacy and trust models used are not known Stakeholders do not do what they have promised in privacy documents
	Privacy model	Privacy as property Personal tailored privacy	Privacy and trust responsibilities are often unclear
Environment	Laws, standards and Golden Rules	New laws needed to: -Force transparency of privacy and trust features -Strengthen the role of person -Restrict hidden collection of the PHI	Ecosystem is highly distributed and cross-border Conflighting laws and privacy and trust models Laws should be global
Ecosystem *The service provider*	Stakeholders' relations and privacy and trust features.	Transparency of business and privacy policies, stakeholders' relations, and features.	Stakeholders' business and policies vary. Stakeholder's relations, privacy and trust features of information systems are not known
	ICT-architecture and technology	Edge and blockchainb architectures Federated computing	Management of encryption keys Regulatory compliance and accountability.
	Business model, Privacy policy Trust features of processes and applications	Data encryption	DS's policy and stakeholser's business policy can be conflighting Measurements of possible harm and the level of trust and privacy
User/DS (Physical view)	Users and the DS personal privacy and trust models. Expression of user's privacy and trust needs	Personal privacy policies Tools to collect data and calculate the actual level of trust and privacy Evaluations of expected benefits and possible harms. Smart contracts Data encryption	No reason to trust Lack of: -Privacy and trust related data -Regulatory support -Practival tool for privacy management -Power to make contract ór negotiate No audit trails
Data and sensors (perception)	Raw data from sensors Self-disclosed PHI	Lite point-to point- encryption of data at sensor level	Data integrity, reliability and availability Lack of computational power for encryption

As the service user in the pHealth ecosystem is fully dependent on service providers' fairness and knowledge concerning privacy and trust features of the ecosystem (Chapter 3), the authors propose for the trust model a solution where trust is a legally binding fiducial duty. Thereby, the service provider and other stakeholders have the legal duty not to prioritize their own business benefits but to take into account service users privacy needs [2,27]. It is also necessary that the service provider publish not only the trust and privacy features of its own information system but also proof of accountability. For this purpose, the service provider must enable the service user to access the audit trail concerning the use of collected PHI. New laws are also needed to strengthen the position of the service user. First, a transparency law is inevitable, which enables the service user to know how and by whom his or her PHI is collected and used and to be aware of what behavioral health data is collected. Secondly, a law for privacy as informational property and a law that supports legal, binding smart collection contracts are needed. The service user should have the choice of a paid pHealth application without health data collection and behavioral tracking.

New information architectures, such as blockchain-based information systems and edge architecture, offer increased privacy compared with currently widely used Cloud platform solutions. Therefore, they are good candidates for future pHealth systems. Federated learning (FL) is another interesting architectural solution. Encryption as a default principle should be used everywhere where it is possible (e.g., homomorphic encryption or differential privacy).

7. A Proposal for Privacy Enabled and Trustworthy for pHealth Ecosystem

Based on previous analysis and the holistic view (Chapter 6), the authors have developed a proposal (an example) of how a high level of privacy and trust can be reached in the pHealth ecosystem. It is assumed that any person has the right to control themselves, including data that describes their own thoughts, behaviors, emotions, values, and personal health-related information [50], and privacy is understood as the amount of power a person has against others control and manipulation over them. The proposal is called a hybrid solution by the authors because it is not aimed at superseding current general privacy protection laws such as the EU GDPR and laws regulating the collection and use of clinical data in health care. The authors' proposal combines PHI as personal property, trust as a fiduciary duty for the service provider and other stakeholders processing PHI in the ecosystem, and a legally binding smart contract that is stored in a blockchain-based repository [27,102]. Property is a special personal property that cannot be traded to any private organization and is not monetarized [103]. Property is an allocation of power to the DS to define what is a fair collection and use of data and how PHI can be used and shared. This power also enables the DS to exclude others [104]. The property should be supported by a new property law. Other elements in this proposal are transparency, edge architecture, data encryption at the sensor, and communication levels.

8. Discussion

Even though information privacy and a high level of trust are prerequisites for successful pHealth, researchers have shown that in ecosystems, current privacy approaches and solutions do not offer a level of privacy acceptable for the service user, so trust is just an illusion. This indicates that future pHealth cannot be built on current privacy models and technology [27]. Furthermore, even the most modern privacy laws, such as the EU-GDPR, rely on insufficient privacy as the notice and choice concept (aka consent model) and on risk analysis that is inadequate in a future pHealth environment [105,106]. Concerning trust, service users are widely expected to blindly trust companies' promises [75]. This all means that, until today, policy makers and technology firms have failed to provide people with reasons to trust information systems and have left users of digital networks and services vulnerable. There are many new technical, architectural, and mathematical privacy and trust solutions, but the authors state that none of them alone is sufficient because privacy and trust in ecosystems are interconnected and holistic system problems.

In this paper, the authors have developed a user-centric five-level conceptual model for privacy and trust in the pHealth ecosystem and a formula for its privacy and trust factors. For each level of the model, the authors have analysed privacy and trust challenges and their possible solutions. The results are shown in the template to provide a holistic view of privacy and trust. The template and the formula have many use cases. The service user can use them to evaluate the level of privacy and trust in pHealth. Furthermore, the service provider can use the template and formula to assess what knowledge should be disclosed to the user. Finally, a developer of a pHealth information system can use the template to plan the required privacy and trust services.

The authors have also made proposals for a future ethical, trusted, and privacy-enabled pHealth ecosystem. Here, PHI and health-related behaviors and emotions are the service user's/DS's personal property. Therefore, the DS has the power to express its own privacy and trust needs to the service provider and other ecosystem stakeholders. Transparency and accountability make it possible for the service user to estimate the actual level of privacy and trust in the ecosystem. For estimating the level of trust, the authors propose the use of computational methods [48]. In the proposed solution, users' privacy and trust needs are stored in the form of computer-understandable policies and smart contracts on the blockchain. The legal binding duty concept in the model (fiducial duty) can guarantee fair information processing in the whole ecosystem.

Nevertheless, there are also challenges to be solved. According to Notario et al., ethical concepts, privacy, and trust principles and laws are typically described using high-level terms, and it is difficult to translate them into technical requirements and to support service users concerns and expectations [107]. Some researchers have argued that blockchain technology does not need trust to operate because there is no centralized trust anchor. Instead, according to De Flilippi, blockchain technology produces confidence (and not trust) [108]. Trust in the blockchain is nevertheless necessary because users need trust in the developers and the implementation of algorithms, mathematical knowledge, and cryptographic tools. The authors state that organizational trust and trust in technology are essential elements of ecosystems. What is needed is a commonly accepted definition of the meaning of organizational trust [93].

A big challenge in the authors' proposal is that it requires new internationally accepted regulations and laws. Nowadays, there is no guarantee that policy makers have the intention to enact necessary legislation and force big internet vendors to support and implement laws that can strongly impact their current money-making model. Instead, the responsibility to manage online privacy has been increasingly transferred to service users [109]. Another challenge is to make organizations understand that only systems that behave ethically can be trusted [39]. Some researchers have also argued that a law for data as personal property may be difficult to construct, and this kind of property approach will cause economic losses and less innovation. The authors see that the hybrid approach discussed in this paper is, from the service user's/DS's point of view, a more preferable solution than PHI as a public/common good and current laws.

The authors state that despite researchers' efforts to develop innovative technological privacy solutions, they alone will hardly make future pHealth ecosystems ethical and trustworthy and guarantee information privacy. Instead, it is necessary to start the development of next-generation pHealth ecosystems using a holistic view and a system-theoretical, context-aware, architecture-centred, ontology-based, and policy-driven approach [110] as standardized in ISO 23903:2021 Health informatics: interoperability and integration reference architecture: model and framework [111]. Therefore, the privacy and trust approaches and solutions discussed in this paper will be deployed. It is also necessary to understand privacy and trust in ecosystems at the system level and create new laws to strengthen a person's position. The new solution should also support transparency and explainability. In the long run, global harmonization of how privacy and trust are understood and international regulations are also needed. In agreement with Schneiderman, the authors state that the future pHealth ecosystem shall be created and operated to respect, promote, and protect internationally recognized human rights [112].

Author Contributions: P.R. is the main writer of the original draft; B.B. participated in the development of the draft and made meaningful work in reviewing and editing the article. All authors have read and agreed to the published version of the manuscript.

Funding: This research received no external funding.

Institutional Review Board Statement: Not applicable.

Informed Consent Statement: Not applicable.

Data Availability Statement: Not applicable.

Conflicts of Interest: The authors declare no conflict of interest.

References

1. Cohen, J.E. *Between Truth and Power*; Oxford University Press: Oxford, UK, 2019; ISBN 978-0-91-763754-8.
2. Ruotsalainen, P.; Blobel, B. Privacy and Trust in pHealth—Past, Present and Future. In Proceedings of the pHealth 2022, Oslo, Norway, 8–10 November 2022; Blobel, B., Yang, B., Giacomini, M., Eds.; IOS Press: Amsterdam, The Netherlands, 2022. [CrossRef]
3. Sun, Y.; Zhou, J.; Ji, M.; Pei, L.; Wang, Z. Development and Evaluation of Health Recommender Systems: Systematic Scoping Review and Evidence Mapping. *J. Med. Internet Res.* **2023**, *25*, e38184. [CrossRef] [PubMed]
4. Gellerstedt, M. The digitalization of health care paves the way for improved quality of life. *Syst. Cybern. Inform.* **2016**, *14*, 1–10.
5. Aalbers, G.; Hendrickson, A.T.; MPVanden, A.M.; Keijsers, L. Smartphone-Tracked Digital Markers of Momentary Subjective Stress in College Students: Idiographic Machine Learning Analysis. *JMIR Mhealth Uhealth* **2023**, *11*, e37469. [CrossRef] [PubMed]
6. Rose, C. Ubiquitous Smartphones, Zero Privacy. *Rev. Bus. Inf. Syst. Fourth Quart.* **2012**, *16*, 187–192. [CrossRef]
7. Wei, Z.; Zhao, B.; Su, J. PDA: A Novel Privacy-Preserving Robust Data Aggregation Scheme in People Centric Sensing System. *Int. J. Distrib. Sens. Netw.* **2013**, *9*, 147839. [CrossRef]
8. Zuboff, S. *The Age of Surveillance Capitalism*; Profile Books Ltd.: London, UK, 2019; ISBN 9781781256855.
9. Lamdan, S. *Data Cartels*; Stanford University Press: Stanford, CA, USA, 2023; ISBN 978-1-5036-3371-1.
10. Ziegeldorf, J.H.; Morchom, O.C.; Wehle, K. Privacy in the Internet of Things: Threats and Challenges, Security and Communication networks. *Secur. Commun. Netw.* **2013**, *7*, 2728–2742. [CrossRef]
11. Berger, S.; Rossi, F. AI and neurology: Learning from AI ethics and an expanded Ethics Landscape. *Commun. ACM* **2023**, *66*, 58–68. [CrossRef]
12. van Hoboken, J. *Chapter 10 in Book Human Rights in the Age of Platforms*; Jorgensen, R.F., Ed.; The MIT Press: Cambridge, MA, USA, 2019. Available online: https://mitpress.mit.edu/9780262039055/human-rights-in-the-age-of-platforms/ (accessed on 17 April 2023); ISBN 9780262353946.
13. Hazel, S. Personal Data as Property (7 August 2020). Syracuse Law Review, Forthcoming. Available online: https://doi.org/10.2139/ssrn.3669268 (accessed on 17 April 2023).
14. Piasecki, J.; Cheah, P.Y. Ownership of individual-level health data, data sharing, and data governance. *BMC Med. Ethics* **2022**, *23*, 104. [CrossRef]
15. Grossmann, C.; Goolsby, W.A.; Olsen, L.A.; McGinnis, J.M. *Clinical Data as the Basic Staple of Health Learning: Creating and Protecting a Public Good: Workshop Summary*; The National Academies Press: Washington, DC, USA, 2010. [CrossRef]
16. Taylor, L. The ethics of big data as a public good: Which public? Whose good? *Phil. Trans. R. Soc. A* **2016**, *374*, 20160126. [CrossRef]
17. Schwartz, P.M. Property, Privacy, and Personal Data. Available online: https://ssrn.com/abstract=721642 (accessed on 17 April 2023).
18. Health Data as a Global Public Good. Available online: https://health.ec.europa.eu/ehealth-digital-health-and-care/european-health-data-space_en (accessed on 17 April 2023).
19. Dickens, A. From Information to Valuable Asset: The Commercialization of Health Data as a Human Rights Issue. *Health Hum. Rights J.* **2020**, *22*, 67–69.
20. Health Data as a Global Public Good. Available online: https://cdn.who.int/media/docs/default-source/world-health-data-platform/events/health-data-governance-summit/preread-2-who-data-governance-summit_health-data-as-a-public-good.pdf?sfvrsn=2d1e3ad8_8 (accessed on 17 April 2023).
21. Gstrein, O.J.; Beaulien, A. How to protect privacy in a datafied society? A presentation of multiple legal and conceptual approaches. *Philos. Technol.* **2022**, *35*, 3. [CrossRef] [PubMed]
22. Friedewald, R.F.; Wrigth, D. Seven types of privacy. In *European Data Protection: Coming of Age*; Gutwirth, S., Leenes, R., de Hert, P., Poullet, Y., Eds.; Springer Science+Business Media: Dordrecht, The Netherlands, 2013. [CrossRef]
23. McKnight, D.H.; Choudhury, V.; Kacmar, C. Developing and Validating Trust Measures for e-Commerce: An Integrative Typology. In *The Blackwell Encyclopaedia of Management*; Davis, G.B., Ed.; Management Information Systems; Blackwell: Malden, MA, USA, 2002; Volume 7, pp. 329–331.
24. Ruotsalainen, P.; Blobel, B. How a Service User Knows the Level of How a Service User Knows the Level of Privacy and to Whom Trust in pHealth Systems? *Stud. Health Technol. Inf.* **2021**, *285*, 39–48.
25. Gupta, P.; Akshat Dubey, A. E-Commerce-Study of Privacy, Trust and Security from Consumer's Perspective. *Int. J. Comput. Sci. Mob. Comput.* **2016**, *5*, 224–232.
26. Rubenfield, J. *The End of Privacy*; Yale Law School, Faculty Scholarship Series: New Haven, CT, USA, 2008.
27. Ruotsalainen, P.; Blobel, B. Health Information Systems in the Digital Health Ecosystem—Problems and Solutions for Ethics, Trust and Privacy. *Int. J. Environ. Res. Public Health* **2020**, *17*, 3006. [CrossRef]
28. Rubinstein, I.S. Big Data: The End of Privacy or a New Beginning? In *International Data Privacy Law*; Oxford University Press: Oxford, UK, 2013; Volume 3.
29. Ruotsalainen, P.; Blobel, B. Privacy s Dead–Solutions for Privacy-Enabled Collections and Use of Personal Health Information in Digital Era. *Stud. Health Technol. Inform.* **2020**, *273*, 63–74. [CrossRef]
30. Sharma, S.; Chen, K.; Sheth, A. Towards Practical Privacy-Preserving Analytics for IoT and Cloud-Based Healthcare Systems. *IEEE Internet Comput.* **2018**, *22*, 42–51. [CrossRef]

31. Hansen, J.; Wilson, P.; Verhoeven, E.; Kroneman, M.; Kirwan, M.; Verheij, R.; van Veen, E.-B. *Assessment of the EU Member States' Rules on Health Data in the Light of GDPR*; EU DG Health and Food Safety, Publication Office of the European Union: Luxemburg, 2021; ISBN 978-92-9478-785-9. [CrossRef]
32. Joinson, A.; Houghton, D.J.; Vasalou, A.; Marder, B.L. Digital Crowding: Privacy, Self-Disclosure, and Technology. In *Privacy Online*; Springer Science and Business Media LLC: Berlin/Heidelberg, Germany, 2011; pp. 33–45.
33. DeCew, J.; Zalta, E.N. (Eds.) Privacy, the Stanford Encyclopedia of Philosophy; Zalta, E.N., Ed. Available online: https://plato.stanford.edu/archives/spr2018/entries/privacy/ (accessed on 17 April 2023).
34. WHO. Universal Declaration of Human Rights. Available online: https://www.un.who.org/en/universal-declaration-human-rig (accessed on 17 April 2023).
35. Bélanger, F.; Crossler, R.E. Privacy in the Digital age: A Review of Information Privacy Research in Information systems. *MIS Q.* **2011**, *35*, 1017–1041. [CrossRef]
36. Floridi, L. Ontological interpretations of informational privacy. *Ethics Inf. Technol.* **2006**, *7*, 185–200. [CrossRef]
37. Smith, H.J.; Dinev, T.; Xu, H. Information privacy research: An interdisciplinary review. *MIS Q.* **2011**, *35*, 989–1015. [CrossRef]
38. Waldman, A.E. *Privacy as Trust*; Cambridge University Press: Cambridge, UK, 2018; ISBN 978-1-316-63694-7. [CrossRef]
39. Goldberg, I.; Hill, A.; Shostack, A. *Trust, Ethics, and Privacy*; Boston University Law Review, Boston University, School of Law: Boston, MA, USA, 2001; Volume 81, pp. 407–421.
40. Schwarz, P.M.; Treanor, W.M. The New Privacy, 101 MICH. L. REV. 2163. 2003. Available online: https://repository.law.umich.edu/mlr/vol101/iss6/3 (accessed on 17 April 2023).
41. Marguilis, S.T. Privacy as a Social Issue and Behavioral Concept. *J. Soc. Issues* **2003**, *59*, 243–261. [CrossRef]
42. Becker, M. Privacy in the digital age: Comparing and contrasting individual versus social approaches towards privacy. *Ethics Inf. Technol.* **2019**, *21*, 307–317. [CrossRef]
43. Zwick, D. *Models of Privacy in the Digital Age: Implications for Marketing and E-Commerce*; University of Rhode Island: Kingston, RI, USA, 1999; Available online: https://www.researchgate.net/profile/Nikhilesh-Dholakia/publication/236784823 (accessed on 17 April 2023).
44. Bhatia, J.; Breaux, T.D. Empirical Measurement of Perceived Privacy Risk. *ACM Trans. Comput.-Hum. Interact.* **2018**, *25*, 1–47. [CrossRef]
45. Dinev, T.; Xu, H.; Smith, J.H.; Hart, P. Information privacy and correlates: An empirical attempt to bridge and distinguish privacy-related concepts. *Eur. J. Inf. Syst.* **2013**, *22*, 295–316. [CrossRef]
46. Wisniewski, P.J.; Page, X. Chapter 2: Privacy Theories and Frameworks. In *Modern Socio-Technical Perspectives on Privacy*; Bart, P., Knijnenburg, B.P., Page, X., Wisniewski, P., Lipford, H.R., Proferes, N., Romano, J., Eds.; Springer International Publishing: Cham, Switzerland, 2022; pp. 15–41.
47. Motti, V.G.; Berkovsky, S. Chapter 10 Healthcare Privacy. In *Modern Socio-Technical Perspectives on Privacy*; Bart, P., Knijnenburg, B.P., Page, X., Wisniewski, P., Lipford, H.R., Proferes, N., Romano, J., Eds.; Springer International Publishing: Cham, Switzerland, 2022; pp. 203–231.
48. Ruotsalainen, P.; Blobel, B.; Pohjolainen, S. Privacy and Trust in eHealth: A Fuzzy Linguistic Solution for Calculating the Merit of Service. *J. Pers. Med.* **2022**, *12*, 657. [CrossRef]
49. Sætra, H.K. Privacy as an aggregate public good. *Technol. Soc.* **2020**, *63*, 101422. [CrossRef]
50. DaCosta, S. Privacy-as-Property: A New Fundamental Approach to The Right to Privacy and The Impact This Will Have on the Law and Corporations. CMC Senior Theses. 2635. 2021. Available online: https://scholarship.claremont.edu/cmc_theses/2635 (accessed on 17 April 2023).
51. Acquisti, A.; Brandimarte, L.; Loewenstein, G. Privacy and Human Behavior in the Age of Information. *Science* **2015**, *347*, 509–514. [CrossRef]
52. Beldad, A.; de Jong, M.; Steehouder, M. How shall I trust the faceless and the intangible? A literature review on the antecedents of online trust. *Comput. Hum. Behav.* **2010**, *26*, 857–869. [CrossRef]
53. Nojoumian, M. Rational Trust Modelling, Decision and Game Theory for Security. In Proceedings of the 9th International Conference, GameSec 2018, Seattle, WA, USA, 29–31 October 2018; Bushnell, L., Poovendran, R., Başar, T., Eds.; Lecture Notes in Computer Science. Springer International Publishing: Berlin/Heidelberg, Germany, 2017. [CrossRef]
54. Ruotsalainen, P.; Blobel, B. Transformed Health Ecosystems Challenges for Security, Privacy, and Trust. *Front. Med.* **2022**, *9*, 827253. [CrossRef]
55. Ikeda, S. Is it a rational trust. In *Modern Socio-Technical Perspectives on Privacy*; Knijnenburg, B.P., Page, X., Wisniewski, P., Lipford, H.R., Proferes, M., Romano, J., Eds.; Springer: Berlin/Heidelberg, Germany, 2022. [CrossRef]
56. Pedersen, N.J.L.; Ahlström-Vil, K.; Kappe, K. Rational trust. *Synthese* **2014**, *191*, 1953–1955. [CrossRef]
57. Saariluoma, P.; Karvonen, H.; Rousi, R. Techno-Trust and Rational Trust in Technology–A Conceptual Investigation. In *Human Work Interaction Design. Designing Engaging Automation*; HWID 2018. IFIP Advances in Information and Communication Technology; Springer: Cham, Switzerland, 2019; Volume 544. [CrossRef]
58. McKnight, D.H. Trust in Information Technology. In *The Blackwell Encyclopaedia of Management*; Davis, G.B., Ed.; Management Information Systems; Blackwell: Malden, MA, USA, 2005; Volume 7, pp. 329–331.
59. Balfe, N.; Sharples, S.; Wilson, J.R. Understanding Is Key: An Analysis of Factors Pertaining to Trust in a Real-World Automation System. *Hum. Factors* **2018**, *60*, 477–495. [CrossRef]

60. Yueh, H.-P.; Huang, C.-Y.; Lin, W. Examining the differences between information professional groups in perceiving information ethics: An analytic hierarchy process study. *Front. Psychol.* **2022**, *13*, 954827. [CrossRef] [PubMed]
61. Reitz, J.M. Online Dictionary for Library and Information Sciences. 2014. Available online: https://www.abc-clio.com/ODLIS/odlis_i.aspx (accessed on 17 April 2023).
62. Terrell, B. "Computer and Information Ethics", The Stanford Encyclopedia of Philosophy (Winter 2017 Edition), Zalta, E.N., Ed. Available online: https://plato.stanford.edu/archives/win2017/entries/ethics-computer/ (accessed on 17 April 2023).
63. European Commission, Ethics by Design and Ethics of Use Approaches for Artificial Intelligence, 25 November 2021. Available online: https://ec.europa.eu/info/funding-tenders/opportunities/docs/2021-2027/horizon/guidance/ethics-by-design-and-ethics-of-use-approaches-for-artificial-intelligence_he_en.pdf (accessed on 17 April 2023).
64. Guggenberger, T.M.; Möller, F.; Haarhaus, T.; Gür, I.; Otto, B. Ecosystem Types in Information Systems, Twenty-Eight European Conference on Information Systems (ECIS2020), Marrakesh, Morocco. Available online: https://aisel.aisnet.org/ecis2020_rp/45/ (accessed on 17 April 2023).
65. Benedict, M. Modelling Ecosystems in Information Systems—A Typology Approach. In Proceedings of the Multikonferenz Wirtschaftsinformatik 2018, Lüneburg, Germany, 6–9 March 2018.
66. Dobkin, A. Information fiduciaries in Practice: Data privacy and user expectations. *Berkeley Technol. Law J.* **2018**, *33*, 1. [CrossRef]
67. Balkin, J.M. Information Fiduciaries and the First Amendment. *UC Davis Law Rev.* **2016**, *49*, 1183.
68. Saura, J.R.; Ribeiro-Soriano, D.; Palacios-Marqués, D. Assessing behavioral data science privacy issues in government artificial intelligence deployment. *Gov. Inf. Q.* **2022**, *39*, 101679. [CrossRef]
69. O'Connor, Y.; Rowan, W.; Lynch, L.; Heavin, C. Privacy by Design: Informed Consent and Internet of Things for Smart Health. *Procedia Comput. Sci.* **2017**, *113*, 653–658. [CrossRef]
70. Knijnenburg, B.P. *A User-Tailored Approach to Privacy Decision Support*; University of California: Los Angeles, CA, USA, 2015; Available online: https://escholarship.org/uc/item/9282g37p (accessed on 17 April 2023).
71. Yue, X.; Wang, H.; Jin, D.; Li, M.; Jiang, W. Healthcare Data Gateways: Found Healthcare Intelligence on Blockchain with Novel Privacy Risk Control. *J. Med. Syst.* **2016**, *40*, 218. [CrossRef]
72. Hanish, S.; Arias-Cabarcos, P.; Parra-Arnau, J.; Strufe, T. Privacy-Protecting Techniques for Behavioral Data: A Survey. *arXiv* **2021**, arXiv:2109.04120v1.
73. Huckvale, K.; Prieto, J.T.; Tilney, M.; Benghozi, P.-J.; Car, J. Unaddressed privacy risks in accredited health and wellness apps: A cross-sectional systematic assessment. *BMC Med.* **2015**, *13*, 214.
74. Papageorgiou, A.; Strigkos, M.; Politou, E.; Alepis, E.; Solanas, A.; Patsakis, C. Security and Privacy Analysis of Mobile Health Applications: The Alarming State of Practice. *IEEE Access* **2018**, *6*, 9390–9403. [CrossRef]
75. Kerasidou, C.X.; Kerasidou, A.; Buscher, M.; Wilkinson, S. Before and Beyond Trust: Reliance in Medical AI. *J. Med.* **2020**, *48*, 852–856. Available online: https://jme.bmj.com/content/48/11/852 (accessed on 17 April 2023). [CrossRef]
76. Richards, N.; Hartzog, W. Taking Trust Seriously in Privacy Law. *Stanf. Tech. Law Rev.* **2016**, *19*, 431. [CrossRef]
77. Wilkinson, D.; Sivakumar, S.; Cherry, D.; Knijnenburg, B.P.; Raybourn, E.M.; Wisniewski, P.; Sloan, H. Work in Progress: User-Tailored Privacy by Design. In Proceedings of the USEC'17, San Diego, CA, USA, 26 February 2017; ISBN 1-1891562-47-9. [CrossRef]
78. Knijnenburg, B.P. Chapter 16 User-Tailored Privacy. In *Modern Socio-Technical Perspectives on Privacy*; Bart, P., Knijnenburg, B.P., Page, X., Wisniewski, P., Lipford, H.R., Proferes, N., Romano, J., Eds.; Springer: Berlin/Heidelberg, Germany, 2022. [CrossRef]
79. Li, M.; Yu, S.; Zheng, Y.; Ren, K.; Lou, W. Scalable and Secure Sharing of Personal Health Records in Cloud Computing Using Attribute-Based Encryption. *IEEE Trans. Parallel Distrib. Syst.* **2012**, *24*, 131–143.
80. Ruotsalainen, P.; Blobel, B. *Digital pHealth–Problems and Solutions for Ethics Trust and Privacy, pHealth 2019*; Blobel, B., Giacomini, M., Eds.; IOS Press: Amsterdam, The Netherlands, 2019; pp. 31–46. [CrossRef]
81. Uriarte, R.B.; Zhou, H.; Kritikos, K.; Shi, Z.; Zhao, Z.; De Nicola, R. Distributed service-level agreement management with smart contracts and blockchain. *Concurr. Comput. Pract. Exp.* **2020**, *33*, e5800. [CrossRef]
82. Gursels, S. Privacy and Security Can you engineer privacy? *Commun. ACM* **2014**, *57*, 20–23. [CrossRef]
83. Lopez, G.P.; Montresor, A.; Epema, D.; Datta, A.; Higashino, T.; Iamniychi, A.; Barcellos, M.; Felber, P.; Riviere, E. Edge-centric computing: Vision and Challenges. *ACM SIGCOMM Comput. Commun. Rev.* **2015**, *45*, 37–42. [CrossRef]
84. Cao, X.; Tang, G.; Guo, D.; Li, Y.; Zhang, W. Edge Federation: Towards an Integrated Service Provisioning Model. *IEEE/ACM Trans. Netw.* **2020**, *28*, 1116–1129. [CrossRef]
85. Ritter, J.; Anna Mayer, A. Regulating Data as Property: A New Construct for Moving Forward. *Duke Law Technol. Rev.* **2018**, *16*, 220–277. Available online: https://scholarship.law.duke.edu/dltr/vol16/iss1/ (accessed on 17 April 2023).
86. Samuelson, P. Privacy As Intellectual Property? *Stanf. Law Rev.* **2000**, *52*, 1125. [CrossRef]
87. Koos, S. Protection of Behavioural Generated Personal Data of Consumers. In Proceedings of the 1st Workshop Multimedia Education, Learning, Assessment and Its Implementation in Game and Gamification, Medan, Indonesia, 26 January 2019. [CrossRef]
88. Blanco, S. Trust and Explainable AI: Promises and Limitations. In Proceedings of the ETHICOMP 2022, Turku, Finland, 26–28 July 2022; Koskinen, J., Kimppa, K.K., Heimo, O., Naskali, J., Ponkala, S., Rantanen, M.M., Eds.; University of Turku: Turku, Finland, 2022; pp. 246–257; ISBN 978-951-29-8989-8.

89. Rossi, A.; Lenzini, G. Transparency by design in data-informed research: A collection of information design patterns. *Comput. Law Secur. Rev.* **2020**, *37*, 105402. [CrossRef]
90. EU-GDPR. Available online: Htpps://eur-lex.europa.eu/legal-content/EN/TXT/?uri=CELEX%3A02016R0679-2016950&qid=1532348683434 (accessed on 17 April 2023).
91. Barret, L. Confiding in Con Men: U.S. Privacy Law, the GDPR, and Information Fiduciaries, 42 SEATTLE U. L. REV. 2019; p. 1057. Available online: https://digitalcommons.law.seattleu.edu/sulr/vol42/iss3/5/ (accessed on 17 April 2023).
92. Mayer, R.C.; Davis, J.H.; Schoorman, F.D. An Integrative Model of Organizational Trust. *Acad. Manag. Rev.* **1995**, *20*, 709–734. Available online: http://www.jstor.org/stable/258792.137-154 (accessed on 17 April 2023). [CrossRef]
93. Lumioneau, F.; Schilke, O.; Wang, W. Organizational trust in the age of the fourth industrial revolution: Shifts in the nature, production, and targets of trust. *J. Manag. Inq.* **2022**, *32*. [CrossRef]
94. Hand, D.J. Aspects of Data Ethics in a Changing World: Where Are We Now? *Big Data* **2018**, *6*, 176–190. [CrossRef] [PubMed]
95. Holt, J.; Malčić, S. The Privacy Ecosystem: Regulating Digital Identity in the United States and European Union. *J. Inf. Policy* **2015**, *5*, 155–178. Available online: https://www.jstor.org/stable/10.5325/jinfopoli.5.2015.0155 (accessed on 17 April 2023). [CrossRef]
96. Elrik, E.L. The ecosystem concept: A holistic approach to privacy, protection. *Int. Rev. Law Comput. Technol.* **2021**, *35*, 24–45. [CrossRef]
97. Ferrario, A.; Loi, M. How Explainability Contributes to Trust in AI. In Proceedings of the 2022 ACM Conference on Fairness, Accountability, and Transparency (FAccT'22), Seoul, Republic of Korea, 21–24 June 2022; ACM: New York, NY, USA, 2022; p. 10. [CrossRef]
98. Lederer, S.; Mankoff, J.; Dey, A.K. *A Conceptual Model and Metaphor of Everyday Privacy in Ubiquitous Computing Environments*; Report No, UCB/CSD-2-1288; University of California: Berkeley, CA, USA, June 2002.
99. Wiedemann, K.-P.; Hennings, N.; Varelmann, D.; Reeh, M.-O. Determinants of Consumer Perceived Trust in IT-Ecosystems. *J. Theor. Appl. Electron. Commer. Res.* **2010**, *5*, 137–154. [CrossRef]
100. Najib, W.; Sulityo, S. Widyawan, Surveys on Trust Calculation Methods in Internet of Things. *Procedia Comput. Sci.* **2019**, *161*, 1300–1307. [CrossRef]
101. Truong, N.B.; Um, T.-W.; Lee, G.M. A Reputation and Knowledge Based Trust Service Platform for Trustworthy Social Internet of Things. In Proceedings of the 19th International ICIN Conference–Innovations in Clouds Internet and Networks, Paris, France, 1–3 March 2016.
102. Sattler, A. From Personality to Property? Revisiting the Fundamentals of the Protection of Personal Data. 2018. Available online: https://www.wizdom.ai/publication/10.1007/978-3-662-576465_3/title/from_personality_to_property_revisiting_the_fundamentals_of_the_protection_of_personal_data (accessed on 17 April 2023).
103. Cole, C.L.; Sengupta, S.; Rossetti (ne'e Collins), S.; Vawdrey, D.K.; Halaas, M.; Maddox, T.M.; Gordon, G.; Dave, T.; Payne Philip, R.O.; Williams, A.E.; et al. Ten principles for data sharing and commercialization. *J. Am. Med. Inform. Assoc.* **2021**, *28*, 646–649. [CrossRef] [PubMed]
104. Richter, H. The Power Paradigm in Private Law, Towards a Holistic Regulation of Personal Data. In *Personal Data in Competition, Consumer Protection and Intellectual Property Law*; Springer: Berlin/Heidelberg, Germany, 2018; pp. 527–577. [CrossRef]
105. Gerber, N.; Reinheimer, B.; Volkamer, M. Investigating People's Privacy Risk Perception. *Proc. Priv. Enhancing Technol.* **2019**, *3*, 267–288. [CrossRef]
106. Mitchell, V.-M. Consumer perceived risk: Conceptualizations and models. *Eur. J. Mark.* **1999**, *33*, 163–195. [CrossRef]
107. Notario, N.; Crespo, A.; Martín, Y.-S.; Jose, M.; Alamo, J.M.; Daniel Le Métayer, D.L.; Antignac, T.; Kung, A.; Kroener, I.; Wright, D. PRIPARE: Integrating Privacy Best Practices into a Privacy Engineering Methodology. In *2015 IEEE CS Security and Privacy Workshops*; IEEE: Piscataway, NJ, USA, 2015; pp. 151–158. [CrossRef]
108. De Filippi, P.; Manna, M.; Reijers, W. Blockchain as a confidence machine: The problem of trust & challenges of governance. *Technol. Soc.* **2020**, *62*, 101284. [CrossRef]
109. Shariff, A.; Green, J.; Jettinghoff, W. The Privacy Mismatch: Evolved Intuitions in a Digital World. *Curr. Dir. Phycol. Sci.* **2021**, *30*, 159–166. [CrossRef] [PubMed]
110. Blobel, B.; Oemig, F.; Ruotsalainen, P.; Lopez, D.M. Transformation of Health and Social Care Systems—An Interdisciplinary Approach Toward a Foundational Architecture. *Front. Med.* **2022**, *9*, 802487. [CrossRef] [PubMed]
111. ISO 23903:2021; International Organisation for Standardisation. Health Informatics–Interoperability and Integration Reference Architecture–Model and Framework. ISO: Geneva, Switzerland, 2021.
112. Schneiderman, B. Bridging the Gap Between Ethics and Practice: Guidelines for Reliable, Safe, and Trustworthy Human-Centered AI Systems. *ACM Trans. Interact. Syst.* **2020**, *10*, 1–31. [CrossRef]

Disclaimer/Publisher's Note: The statements, opinions and data contained in all publications are solely those of the individual author(s) and contributor(s) and not of MDPI and/or the editor(s). MDPI and/or the editor(s) disclaim responsibility for any injury to people or property resulting from any ideas, methods, instructions or products referred to in the content.

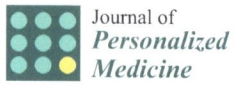

Article

Assessing the Potential Risks of Digital Therapeutics (DTX): The DTX Risk Assessment Canvas

Kerstin Denecke [1,*], Richard May [2], Elia Gabarron [3,4] and Guillermo H. Lopez-Campos [5]

1. Department Engineering and Computer Science, Institute Patient-Centered Digital Health, Bern University of Applied Sciences, 3012 Bern, Switzerland
2. Department of Automation and Computer Science, Harz University of Applied Sciences, 38855 Wernigerode, Germany; rmay@hs-harz.de
3. Norwegian Centre for E-Health Research, University Hospital of North Norway, 9019 Tromsø, Norway; elia.gabarron@hiof.no
4. Department of Education, ICT and Learning, Østfold University College, 1757 Halden, Norway
5. Wellcome-Wolfson Institute for Experimental Medicine, Queen's University Belfast, Belfast BT9 7BL, UK; g.lopezcampos@qub.ac.uk
* Correspondence: kerstin.denecke@bfh.ch

Citation: Denecke, K.; May, R.; Gabarron, E.; Lopez-Campos, G.H. Assessing the Potential Risks of Digital Therapeutics (DTX): The DTX Risk Assessment Canvas. *J. Pers. Med.* 2023, 13, 1523. https://doi.org/10.3390/jpm13101523

Academic Editors: Bian Yang, Bernd Blobel and Mauro Giacomini

Received: 5 October 2023
Revised: 18 October 2023
Accepted: 19 October 2023
Published: 23 October 2023

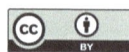

Copyright: © 2023 by the authors. Licensee MDPI, Basel, Switzerland. This article is an open access article distributed under the terms and conditions of the Creative Commons Attribution (CC BY) license (https://creativecommons.org/licenses/by/4.0/).

Abstract: Motivation: Digital therapeutics (DTX), i.e., health interventions that are provided through digital means, are increasingly available for use; in some countries, physicians can even prescribe selected DTX following a reimbursement by health insurances. This results in an increasing need for methodologies to consider and monitor DTX's negative consequences, their risks to patient safety, and possible adverse events. However, it is completely unknown which aspects should be subject to surveillance given the missing experiences with the tools and their negative impacts. Objective: Our aim is to develop a tool—the DTX Risk Assessment Canvas—that enables researchers, developers, and practitioners to reflect on the negative consequences of DTX in a participatory process. Method: Taking the well-established business model canvas as a starting point, we identified relevant aspects to be considered in a risk assessment of a DTX. The aspects or building blocks of the canvas were constructed in a two-way process: first, we defined the aspects relevant for discussing and reflecting on how a DTX might bring negative consequences and risks for its users by considering ISO/TS 82304-2, the scientific literature, and by reviewing existing DTX and their listed adverse effects. The resulting aspects were grouped into thematic blocks and the canvas was created. Second, six experts in health informatics and mental health provided feedback and tested the understandability of the initial canvas by individually applying it to a DTX of their choice. Based on their feedback, the canvas was modified. Results: The DTX Risk Assessment Canvas is organized into 15 thematic blocks which are in turn grouped into three thematic groups considering the DTX itself, the users of the DTX, and the effects of the DTX. For each thematic block, questions have been formulated to guide the user of the canvas in reflecting on the single aspects. Conclusions: The DTX Risk Assessment Canvas is a tool to reflect the negative consequences and risks of a DTX by discussing different thematic blocks that together constitute a comprehensive interpretation of a DTX regarding possible risks. Applied during the DTX design and development phase, it can help in implementing countermeasures for mitigation or means for their monitoring.

Keywords: digital therapeutics; adverse event; patient safety; surveillance

1. Introduction

After having addressed quality requirements according to ISO/TS 82304-2 for evaluating the deployment of conversational agents in healthcare [1,2], in this paper, we dive deeper into the topic of assessing the risks associated with the use of digital therapeutics (DTX). DTX offer therapeutic interventions to patients delivered through high-quality software programs [3]. Similar to drugs or other treatments, they aim to cure, manage, or prevent disease. DTX can be used alone or in combination with other therapies, medical devices, or pharmaceuticals to improve patient care and health outcomes and are delivered as web-based disease prevention programs [4], conversational agents that deliver cognitive behavioral therapy [5,6], or in other ways.

The global DTX market size was estimated at USD 5.09 billion in 2022 and is expected to grow [7]. Applications related to diabetes and diabetes management dominated the global DTX market and held the largest revenue share of more than 28% in 2022. In 2022, North America held a commanding position in the digital therapeutics market, accounting for 40.7% of the market share. This can be attributed to the increasing implementation of healthcare spending reduction initiatives in the region, combined with a strong commitment to adopting a patient-centered approach to healthcare [7]. Some DTX can automatically adapt to the user's needs and support active patient involvement in their care and disease self-management. For example, Woebot is a mental health chatbot that uses artificial intelligence (AI) and cognitive behavioral therapy techniques to provide mental health support to users [5]. EndeavorRx [8] is a DTX that aims to improve attention function in children aged 8–12 years with primarily inattentive or combined Attention Deficit Hyperactivity Disorder (ADHD) who have a demonstrated attention problem. It is the first FDA-approved ADHD treatment delivered through a video game.

Depending on their intended use, risk classification, and the regulations of the country in which a DTX is marketed, some DTX are classified as medical devices. For such DTX, some countries have already implemented a prescription and reimbursement process [9]. As of October 2023, the DTX Alliance lists nine countries in which DTX are available with a regulatory and reimbursement process in place (https://dtxalliance.org/ (accessed on 25 September 2023)). These include the United States, Japan, Singapore, South Korea, the UK, Australia, China, France, and Germany. For example, a regulatory and reimbursement pathway for DTX in the German market has been established [10] and the "fast-track" regulatory process for DTX was launched in 2019.

As they are used by individuals with or without the supervision of a healthcare practitioner, the quality of DTX is essential to avoid harming patients. However, we can recognize a lack of research on harm and the adverse effects of DTX and its current methodological imprecision [11]. A reason might be that it is still unclear which adverse reactions, responses, or risks can occur in the context of DTX. For example, one app that provides cognitive behavioral therapy for insomnia patients—which has been approved for reimbursement upon prescription in Germany—asks patients to keep a diary in the morning and evening using the app. However, no information is provided as part of the usage instructions and list of adverse effects that the blue light from the device might affect sleep and sleep quality. The effect has already been researched but obviously has not been reflected when developing the app [12]. This raises the question of whether developers of DTX are sufficiently reflecting on possible adverse reactions, responses, or risks (e.g., app–app interactions). Additionally, there is still no knowledge available about which negative consequences and risks can occur outside the controlled environment of clinical trials. Similar to drug–drug interactions, DTX can potentially interact with other digital health tools in a non-controlled environment [13]. Research and critical reflections on this are still missing.

To overcome this situation and ensure more patient safety, we believe it is necessary to carefully reflect on potential risks before DTX are released to market or tested on a large scale with patients. This paper therefore introduces a tool, a Risk Assessment Canvas for DTX. Its aim is to support a critical reflection on aspects that should be considered during the DTX development phase and for risk surveillance purposes when releasing DTX to the market, when prescribing a specific DTX to prepare for the broad range of negative effects and risks the use of DTX may cause, or for warning individuals before using a DTX. In previous work, we already recognized that the ISO Technical specification 82304-2 (ISO/TS 82304-2) Health software—Part 2: Health and wellness apps—Quality and reliability [2] provides relevant information to ensure high-quality conversational agents in healthcare [1].

In that paper, we linked quality requirements specified in the ISO/TS 82304-2 to global evaluation metrics defined for conversational agents in healthcare. Only a limited overlap was recognized, namely for the metrics related to ease of use, security, and accessibility. In this work, we will again use this technical specification in addition to other sources of information to identify relevant aspects for the risk assessment of DTX.

2. Materials and Methods

In this paper, we are suggesting a "DTX Risk Assessment Canvas" as a tool that supports a critical reflection on adverse reactions, events, and risks of a specific DTX. We are taking the Business Model Canvas developed by Osterwalder and Pigneur [14] as the basis for the development. It consists of nine "building blocks" that can be used to describe a business model. It is argued that a business model can be defined as a model that "describes the rationale for how an organization creates, delivers and captures value" [14] and that this definition can be captured by participants discussing all the "building blocks" of a business model. By discussing the different building blocks of a business model, such as key partners, channels, or revenue streams, it is possible to develop a comprehensive understanding of the way in which a company or organization is supposed to create, deliver, and capture value. In its original form, the business model canvas is used for a collaborative discussion. It has been adapted to other domains such as ethics [15].

Taking the business model canvas as a starting point, we defined building blocks to enable an interdisciplinary group of researchers, developers, practitioners, and potential users of a specific DTX to discuss and reflect on how this DTX might result in risks for users, the care process they are involved in, and the patient's health. Similar to the business model canvas, we believe that by discussing the different aspects related to a DTX, such as risks, harms, or problematic use, it is possible to develop a comprehensive understanding of the adverse reactions, events, and risks of a DTX. This will help in developing countermeasures or establishing surveillance methodologies.

To achieve this, we collected different aspects that could contribute to adverse reactions, events, and risks of a DTX. The aspects or building blocks of the canvas were constructed in a two-way process: first, one author (KD) defined the building blocks. This was undertaken based on previous work related to quality of conversational agents in healthcare: KD considered the ISO/TS 82304-2, which was first published in August 2020 [2]. It is based upon guidelines and requirements for apps. Its purpose is to ensure that health and wellness apps are safe, reliable, and effective. The technical specification is intended for use by app manufacturers as well as app assessment organizations in order to communicate the quality and reliability of a health app. It groups quality aspects into 5 categories: product information, healthy and safe, easy to use, secure data, and robust build. It has already been considered for collecting aspects for an evaluation framework for conversational agents in healthcare. Therefore, KD assessed the quality requirements listed in this specification and selected aspects that might be of interest for assessing aspects related to the risks associated with a DTX. Additionally, she studied the relevant literature and the product information of the DTX listed in the DTX repository of the German Authorities for regulating drugs and medical devices (https://diga.bfarm.de/de/verzeichnis (accessed on 25 September 2023)). At the time of reviewing these, 54 DTX were listed in the repository. Relevant aspects were collected and aggregated into groups that formed at the end the thematic blocks of the canvas.

In a second step, 6 experts in health informatics and mental health provided feedback and tested the understandability of the canvas by individually applying it to a DTX of their choice. None of the experts were introduced to the canvas before the test. They were provided with a brief introduction to the DTX Risk Assessment Canvas and its objectives, including its expected use. They were asked to consider a concrete DTX and reflect on the aspects listed in the canvas. Additionally, they were asked to provide feedback on the process of applying the canvas. The experts' input was used to adapt the canvas and the guiding questions. The resulting canvas will be described in Section 3.

3. Results

3.1. DTX Risk Assessment Canvas

The DTX Risk Assessment Canvas is organized into 15 thematic blocks. They are grouped together into three thematic groups (see Figure 1): DTX (Section 3.1.1), users of the DTX (Section 3.1.2), and effects of the DTX (Section 3.1.3). For each block, guiding questions have been formulated to encourage researchers, developers, and practitioners to reflect on the individual thematic blocks (Table 1 and Figure A1).

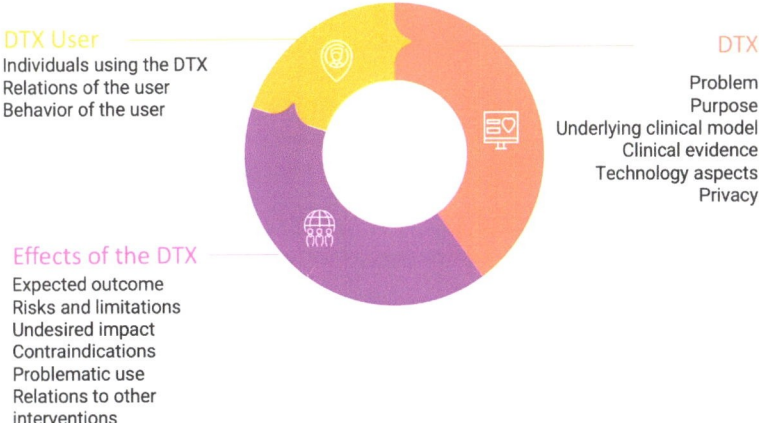

Figure 1. Overview of the three thematic groups and 15 thematic blocks of the DTX Risk Assessment Canvas.

Table 1. The DTX Risk Assessment Canvas including the guiding questions.

	Guiding Questions
	DTX
Problem	What is the medical condition the DTX addresses? What is it supposed to help with?
Purpose	What is the intended purpose of the DTX? (e.g., coaching, diagnosing, information provision, self-management support) What is the DTX expected to support, to improve, or to achieve support (e.g., having a relationship with a care provider or availability of a support person)? Is there a declared purpose as foreseen by the medical device regulation?
Underlying clinical model	Is the DTX modelled based on a non-digital health intervention (e.g., cognitive behavior therapy)? Which one? Which negative impacts are known for this non-digital health intervention? What is the clinical evidence of this non-digital health intervention (i.e., efficacy and safety results measured by a clinical trial)?
Clinical evidence	What is the underlying clinical evidence of the DTX as measured in a clinical trial? Does it differ from the clinical evidence of the related non-digital health intervention (if there is a non-digital health intervention based on which the DTX was modeled)?
Technology aspects that may impact outcome or the individual	What are technology aspects of the DTX that may impact the outcome of the DTX or its user (user interface design, personalization techniques, gamification, automatic adaptation, or learning...)? E.g., using gamification to increase adherence to the DTX could have a negative impact on persons with addictive behavior.
Privacy	Are data collected and processed by the DTX? What happens to the data? Does data storage and processing consider country-specific regulations (e.g., GDPR)? Are there any data privacy issues that could result in negative impacts on the user?

Table 1. *Cont.*

	Guiding Questions
	User of the DTX
Individuals using the DTX	Who uses the DTX? (e.g., men, women, age, race, profession, health status...) Does the expected user group have specific characteristics regarding their health?
Relations of the user	What relations does the user have that are somehow related to the DTX? (e.g., relatives and family, healthcare professionals, social workers...).
Behavior of the user	How might the user's behavior change because of the use of the DTX? How are users expected to interact with the DTX?
	Effects of DTX
Expected outcome	What is the expected outcome of the DTX? Has the outcome already been studied in a clinical trial?
Risks and limitations	Are there specific user groups for whom the DTX creates risks or who cannot use the DTX? Are there care settings in which the DTX should not be applied?
Contraindications	Are there medical conditions for which the use of the DTX should be avoided? Are there other treatments that provide a contraindication for using the DTX?
Undesired impact	What are the potential undesired impacts of the DTX? What happens in case of system failure? Which technology aspects might impact the outcome of the DTX (e.g., blue light can cause sleep problems)? What could go wrong? What failure could happen? How may relations of the user change through the use of the DTX? (e.g., patient–doctor relationship, family).
Problematic use	What could be a problematic use of the DTX? Can it be misused?
Relations to other interventions	What interactions with other interventions (digital or non-digital) can occur? What interactions can have an impact on the outcome of the intervention delivered through the DTX?

3.1.1. Thematic Blocks Related to the DTX

The group DTX considers aspects related to the digital solution that are described by six thematic blocks: problem, purpose, clinical model, clinical evidence, technology aspects, and privacy [16]. First, the problem the DTX addresses should be specified when reflecting the possible risks of a DTX. Guiding questions include: which medical condition is addressed or what is the DTX supposed to support? This aspect is of relevance since there may be risks associated with the medical condition the DTX is targeting. For example, Yang and Li studied the "dark side" of gamification for healthcare management support and found "that both privacy invasion and social overload are positively associated with users' gamification exhaustion" [17].

The second aspect to be reflected related to the DTX is the purpose. We define purpose as the aim or goal of the DTX. The purpose of a DTX has to be described, in particular when assigning a DTX to one of the medical device classes defined by the medical device regulations [18]. However, since the canvas is also relevant for DTX that are not considered medical devices, we consider specifying the purpose as relevant for all DTX. The purpose may impact the care process where a DTX will be integrated and where risks could be associated with.

Two other thematic blocks related to the solution consider the underlying clinical model and the clinical evidence. Sometimes an existing clinical model is digitized in a DTX, so the risks or negative impacts of this clinical model could also be relevant to the digital version. For example, the chatbot Woebot integrates the clinical model of cognitive behavioral therapy [5,19]. Possible risks associated with this type of therapy might have already been studied for its non-digital delivery.

A non-digital health intervention is assessed regarding efficacy and safety in clinical trials (phase III). This is summarized as clinical evidence. A similar concept has been defined for medical devices: According to the International Medical Device Regulators

Forum, clinical evidence is "the clinical data and the clinical evaluation report pertaining to a medical device." [20]. Given the missing knowledge of safety aspects related to DTX, the DTX Risk Assessment Canvas asks to reflect on the non-digital health intervention that may underly a DTX (i.e., the clinical model) and its effects and evidence. Our canvas therefore asks for reflecting on the clinical evidence of the DTX.

Another important aspect regarding the DTX itself is technology aspects that may have an impact on the outcome of the DTX or its users. Within this thematic block, it is important to reflect on aspects such as personalization techniques, the realization of interactions between the user and the DTX (e.g., an empathetic chatbot who claims to be a best friend could have an impact on social contacts in the real world), or technology aspects such as blue light transmitted by the screen of the smartphone or the PC screen.

The sixth thematic block related to the DTX itself considers privacy which is strongly related to data processing and storage as well as associated security mechanisms [16]. Data misuse or reuse for different purposes may have negative impacts on the users of a DTX [21], even in the context of their safety.

3.1.2. Thematic Blocks Related to the User of a DTX

A second group of aspects in the canvas addresses three aspects related to the user of a DTX: user, relations of the user, behavior of the user. The idea behind the user block is to help in identifying aspects related to the health or sociodemographic aspects of the user that may be problematic when using a DTX. It aims to capture details such as cultural aspects of the expected user group.

In certain situations, the use of a DTX may also impact the relationships with other individuals associated with the DTX user such as relatives or friends. Related to this, risks or undesired impacts can occur (which are then reflected in the third thematic block under "undesired impact"). Therefore, the second thematic block in this group concerns the relations of the user.

The third thematic block asks to reflect on the behavior of the user. Here we are asking to think about potential changes in the user's behavior because of the use of a DTX and for the expected interaction with the DTX. As exemplified, the above mentioned therapeutic video game EndeavorRx [8] for children with primarily inattentive or combined Attention Deficit Hyperactivity Disorder led to an increased aggressivity in some kids. It could have been reflected in advance, i.e., before releasing the DTX, that playing videogames can lead to negative behavior changes in kids. Even though this could not be changed, it could be indicated as a possible effect to be surveilled as part of the surveillance process of this DTX.

3.1.3. Thematic Blocks Related to the Effects of a DTX

The third group deals with the effects of a DTX and consists of six thematic blocks: Expected outcome, risks and limitations, contraindications, undesired impact, problematic use, and relations to other interventions. First, the expected outcome should be reflected. What is the DTX expected to support, to improve, or to achieve? We are also asking whether the outcome has already been studied in a clinical trial.

Second, risks and limitations should be collected. A DTX could create risks for a specific user group or specific users might be prevented from using a DTX. For example, people with visual impairment may have problems with interacting with a text-based conversational agent (or when they use it, the risk for wrong usage behavior could increase). Potential harms caused by gamification elements should be considered here when gamification is a technology aspect of the DTX. There might be also care settings in which a DTX should not be applied. These aspects are asked to be reflected.

Third, contraindications are collected. In this item, contraindications of the underlying clinical model should be reflected. Although it might be still unknown whether the DTX will have the same contraindications as the underlying clinical model, a critical reflection might already be useful to create an awareness of potential risks.

Fourth, reflections on problematic use of the DTX are requested by the canvas. Can the DTX be misused by users or used in a way that leads to health issues or other negative impacts? These considerations are important to develop mitigation strategies for problematic use or—when the DTX is supposed to be integrated in a care process—to create sensitivity to the potential risk of misuse by the care provider.

The fifth thematic block related to the effects of the DTX addresses interactions with other interventions (digital or non-digital, regulated or unregulated interventions). For example, the exposure to other digital contents might affect the use or outcome of a DTX [22]. An example of this type of interaction would be interactions of the user with social media and their influence on the outcomes of a DTX addressing the eating disorder of the user [23].

Sixth, it should be reflected which inferences of potential undesired impacts the DTX may have. For this reflection, the information on the user and the DTX as collected by the thematic blocks in the other two groups as well as of the other five thematic blocks of this group are relevant to be considered. This thematic block is probably the core of the canvas. As exemplified, a DTX can impact the relationship with the healthcare provider. This clearly depends on the integration into the care flow. When a user uses a DTX accompanying the standard therapy without letting the treating healthcare provider know, adverse events cannot be recognized; trust in the healthcare provider could be impacted, etc. The technological aspects collected in the first block can lead to undesired impacts. Besides this, we are asking to think about situations of system failure, specifically which failures could occur in a real-world setting.

3.1.4. Expected Use of the DTX Risk Assessment Canvas

We expect the use of the DTX Risk Assessment Canvas to be in a participatory discussion process among developers of the DTX, healthcare professionals and other groups of persons that might be involved in the process the DTX is supposed to be used in, and researchers. The participants discuss the aspects defined by the 15 thematic blocks. Further, potential users of the DTX under consideration could be involved in this reflection process. Specifically, the canvas is used by the group to reflect on risks associated with the DTX. First, the group will collect and aggregate the information on the DTX (thematic group 1) and its users (thematic group 2). Once this has been undertaken, the third thematic group is used to assess potential risks. Another option is that the participants are reflecting on the 15 thematic blocks in an individual manner and meet afterwards to discuss and aggregate their individually collected thoughts in the group discussion. To support this process, we are providing a sheet with the 15 thematic blocks to be filled (Figure A2) and a sheet with the guiding questions per block (Figure A1).

When applied during the conceptual or development phase of a DTX, the collected possible risks and adverse events can be considered in order to implement possible mitigation strategies. For harms and risks where no mitigation strategy can be found, a clear announcement in terms of possible contraindications or risks associated with DTX use should be provided to all users of a DTX. Also, surveillance measures can be put in place to at least monitor the risks.

To facilitate working with the canvas in multidisciplinary teams, we created a glossary of terms with definitions of the most important terms (Table A1). Since the participants in the risk assessment process can originate from different fields, it has to be ensured that a common terminology is used.

4. Discussion

4.1. Relevance to Prior Work

With regulations released in recent years (e.g., the EU Medical Device Regulation), there are DTX that are classified as medical devices and are now subject to similar development and approval processes as drugs and medical devices. They are tested on selected volunteers and patients prior to market launch to verify their efficacy and safety. Their effectiveness of use must be proven through systematic clinical trials [24] that assess the outcome in controlled settings to reduce bias. In fact, the most often chosen study design for DTX is randomized controlled trials (RCT) [25]. When reading through the instructions of use for the DTX currently approved for prescription in Germany [9], we can recognize that the surveillance of a DTX relies upon active reporting from the users and eventually healthcare providers. All apps listed in the German repository confirm that no adverse effects were recognized in the trial or testing phase (September 2023). Even obvious contraindications such as the one described in the introduction (blue light having an impact on sleep quality [26]) remain undescribed in the usage instructions.

In pharmacological treatment, assessment of harm takes place in all phases of the clinical trials, from the early preclinical and basic science phases of the development (Phase I) to the postmarketing stage (Phase IV). In contrast, DTX are typically studied in single-phased RCTs aimed at evaluating their efficacy or observation studies focused on assessing their clinical efficacy and comparison with current treatments, omitting in-depth harm assessments during treatment development [27]. Beyond this, the need for conducting a clinical trial and assessing adverse effects and efficacy does only apply for DTX that are classified as medical devices. Ensuring user safety would be necessary for any DTX available to individuals.

For drugs, a monitoring process called pharmacovigilance has become mandatory in order to collect risks and adverse effects after the market release of a drug. A similar approach was suggested with upcoming Artificial Intelligence (AI) applications in healthcare. The concept of "Algorithmovigilance" introduced by P. Embi in 2021 is an approach to evaluate systematically AI-enabled health interventions [28]. It focuses basically on the AI algorithms, their development, and related biases. Recently, we defined the field of digitalovigilance as a research field for collecting, detecting, assessing, monitoring, and preventing adverse effects caused by DTX [13]. However, only risks or events that are known can be surveilled in such a process.

The DTX Risk Assessment Canvas therefore aims to support analyzing the complexities and challenges related to DTX. DTX often involve a combination of technology, healthcare processes, patient engagement, and data management. The canvas provides a structured framework to consider and reflect on these multifaceted aspects. It also helps in assessing the impacts of a DTX in a landscape of diverse stakeholders. We intentionally did not include regulatory and ethical considerations related to DTX in order to focus on the technical-related risks and adverse events. There are other tools and frameworks available to address these aspects. For example, the Digital Therapeutics Alliance formulated a DTX Industry Code of Ethics [29]. The Ethics Canvas provided by the ADAPT Centre and Trinity College Dublin is a tool that supports reflection on the ethical aspects of solutions (not necessarily digital health solutions) [30].

A common process for assessing the value of a health technology is health technology assessment (HTA): *"HTA is a multidisciplinary process that uses explicit methods to determine the value of a health technology at different points in its lifecycle. The purpose is to inform decision-making in order to promote an equitable, efficient, and high-quality health system"* [31]. Traditional HTA does not cover all factors relevant to digital tools, such as accessibility and data security and protection [32]. To address this issue, Haverinen et al. adapted the HTA framework for realizing the HTA process for digital healthcare services. The framework was named Digi-HTA [33]. It contains aspects that are related to ours in the DTX Risk Assessment Canvas; for example, it asks for safety issues related to robotics and AI. As in the traditional HTA process, the effectiveness is of importance as well. In our framework, we included clinical evidence. However, the Digi-HTA includes aspects such as usability and interoperability as well as costs, which are not part of our canvas. The overlapping aspects show the relevance of aspects such as data security or technology aspects on patient safety. In addition to the Digi-HTA, other resources have been developed for digital health technology assessment across different regions in the world: the Digital Technology Assessment Criteria for Health and Social Care (DTAC) in the UK, the Digital

Health Assessment Framework (DHAF) in the US, NorDEC in Nordic countries in Europe, and the overarching ORCHA. As was previously discussed in the context of Digi-HTA, these HTA solutions cover areas that are not covered in our canvas. Table 2 presents the similarities and differences between these different digital health technology assessment tools and our DTX Risk Assessment Canvas. The overlapping domains across all these tools are privacy, clinical evidence, and functionality and purpose, whereas other relevant domains in regulatory DHTA such as usability or interoperability are not covered in the DTX Risk Assessment Canvas. Many of these other approaches represent a comprehensive process to be realized when the implementation of the digital solution has been completed, while our DTX Risk Assessment Canvas is supposed to be used in the development and design phase to address relevant aspects already in the development phase. Beyond this, our canvas should also be used for DTX that are not considered medical devices to ensure user safety. Digi-HTA and HTA processes are normally only applied to medical devices since the assessment process is very comprehensive and time-consuming.

Table 2. This table presents the similarities and differences between different digital health technology assessment (DHTA) tools and the proposed DTX Risk Assessment Canvas.

Digital Health Technology Assessment Tool	No. Domains	Domains Details	Overlapping Concepts with DTX Risk Assessment Canvas
DTX Risk Assessment Canvas	3	DTX description User of the DTX Effects of the DTX	
The Digital Technology Assessment Criteria for Health and Social Care (DTAC) (UK) [1]	5	Clinical Safety Data Protection Technical security Interoperability criteria Value proposition (not assessed)	Privacy, clinical evidence, functionality and purpose, and intended users
ORCHA Baseline review (OBR) [2]	3	Clinical or professional assurance Data and privacy Usability and accessibility	Privacy, clinical evidence, and functionality and purpose
Digi-HTA [33]	11	Company information Product information Technical stability Usability and accessibility Interoperability Cost Effectiveness Clinical safety Data security and protection Artificial intelligence Robotics	Privacy, clinical evidence, and functionality and purpose
Digital Health Assessment Framework (DHAF) (US) [3]	4	Data and Privacy Clinical assurance and safety Usability and accessibility Technical security and stability	Privacy, clinical evidence, and functionality and purpose
NorDEC (Nordic countries Europe) [4]	5	Data and Privacy Professional Assurance and clinical safety Usability and accessibility Security and technical stability Interoperability	Privacy, clinical evidence, and functionality and purpose

[1] https://transform.england.nhs.uk/key-tools-and-info/digital-technology-assessment-criteria-dtac/ (accessed on 17 September 2023), [2] https://orchahealth.com (accessed on 17 September 2023), [3] https://dhealthframework.org (accessed on 17 September 2023), [4] https://norddec.org (accessed on 17 September 2023).

There are also technical specifications for health and wellness apps addressing aspects around quality and reliability developed by the ISO committee. We considered these specifications in the definition of the thematic blocks and guiding questions. We retrieved some input for our DTX Risk Assessment Canvas. For example, the ISO/TS 82304-2 contains the subcategories "health risks" and "health benefit" as well as "privacy" and "security". However, the technical specification is intended to be used by developers, manufacturers, and regulatory bodies to assess and improve the performance of health software applications. It offers guidance on various aspects of app development, such as user interface design, data security, interoperability, and usability. It is a comprehensive guideline covering multiple aspects. In contrast, our DTX Risk Assessment Canvas is more focused on the negative consequences and adverse events of DTX and also considers the processes a DTX is supposed to be used in.

4.2. Strengths and Limitations

This is, to our knowledge, the first attempt at supporting a critical reflection on possible adverse events for DTX. In this way, we offer a guidance for reflection that could hopefully support the development of countermeasures for potential serious adverse events, or at least a warning towards the users. The DTX Risk Assessment Canvas is based on the literature, the ISO/TS 82304-2, and on existing evidence in terms of DTX and their contraindication and adverse events, as well as expert knowledge.

So far, the canvas is a proof of concept prototype that was tested by a limited number of users. It is clear that this cannot ensure the understandability and completeness of the canvas. A more comprehensive evaluation is needed to ensure understandability. However, the canvas is intended to provide a basis for thinking about and discussing possible adverse reactions. This does not necessarily require that for all possible aspects questions are contained in the canvas.

5. Conclusions

In an increasingly digitalized world, the role of digitalovigilance for the detection and study of the potential interactions between the different digital health components will be key to the safe use of DTX and their integration in care processes.

Future research will have to study effects on patient safety and outcomes when different DTX are combined and evaluated together, similar to the way combined drug therapies are currently used. Although a complete assessment of the adverse effects of DTX and their interactions is impossible, it is important to recognize and consider them. The DTX Risk Assessment Canvas provides a tool to reflect the possible risks and negative consequences of a DTX by discussing different thematic blocks that together constitute a comprehensive interpretation of a DTX regarding aspects relevant to be considered within surveillance of a DTX. It is expected that it will raise awareness for the need for a systematic assessment of risks associated with the use of DTX and for the discipline "digitalovigilance", ensuring continuous monitoring of such negative impacts going beyond the regulatory minimum. Consequently, our next steps are to first validate the usage of the canvas in workshops and to derive from this validation phase a workshop concept that can be used by persons developing a DTX. Additionally, the validation phase would result in an improved knowledge of the possible risks of a DTX, which helps in developing monitoring measures. We expect the best time to use the canvas is during the design stage since many options in terms of development and realization are still open, which will allow the implementation of countermeasures to the potential risks right from the beginning. However, it could also be applied in later development stages or during use time to tailor surveillance methods. This still has to be studied.

Author Contributions: Conceptualization, K.D. and G.H.L.-C.; methodology, K.D.; initial canvas development, K.D.; validation of canvas, G.H.L.-C., E.G. and R.M.; writing—original draft preparation, K.D.; writing—review and editing, G.H.L.-C., E.G. and R.M.; All authors have read and agreed to the published version of the manuscript.

Funding: This research received no external funding.

Institutional Review Board Statement: Not applicable.

Informed Consent Statement: Not applicable.

Data Availability Statement: Not applicable.

Conflicts of Interest: The authors declare no conflict of interest.

Appendix A

Table A1. Definitions of Terms Attached to the Canvas.

Term	Definition
Adverse event	An adverse event is an unexpected and undesirable occurrence or outcome that happens during or after a medical treatment, intervention, or the use of a DTX. Adverse events can range from mild side effects to severe complications and may include reactions to medications, medical procedures, medical device malfunctions, or incidents related to healthcare delivery. The identification, reporting, and analysis of adverse events are crucial in healthcare to monitor and improve the safety and effectiveness of treatments and interventions.
Clinical evidence	Clinical evidence refers to the information and data obtained from clinical research studies and trials that provide insights into the effectiveness, safety, and potential benefits or risks of medical treatments, interventions, therapies, or procedures. This evidence is gathered through systematic scientific research involving human participants under controlled conditions and is a fundamental component of evidence-based medicine.
Clinical model	Therapeutic approach underlying a non-digital health intervention.
Contraindication	A contraindication or counter-indication is a circumstance that prohibits the use of a diagnostic or therapeutic procedure in the case of a given indication or only permits it after strict consideration of the risks involved.
Digital Therapeutic (DTX)	DTX provide patients with evidence-based therapeutic interventions. They are delivered through high-quality software programs.
Gamification	Gamification is the practice of incorporating game-like elements, such as points, challenges, and rewards, into DTX to engage and motivate individuals, encouraging desired behaviors and achieving specific goals. It aims to make tasks or interactions with a DTX more enjoyable and interactive, often enhancing engagement and adherence.
Harm	Harm refers to any adverse effect or negative outcome experienced by individuals as a result of using DTX. This can include physical harm, such as health complications arising from the use of a medical app, as well as privacy breaches, emotional distress, or misinformation that may result from the interaction with DTX.
Impact	Impact in the context of DTX refers to the measurable and often intended outcomes or effects resulting from the implementation and use of DTX. These impacts can be categorized as follows: Expected Impact: These are the anticipated and planned positive outcomes that DTX aim to achieve. Expected impacts may include improved patient outcomes, enhanced access to healthcare services, increased efficiency in healthcare delivery, cost savings, and better management of health conditions. These effects are typically part of the intervention's intended goals and objectives. Undesired impact: These are unanticipated consequences, whether positive or negative, that arise from the use of DTX. Undesired impacts can include unanticipated benefits or risks that were not initially foreseen during the development and implementation of the intervention. These effects may emerge as users engage with the technology, and they may require adjustments or further evaluation to address.

Table A1. Cont.

Term	Definition
Problematic use	Problematic use of a DTX refers to when an individual excessively relies on or becomes overly preoccupied with a DTX or applies it for other purposes then foreseen, leading to negative impacts on their well-being or health outcomes. This can include spending too much time using the tool, prioritizing it over professional advice, experiencing negative emotions related to its use, and even neglecting other aspects of their life, potentially harming their health.
Privacy	Privacy refers to the protection of individuals' personal health information and data collected, processed, or shared through DTX. It involves ensuring that sensitive health-related data are kept confidential and secure.
Risk	Risk refers to the potential for adverse outcomes or harm associated with the use or deployment of DTX. These risks can include issues related to data security and privacy, inaccurate health information, user dependence, and negative health consequences resulting from the intervention.

DTX Risk Assessment Canvas - guiding questions

DTX | **Author** | **Date**

Red – Digital therapeutic

Problem
What is the medical condition the DTX addresses? What is it supposed to help with?

Purpose
information provision, self management support)
What is the DTX expected to support, to improve or to achieve support (e.g. having a relationship with a care provider, or availability of a support person)?
Is there a declared purpose as foreseen by the medical device regulation?

Technology aspects impacting on outcome
What are technology aspects of the DTX that may impact on the outcome of the DTX or its user (user interface design, personalization techniques, gamification, automatic adaptation or learning…)? E.g. gamification to increase adherence to the DTX could have a negative impact on persons with addictive behavior

Privacy
Is data collected and processed by the DTX? What happens to the data? Does data storage and processing consider the country-specific regulations (e.g. GDPR)? Are there any data privacy issues that could result in negative impacts on the user?

Clinical evidence
What is the underlying clinical evidence of the DTX as measured in a clinical trial?
Does it differ from the clinical evidence of the related non-digital health intervention (if there is a non-digital health intervention based on which the DTX was modelled on)?

Underlying clinical model
Is the DTX modelled based on a non-digital health intervention? Which negative impacts are known for this non-digital health intervention? What is the clinical evidence of this non-digital health intervention?

Green – User of the digital therapeutic

Individuals using the DTX
Who uses the DHI? (e.g. men, women, age, race, profession, health status…)
Does the expected user group have specific characteristics regarding their health?

Behavior of the user
How might user's behavior change because of the use of the DTX? How are users expected to interact with the DTX?

Relations of the user
Which relations does the user has that are somehow related to the DTX? (e.g. relatives and family, healthcare professionals, social workers…)

Blue – Effects of the digital therapeutic

Expected outcome
What is the expected outcome of the DTX? Has the outcome already been studied in a clinical trial?

Risks and limitations
Are there specific user groups for whom the DTX creates risks or who cannot use the DTX?
Are there care settings where the DTX should not be applied?

Undesired impact
What are potential undesired impacts? What happens in case of system failure? What could go wrong? What failure could happen?

Contraindications
Are there medical conditions when the use of the DTX should be avoided?
Are there other treatments that provide a contraindication for using the DTX?

Problematic use
What could be a problematic use of the DTX? Can it be misused?

Relations to other interventions
Which interactions with other interventions (digital or non-digital) can occur?
Which interactions can have an impact on the outcome of intervention delivered through the DTX?

DTX – Digital therapeutic

Figure A1. DTX Risk Assessment Canvas and Guiding Questions.

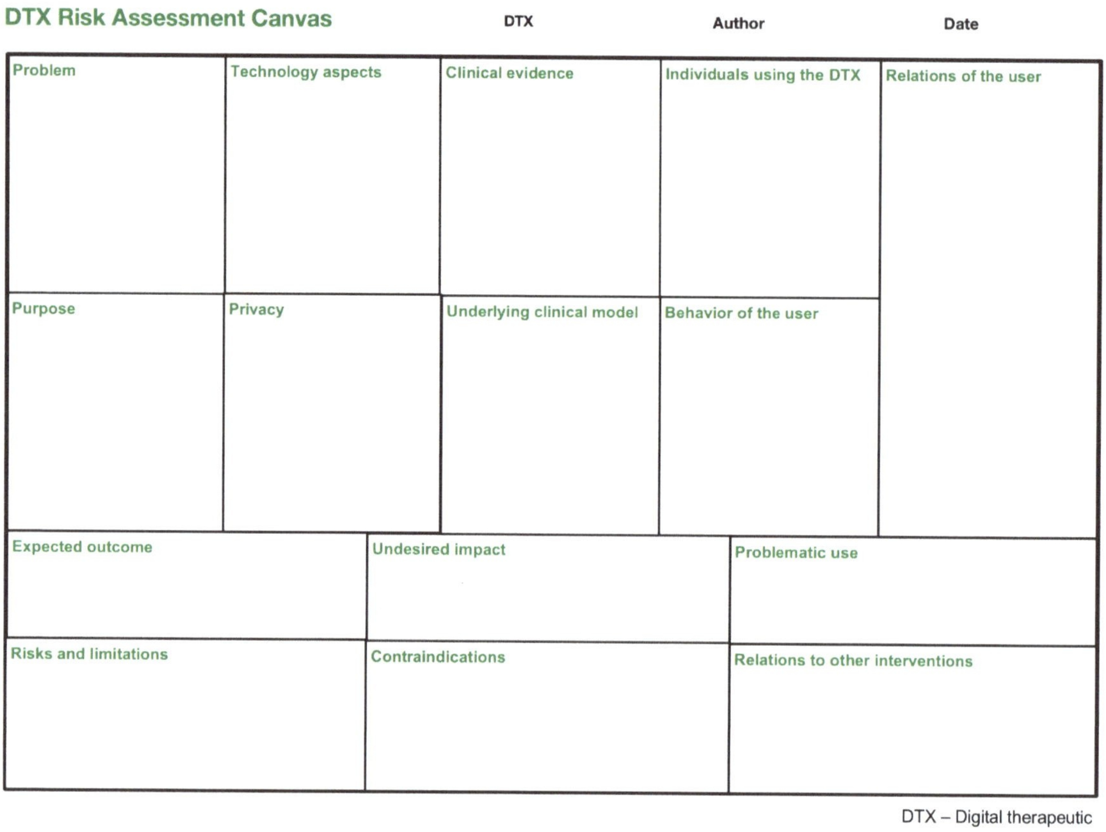

Figure A2. DTX Risk Assessment Canvas Template.

References

1. Denecke, K.B.; Elizabeth, M.; Andre, W.K. What can we learn from quality requirements in ISO/TS 82304-2 for evaluating conversational agents in healthcare? In *Studies in Health Technology and Informatics*; IOS Press: Amsterdam, The Netherlands, 2022; pp. 245–250.
2. ISO/TS 82304-2; Technical Specification: Part 2: Health Software—Health and Wellness Apps—Quality and Reliability. ISO: Geneva, Switzerland, 2021. Available online: https://www.iso.org/standard/78182.html (accessed on 20 September 2023).
3. Crisafulli, S.; Santoro, E.; Recchia, G.; Trifirò, G. Digital Therapeutics in Perspective: From Regulatory Challenges to Post-Marketing Surveillance. *Front. Drug Saf. Regul.* 2022, 2, 900946. [CrossRef]
4. Renton, T.; Tang, H.; Ennis, N.; Cusimano, M.D.; Bhalerao, S.; Schweizer, T.A.; Topolovec-Vranic, J. Web-based intervention programs for depression: A scoping review and evaluation. *J. Med. Internet Res.* 2014, 16, e209. [CrossRef]
5. Darcy, A.; Beaudette, A.; Chiauzzi, E.; Daniels, J.; Goodwin, K.; Mariano, T.Y.; Wicks, P.; Robinson, A. Anatomy of a Woebot® (WB001): Agent guided CBT for women with postpartum depression. *Expert Rev. Med. Devices* 2022, 19, 287–301. [CrossRef]
6. Maher, C.A.; Davis, C.R.; Curtis, R.G.; Short, C.E.; Murphy, K.J. A Physical Activity and Diet Program Delivered by Artificially Intelligent Virtual Health Coach: Proof-of-Concept Study. *JMIR mHealth uHealth* 2020, 8, e17558. [CrossRef] [PubMed]
7. Digital Therapeutics Market Size, Share &Trends Analysis Report. Available online: https://www.grandviewresearch.com/industry-analysis/digital-therapeutics-market (accessed on 17 September 2023).
8. Akili Interactive Labs. 'EndeavorRx'. Available online: https://www.endeavorrx.com/faq/ (accessed on 5 April 2023).
9. Bundesinstitut für Arzneimittel und Medizinprodukte. German Federal Institute for Drugs and Medical Devices. DiGa (Digital Health Applications). Available online: https://www.bfarm.de/EN/Medical-devices/Tasks/DiGA-and-DiPA/Digital-Health-Applications/_node.html (accessed on 20 September 2023).
10. Federal Ministry of Health. Driving the Digital Transformation of Germany's Healthcare System for the Good of Patients. Available online: https://www.bundesgesundheitsministerium.de/en/digital-healthcare-act.html (accessed on 5 April 2023).

11. Bergin, A.D.G.; Valentine, A.Z.; Rennick-Egglestone, S.; Slade, M.; Hollis, C.; Hall, C.L. Identifying and Categorizing Adverse Events in Trials of Digital Mental Health Interventions: Narrative Scoping Review of Trials in the International Standard Randomized Controlled Trial Number Registry. *JMIR Ment. Health* **2023**, *10*, e42501. [CrossRef] [PubMed]
12. Hering, T. Blaues Licht—Einfluss auf Schlafen und Wachen. *MMW Fortschritte Med.* **2020**, *162*, 56–58. [CrossRef] [PubMed]
13. Lopez-Campos, G.; Gabarron, E.; Martin-Sanchez, F.J.; Merolli, M.; Petersen, C.; Denecke, K. Digital interventions and their unexpected outcomes—Time for digitalovigilance. In *Studies in Health Technology and Informatics*; IOS Press: Amsterdam, The Netherlands, 2023.
14. Osterwalder, A.; Pigneur, Y.; Clark, T. *Business Model Generation: A Handbook for Visionaries, Game Changers, and Challengers*; Wiley: Hoboken, NJ, USA, 2010.
15. Reijers, W.; Koidl, K.; Lewis, D.; Pandit, H.J.; Gordijn, B. Discussing ethical impacts in research and innovation: The ethics canvas. In *This Changes Everything—ICT and Climate Change: What Can We Do?* HCC13 2018. IFIP Advances in Information and Communication Technology; Kreps, D., Ess, C., Leenen, L., Kimppa, K., Eds.; Springer International Publishing: Cham, Switzerland, 2018; Volume 537, pp. 299–313. [CrossRef]
16. Denecke, K. Framework for Guiding the Development of High-Quality Conversational Agents in Healthcare. *Healthcare* **2023**, *11*, 1061. [CrossRef] [PubMed]
17. Yang, H.; Li, D. Understanding the dark side of gamification health management: A stress perspective. *Inf. Process. Manag.* **2021**, *58*, 102649. [CrossRef]
18. Aronson, J.K.; Heneghan, C.; Ferner, R.E. Medical Devices: Definition, Classification, and Regulatory Implications. *Drug Saf.* **2020**, *43*, 83–93. [CrossRef] [PubMed]
19. Prochaska, J.J.; Vogel, E.A.; Chieng, A.; Kendra, M.; Baiocchi, M.; Pajarito, S.; Robinson, A. A Therapeutic Relational Agent for Reducing Problematic Substance Use (Woebot): Development and Usability Study. *J. Med. Internet Res.* **2021**, *23*, e24850. [CrossRef] [PubMed]
20. Medical Device Clinical Evaluation Working Group. Clinical Evidence—Key Definitions and Concepts. 2019. Available online: https://www.imdrf.org/sites/default/files/2021-09/imdrf-cons-clinical-evaluation-kdc-190405.pdf (accessed on 20 September 2023).
21. May, R.; Security, K.D.; Care, I.H.S. Security, privacy, and healthcare-related conversational agents: A scoping review. *Inform. Health Soc. Care* **2021**, *47*, 194–210. [CrossRef] [PubMed]
22. Lopez-Campos, G.; Merolli, M.; Martin-Sanchez, F. Biomedical Informatics and the Digital Component of the Exposome. *Stud. Health Technol. Inform.* **2017**, *245*, 496–500. [PubMed]
23. Sanzari, C.M.; Gorrell, S.; Anderson, L.M.; Reilly, E.E.; Niemiec, M.A.; Orloff, N.C.; Anderson, D.A.; Hormes, J.M. The impact of social media use on body image and disordered eating behaviors: Content matters more than duration of exposure. *Eat. Behav.* **2023**, *49*, 101722. [CrossRef]
24. Wang, C.; Lee, C.; Shin, H. Digital therapeutics from bench to bedside. *Npj Digit. Med.* **2023**, *6*, 38. [CrossRef]
25. Huh, K.Y.; Oh, J.; Lee, S.; Yu, K.-S. Clinical Evaluation of Digital Therapeutics: Present and Future. *Healthc. Inform. Res.* **2022**, *28*, 188–197. [CrossRef] [PubMed]
26. Silvani, M.I.; Werder, R.; Perret, C. The influence of blue light on sleep, performance and wellbeing in young adults: A systematic review. *Front. Physiol.* **2022**, *13*, 943108. [CrossRef]
27. Britton, W.B.; Lindahl, J.R.; Cooper, D.J.; Canby, N.K.; Palitsky, R. Defining and Measuring Meditation-Related Adverse Effects in Mindfulness-Based Programs. *Clin. Psychol. Sci.* **2021**, *9*, 1185–1204. [CrossRef] [PubMed]
28. Embi, P.J. Algorithmovigilance-Advancing Methods to Analyze and Monitor Artificial Intelligence-Driven Health Care for Effectiveness and Equity. *JAMA Netw. Open* **2021**, *4*, e214622. [CrossRef] [PubMed]
29. Digital Therapeutics Alliance. DTx Industry Code of Ethics. 2019. Available online: https://dtxalliance.org/wp-content/uploads/2019/11/DTA_DTx-Industry-Code-of-Ethics_11.11.19.pdf (accessed on 20 September 2023).
30. ADAPT Centre & Trinity College Dublin. 'Ethics Canvas'. 2023. Available online: https://www.ethicscanvas.org (accessed on 20 September 2023).
31. O'Rourke, B.; Oortwijn, W.; Schuller, T.; International Joint Task Group. The new definition of health technology assessment: A milestone in international collaboration. *Int. J. Technol. Assess. Health Care* **2020**, *36*, 187–190. [CrossRef] [PubMed]
32. Martínez-Pérez, B.; De La Torre-Díez, I.; López-Coronado, M. Privacy and Security in Mobile Health Apps: A Review and Recommendations. *J. Med. Syst.* **2015**, *39*, 181. [CrossRef]
33. Haverinen, J.; Keränen, N.; Falkenbach, P.; Maijala, A.; Kolehmainen, T.; Reponen, J. Digi-HTA: Health technology assessment framework for digital healthcare services. *Finn. J. eHealth eWelfare* **2019**, *11*, 326–341. [CrossRef]

Disclaimer/Publisher's Note: The statements, opinions and data contained in all publications are solely those of the individual author(s) and contributor(s) and not of MDPI and/or the editor(s). MDPI and/or the editor(s) disclaim responsibility for any injury to people or property resulting from any ideas, methods, instructions or products referred to in the content.

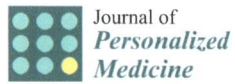

Article

HL7-FHIR-Based ContSys Formal Ontology for Enabling Continuity of Care Data Interoperability

Subhashis Das * and Pamela Hussey

ADAPT Centre & CeIC, Dublin City University (DCU), D09FW22 Dublin, Ireland; pamela.hussey@dcu.ie
* Correspondence: subhashis.das@dcu.ie

Abstract: The rapid advancement of digital technologies and recent global pandemic-like scenarios have pressed our society to reform and adapt health and social care toward personalizing the home care setting. This transformation assists in avoiding treatment in crowded secondary health care facilities and improves the experience and impact on both healthcare professionals and service users alike. The interoperability challenge through standards-based roadmaps is the lynchpin toward enabling the efficient interconnection between health and social care services. Hence, facilitating safe and trustworthy data workflow from one healthcare system to another is a crucial aspect of the communication process. In this paper, we showcase a methodology as to how we can extract, transform and load data in a semi-automated process using a common semantic standardized data model (CSSDM) to generate a personalized healthcare knowledge graph (KG). CSSDM is based on a formal ontology of ISO 13940:2015 ContSys for conceptual grounding and FHIR-based specification to accommodate structural attributes to generate KG. The goal of CSSDM is to offer an alternative pathway to discuss interoperability by supporting a unique collaboration between a company creating a health information system and a cloud-enabled health service. The resulting pathway of communication provides access to multiple stakeholders for sharing high-quality data and information.

Keywords: data integration; EHR; FHIR; interoperability; ontology; knowledge graph; healthcare system

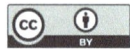

Copyright: © 2023 by the authors. Licensee MDPI, Basel, Switzerland. This article is an open access article distributed under the terms and conditions of the Creative Commons Attribution (CC BY) license (https://creativecommons.org/licenses/by/4.0/).

1. Introduction

In the age of information and communication technology (ICT), digital systems support various sectors, for example, day-to-day business, education, transportation, or tourism. The healthcare sector is one example where the digital footprint is more prominent as well as disruptive, with a vision to transform the healthcare system and service from the local to the global level. The pandemic brought about by the repeated recurrence of variants of COVID-19 has crucially transformed the modality of the functioning of industries and service-providing industries that are natively dependent on ICT tools and technologies. The healthcare and social care sectors have been quick to respond to COVID-19, necessitating, in some cases, a transformation of functioning modality, cognizant of the dual-sided impact on ICT. To that end, the various national healthcare and social care service providers are formulating and integrating digital transformation action plans as the foundational basis in the planning of next-generation social care systems, for example, the United Kingdom National Health Service Plan (NHS) by 2025 [1]. With the increasing maturity of digital platforms and platform-based services in society, the gap between organizational requirements and citizens' needs is becoming diminished as the potential value of remote monitoring and home-based solutions, which are technologically founded, is realized. Such initiatives are resulting in a greater demand for digitized healthcare and social care services, both for service providers and end users. Technologically driven solutions, for example, can provide the scheduling of online interactions, the remote monitoring of health conditions, and a more efficient access for sharing information with healthcare professionals to address demands and plan care interventions. To meet such demands, the analysis of only electronic health records (EHRs) is insufficient. The inclusion and consideration of user needs and the social embedding of the context of care delivery can be crucial. For the above aspect, some important parameters can include purchasing agility, socio-economical living standards, digital literacy and healthcare information access and consent. To securely access information from one setting to another, healthcare management architecture such as well-defined access control, data modeling and conceptual reference frameworks are needed. Recent evidence signposts the fiscal implications and importance of standards. For example, the inadequacy and malfunctioning of IT systems and equipment cost the healthcare industry an amount equivalent to almost 8000 full-time doctors, or nearly GBP 1 billion in the UK [2]. Additionally, the 21st Century Cures Act: Interoperability, Information Blocking, and the ONC Health IT program was proposed by the US government Office of the National Coordinator (ONC) [3].

From a European standard perspective, the Rolling Plan for ICT Standardization (2022) by the European Commission prioritizes healthcare interoperability, cross-border treatment, and the involvement of societal stakeholders in the development of EHR systems within the European Health Data Space (EHDS). Therefore, standards such as the ISO 23903:2021 Health informatics—Interoperability and integration reference architecture—Model and framework shall become mandatory [4]. The accuracy of data integration and interoperability cannot be decided at data level, but must be modeled according to the ISO 23903 model and framework [4]. This foundational standard focuses on ecosystems which offer a harmonized representation to realize interoperability and advance systems that are flexible, scalable, and follow a systems-oriented, architecture-centric, ontology-based, and policy-driven approach [5]. ISO 23903:2021 also provides a clear rationale as to why multi-domain interoperability not only requires the improvement of a data model, informal model, and ICT-domain-specific knowledge, but also highlights the need to define the business model perspective [4,6]. To represent an advanced interoperability and integration of different domain knowledge use cases, the requirement of using a top-level ontology 78-driven approach is specified in ISO 21838 [7].

Internationally, the reference of a conceptual modeling formalism to represent and support concepts relevant for the continuity of care (i.e., ContSys) is ISO: 13940:2015 system of concepts to inter-relate patient needs, which comprise their overall care journey [8]. In scientific terms, ContSys grounds the healthcare continuity of care into clinical processes toward facilitating the reuse of health and social care information for non-native purposes, such as knowledge management activities. To that end, it formalizes the connection between patients who are subjects of care and healthcare professionals. The Health Level 7 (HL7) Fast Healthcare Interoperability Resources (FHIR) [9] provides a set of modular components (FHIR resources) along with detailed requirements for use to store data in order to address queries on a wide range of healthcare-related problems. Less noticeable in these resources is a formal semantic data model, which can be used for integrating datasets from across different healthcare facilities. The latest research has shown various advantages of knowledge graphs (KGs) for the utilization of her data and the provision of explicit explainable results to address healthcare queries over time. KGs represent the knowledge, relationship, and data entities in a formal ontological structure so that the healthcare concepts in the knowledge graph are explicit [10]. In this paper, we present a hybrid model and subsequent steps to manifest how the OWL 2 (web ontology language v2) ontology model can enable data integration from different existing legacy database systems using a semi-automated mapping. Our proposed common semantic standardized data model (CSSDM) aligns with ISO 23903:2021 Health informatics—Interoperability and integration reference architecture—Model and framework [4].

The remainder of the paper is organized as follows. Section 2 details the research background of the work findings on a comprehensive review of relevant scientific literature in healthcare information model and health informatics standards. Section 3 elucidates the overview of the proposed CSSDM methodology. Section 4 provide a glimpse of the technical implementation of the CSSDM ontology and populated KG model and an illustrative evaluation of its performance against (user) queries. Section 5 summarizes and concludes the paper by stressing the need of standardization and an ontology-based information model to enable the continuity of healthcare services.

This paper is an extended version of the work originally published in the 19th International Conference on Wearable Micro- and Nano-Technologies for Personalized Health (pHealth) conference 2022 titled "FHIR-Based ContSys Ontology to Enable Continuity of Care Data Interoperability" [11]. The extended version elaborated in detail the technical system architecture to generate a personalized knowledge graph.

2. Related Works

To understand social and technical interaction within healthcare networks, socio-technical theories such as actor–network theory (ANT) provides a set of useful guiding principles [12]. The co-participation (i.e., engagement of people) organization in system design can be obtained by using the quadruple helix model (a model involved in the creation of a network of interactions and relationships between university–industry–government–public environments within a knowledge economy designed for creating value) [13]. On the one hand, ontology-based information models allow us to capture complex relations in a formal language, as well as integrate different schemas based on semantic meaning. On the other hand, ontology provides a formal way to capture existing knowledge of the world [14]. Using fundamental ontological principles, we are able to capture all kinds of relations existing in the multi-faceted and complex contextual healthcare network. For example, relationships such as professional relation/role (e.g., doctor, patient, or nurse), spatial relation (e.g., *located-in* or *address*), applied technologies (e.g., mHealth apps, telemedicine), or qualitative performance (e.g., quality of service, drug performance) can be handled by a web ontology language (OWL) model [15]. There is not only the aspect of the social relationship that plays a major role in a complex healthcare system, but there are also other non-social relations. For example, spatial relation, organization structures, interaction among information systems, and other events associated with the healthcare setting that demand and require analysis. We believe that the combination of both ontological principles and social principles can complement each other, thus leading to a better understanding of the socio-technical system (STS) and thereby creating avenues for the implementation of an enhanced and robust model.

The ontological analysis of complex healthcare networks using actor–network theory (ANT) on health facilities has been described in a recent study by Iyamu, T. and Mgudlwa, S. [16]. A study by the eHealth Research Group from the University of Edinburgh highlights the role of ANT in understanding the implementation of information technology developments in healthcare. Although this study was mainly a theoretical analysis, it provided various approaches on how to deal with healthcare networks from an ANT perspective. The Yosemite Project [17], for example, suggested using resource description framework (RDF) as the representative of universal information in order to achieve semantic interoperability of all structured healthcare information. The Yosemite Project's study, however, overlooked human involvement in the design process as well as merging other healthcare schema standards such as the International Organization for Standardization (ISO) system of concepts for the continuity of care (ContSys). As a standard, ContSys is essential for connecting different healthcare settings. ContSys provides an overarching conceptual model, including professional healthcare activity as well as self-care, care by a healthcare third party such as a family member, personal care assistant or homecare service provider, and extends to include all aspects of social care over the life course of an individual subject of care. These existing standards, however, do not align with W3C semantic web technologies and linked data, which, in particular, are the key drivers for creating and maintaining a global interconnected graph of data. More recently, a paper by Shang Y. et al. (2021) [10] emphasized the use of knowledge graphs to connect various nonclinical data with EHR for better decision making. Knowledge graphs represent knowledge and data entities in a formal ontological structure so that the healthcare concepts in the model are explicit. A recently completed H2020 InteropEHRate project [18] also demonstrates an interoperability infrastructure using technologies for health data exchange that is centered on the citizen. This project did not, however, implement or align with specific ISO standards, thus potentially limiting its re-use at an international scale.

According to the survey conducted by the Deloitte Center for Health Solution and on the EU rolling plan for ICT standardization (2022) [19], the main drawbacks of the existing healthcare systems are as follows:

1. Scattered resources and multiple technology platforms.
2. Healthcare professionals were poorly involved in designing and implementing the healthcare information model.
3. A lack of information models, based on native formal ontology language, ignoring the inclusion of social determinants of health concepts in the model.
4. Existing systems rely on system-specific query language such as archetype query language (AQL) [20] for query and retrieval, thus restricting federated queries and the linking of social determinants of health.
5. An inability in many cases of the health care systems to support knowledge graph structures.
6. Healthcare domain investment with healthcare professional-oriented tools and methods to support and render the model interpretation.
7. A lack of interoperable patient records.

The study of Manard, S. et al. (2019) [21] explains well the lack of interoperability in the implemented EHRs systems in primary and specialty care in Europe. A nationwide study by Moore, N. et al. (2021) [22] and the World Economic Forum (WEF) report on sustainability and resilience in the French, Irish, and Spanish Health System (2021) [23]. This evidence reports on the lack of interoperability and associated standardization between ambulatory, hospital, and social (long-term) care providers. In fact, this has long been recognized as a major drawback in terms of service efficiency, cost control, and the quality and sustainability of care provision, both at the central and regional levels, which hinders the better planning and monitoring of patient care and outcomes. Another aspect often missed in healthcare interoperability is avoiding stakeholder viewpoints and thereby relying on certain vendor-specific and service-provider-centric EHR systems or the use of technical jargon (e.g., medication statement) without properly consulting healthcare professionals for its meaning, who are using it for data capture (i.e., model of use). The lack of interoperability is a major obstacle in progress on the digital single market [24]. While implementing interoperability between systems, with particular attention to semantic interoperability in healthcare, there is a tendency to overlook certain pertinent components. This can then passively influence the objective of accomplishing interoperability and capacity to report upon important data such as social determinants of health (SDH). The secondary use of health data can reveal new insights to understand SDH by linking healthcare data with other datasets such as geospatial, economy and finance or population datasets cited by Marmot [25] as a key indicator for addressing poverty. The objective of this research work is to develop a common semantic standardized data model (CSSDM) to achieve interoperability in the continuity of care network and contribute to influencing health and life expectancy [25].

As part of the development of a standards-based roadmap to inform our research, several standards were critiqued to inform our decision-making and development plan. For example, ISO/AWI TR 24305 Health informatics—Guidelines for the implementation of HL7/FHIR based on ISO 13940 and ISO 13606 were reviewed, and it was noted on that neither of the aforementioned resources have to date modified the existing ISO 13940-based model, nor is any semantic formalism in this initial work included [26]. By semantic formalism, we mean the use of knowledge representation (KR) language that is based on description logic (DL), for example, the web ontology language (OWL2) [27] as recommended by W3C. OWL2 encodes knowledge using a specific standardized (XML, RDF) syntax. It provides a given information model with a formal semantics framework, which is usually realized operationally using hypertableau-based reasoning. This decision is based on the fact that OWL is clearly tailored for a specific logic and reasoning method and OWL is the most adequate interchange formalism for KR and automated reasoning (AR) [28].

Subsequent work also highlights the key challenges as a result of the limited involvement of healthcare professionals in designing and implementing the healthcare information model. For the most part, health care models are designed by ICT professionals and often with a minimal involvement of healthcare professionals, with such models consequently becoming more ICT-driven than being domain-driven for the context of use [29]. Non-standardized and self-defined data models can therefore more often face adoption problems for scaling diverse EHR datasets [30]. FHIR as a resource also does not provide any specific implementation guidelines for context of use or functionality. Examples from different countries include the USA, who have their own FHIR profile, compared to a FHIR profile used by Indian hospitals, which indicate that the two FHIR profiles are not interoperable. This would suggest that, in our review of the evidence, there is no published native FHIR OWL specification for use as part of a semantic model. There are, in existence, a small number of ongoing projects attempting to develop a transformation schema in order to transform FHIR JSON to JSON-LD and then convert into a Terse RDF triple language (Turtle) format. They are, however, in our view not fit for data integration as they neither follow any ontological principle as suggested by OntoClean methodology [31], nor clearly make any distinction between the structured attributes and classes. In this paper, we mainly focus on the adoption of a collaborative approach to address these aforementioned gaps. Through working with ISO Health informatics' technical committee (ISO/TC 215) and based on the experience gained from the EU Horizon 2020 interopEHRate project, we provide in the following section a summary of the results of our selected methodology and technical implementation.

3. Methodology

We initiate our proposed methodology with two key assumptions. The first assumption is not to create another new ontology or propose a new working item proposal for another draft standard (i.e., draft international standard (DIS)), but rather use the existing mature and in-use standards with recently published ISO TC215 standards to inform an emerging standards-based road map that may provide potential solutions to the existing healthcare system challenges in order to address semantic interoperability raised in the introduction section. The second assumption is reusability, by which, we mean the usage of what is the best practice from the given domain. For example, using OntoClean methodology as proposed by Guarino and Welty (2002) [31] to build an ontologically well-founded backbone infrastructure to support the formal model. In terms of modeling software and tool adoption, we utilize Protégé, a popular and free ontology editor developed by Stanford Center for Biomedical Informatics Research [32].

Our rationale to choose RDF/XML is based on the following reasoning: the syntax as RDF/XML was the first RDF format created by W3C and it is therefore considered in the evidence as a foundation standard format. This would suggest that in most RDF libraries and triple stores, the output RDF is used in this format by default, thereby suggesting that if one should want to work with legacy RDF systems or would want to use XML libraries to manipulate data (as RDF/XML is valid XML), then the RDF/XML is the most practical format to use.

The main backbone of our methodology is based on ISO/TS 22272 Health Informatics—Methodology [33–35] for the analysis of business and information needs of health enterprises to support standards-based architectures. The projects' main objective is to create a common semantic standardized data (CSSDM) model, which has the functionality to connect an existing legacy system using a semi-automated mapping process as well as a defined OWL data model facility to potentially link with all existing open-linked datasets so that secondary data analysis can be facilitated and run over time.

We have also critically analyzed and accommodated the viewpoint of ISO 23903:2021—Interoperability and integration reference architecture, Care Coordination Measures Atlas [36], and a future inference model [37]. This was achieved through the process modeling of the patient-centric view and considering core foundation requirements to reach an agreed target state as detailed in ISO/TS 22272:2021 [37]. The overall process of engagement with defined resources in CSSDM is shown in Figure 1 and is further expanded upon in the following sections. In Step 1, we engaged in the development of a formal ontology for continuity of care [38], the technical details of which are illustrated in Section 4 of this paper. In this action step, we considered and consulted existing available resources relating to information models, which we identified as relevant in the context of continuity of care. These include national EHR, regional EHR model, HL7 FHIR resources and the ASTM continuity of care records (CCR) model, which were then used to support and inform the development of use cases and clinical workflows mapped against and translated into the formal OWL model.

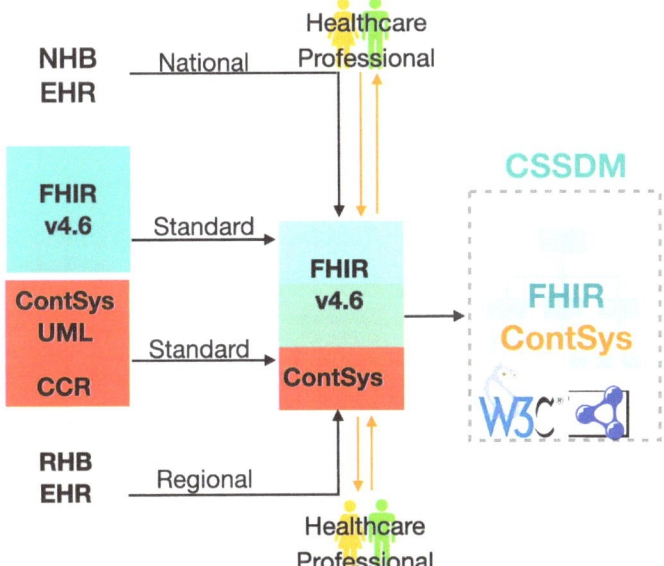

Figure 1. CSSDM process. NHB: National Health Board, FHIR: Fast Healthcare Interoperability Resources, UML: Unified Modeling Language, CCR: Continuity of Care Record, RHB: Regional Health Board, EHR: Electronic health record, W3C: World Wide Web Consortium.

In Step 2, we presented, discussed, and disseminated information on our formal OWL model with clinical domain experts and national and international technical committees, which we engaged with in order to agree and map concepts based on their meanings. These included presenting our work at national conferences and postgraduate educational programs of study with multidisciplinary health care practitioners. Key decisions achieved through this discussion included exploring core concepts such as the subject of care and its equivalent to *FHIR:Patient* and *ObservedCondition*, subsequently mapping with *FHIR:Observation*. In the case of *FHIR:Medication* request, we could not identify an exact mapping in the ContSys resource. We therefore opted to create a subclass of request; the mapping detail is presented in Table 1.

Table 1. ContSys FHIR mapping.

ContSys Concept	FHIR Resources
SubjectOfCare: Healthcare actor with a person role who seeks to receive, is receiving, or has received healthcare	FHIR:Patient: Demographics and other administrative information about an individual or animal receiving care or other health-related services.
ObservedCondition: Health condition observed by a healthcare actor	FHIR:Observation: Measurements and simple assertions made about a patient, device or other subject.
Request: Demand for care where a healthcare professional asks a healthcare provider to perform one or more healthcare provider activity	No one-to-one mapping available
MedicationRequest (new subclass)	FHIR: MedicationRequest: An order or request for both supply of the medication and the instructions for administration of the medication to a patient.

In Step 3, we created a summary of the enriched formal OWL model with the attributes specified in the FHIR resources. Figure 2 shows a snapshot from the ontology editor. On the left-hand side, it provides the location of the particular concept in the class hierarchy, i.e., subject of care is a subclass of role. Alternatively, on the right side of the diagram, all attributes which are borrowed from FHIR resources are illustrated.

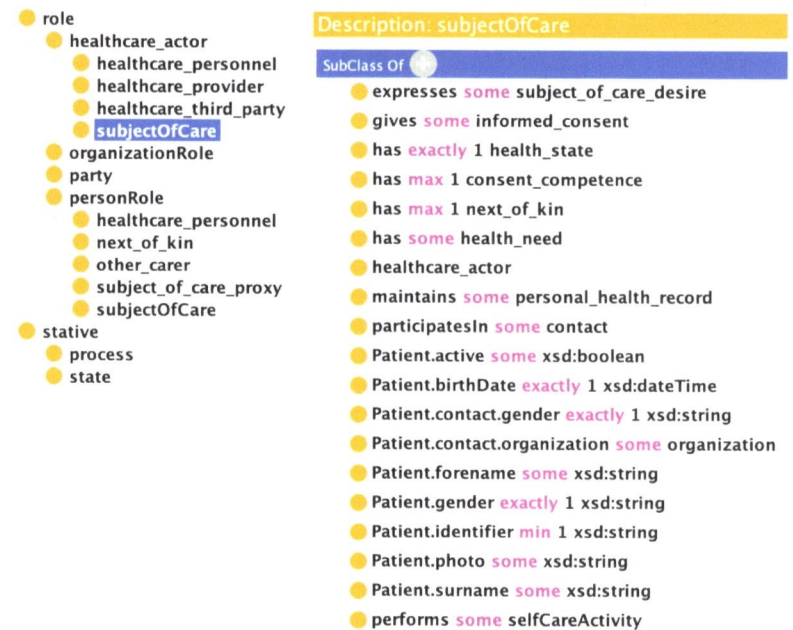

Figure 2. FHIR:Patient attributes inclusion in subject of care.

4. Technical Implementation

The dissemination of information on the CSSDM progress is provided on a phased basis with the ISO and CEN Community over a duration of two years, for example, the publication of formal ontology for continuity of care is available with a supporting blog post on the Contsys Website (see https://ContSys.org/pages/Guest%20blog/FormalOntology accessed on 15 March 2023). For the technical implementation, Figure 3 includes a summary of CSSDM's intended implementation pipeline, which provides details of the tools and techniques on how we have executed our work to date.

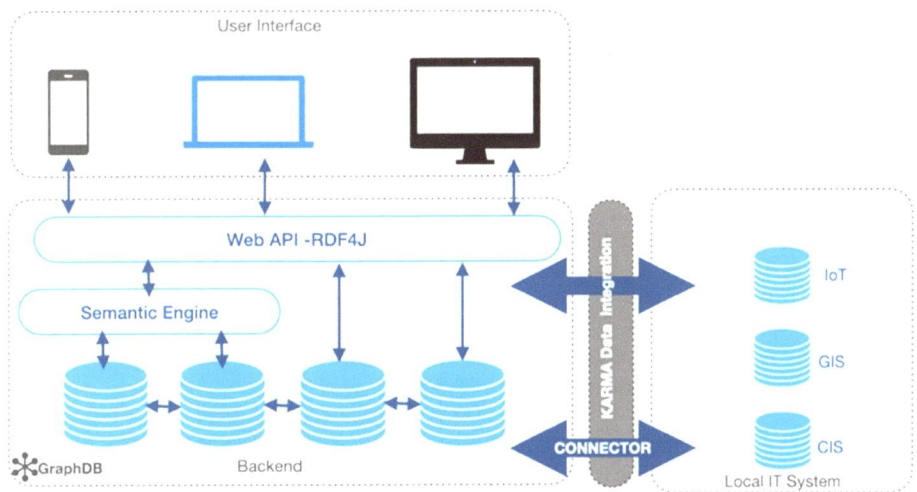

Figure 3. CSSDM system architecture. API: Application Programming Interface, RDF4J: Java-based Resource Description Framework (RDF) framework, IoT: Internet of Things, GIS: Geographic Information System, CIS: Clinical Information System, IT: Information technology.

We have progressed proposals and funding opportunities for further data collection and once ethical approval has been secured, plan to collect more data from different healthcare data sources through our identified service. We anticipate that this will be possible through planned fieldwork, such as workshop and survey activities, as these approaches have worked well for preliminary work conducted in the initial project work of the study.

As the project scales up, the development team will clean the data collected using software such as ontoRefine, which is a data transformation tool, based on OpenRefine integrated in the GraphDB workbench [39]. Protégé offers a free open-source ontology editor and a knowledge management system, which can be used for designing and editing the CSSDM schema. Initial testing suggests that Protégé is a user-friendly graphical interface for defining ontologies. In particular, for defining the terminology and schema mapping Cellfie [40], a Protégé desktop plugin will be used for importing spreadsheet data into OWL ontologies specifically for data integration tasks. As the research program grows, a large dataset will use KARMA for data integration [41]. KARMA as an open-source tool enables data integration from different sources such as XML, CSV, text files, and web application programming interface (API's). KARMA also has the advantage to generate RDB-to-RDF mapping language (R2RML), thus facilitating file mapping, which can be reused again and again in the case of feeding any new or emerging model with new data.

Additional features under consideration for the system architecture of CSSDM as depicted in Figure 3 aim to connect with an existing local IT system called the clinical information system (CIS). This is a particular in-house system of the field site service organization, which has been in place for several years. Geographical information system (GIS) applications can then be used to collect and locate service user and staff details, including emergency management planning and IoT devices to monitor service user's health and well-being. The local IT information system CIS could be connected with the GraphDB via a connector, while KARMA could be used to harmonize the data. This could then facilitate access by staff and service users to information via organizational laptop, desktop, or other mobile devices, which are connected with the system via web API (application programming interface).

For our prototype development, we used a free version of the Ontotext GraphDB [39]. GraphDB's access control is implemented using a hierarchical role-based access control

(RBAC) model [42,43]. This means that while setting up the server, the database administrator can assign specific access roles such as:

- ADMIN: Can perform all operations, i.e., the security never rejects an operation.
- USER: Can save SPARQL queries, graph visualizations, or user-specific settings.
- MONITORING: Allows monitoring operations (queries, updates, abort query/update, resource monitoring).
- REPO MANAGER: Can create, edit, and delete repositories with read and write permissions to all repositories.
- GraphDB also supports lightweight directory access protocol (LDAP).

The abovementioned access control and protocol ensure the security of the healthcare system by preventing any unauthorized third-party access. CSSDM as a model can also be deployed on a commercial cloud service provider system such as Amazon Neptune. In such cases, the security and safety of the system will be handled by a managed service provider such as Amazon Web Services (AWSs).

The safety and reliability of the CSSDM in practice relies on the healthcare system implementer. In our case, it is the industry partner, Davra, an Irish-based startup company, which is responsible for making CSSDM for large-scale deployment. Davra has the following regulatory compliance frameworks: FedRamp, HIPAA compliant, ISO 27001 (which outlines the processes that are required for the acquisition, use, management of and exit from cloud services), HITRUST certification, and NIST 8259 CSF2014 cloud software.

4.1. Data Modeling

The first phase of this project was mainly focused on the data modeling activity in order to generate the initial CSSDM ontological schema. The formal ontology for continuity of care comprises a total of around 138 classes. Out of the identified 138 classes, the main classes needed to capture our defined scenario, which we considered, were limited to a small number of classes:

- *Healthcare actor*: Organization or person participating in healthcare. The involvement of the healthcare actor will be either direct (for example, the actual provision of care) or indirect (for example, at organizational level).
- *Subject of care*: Healthcare actor with a person role who seeks to receive, is receiving, or has received healthcare. Synonym: subject of healthcare; service user; patient; client; relevant person [44].
- *Healthcare profession*: One having a healthcare professional entitlement recognized in a given jurisdiction. The healthcare professional entitlement entitles a healthcare professional to provide healthcare independent of a role in a healthcare organization.
- *Observation*: Observations are a central element in healthcare used to support diagnosis, monitor progress, determine baselines and patterns and even capture demographic characteristics.

For this reason, we opted to reuse HL7 FHIR observation resource in the ontology, which provided a detailed data structure for capturing patient daily observations. The class relationship with observation class is depicted in Figure 4. It represents class relationships among the nine classes, which contain data, and how they are interrelated with each other. We use the Ontotext GraphDB tool to generate this class diagram as an example. The class relationships diagram is based on real statements (i.e., instance level) between classes and not solely on the ontology schema.

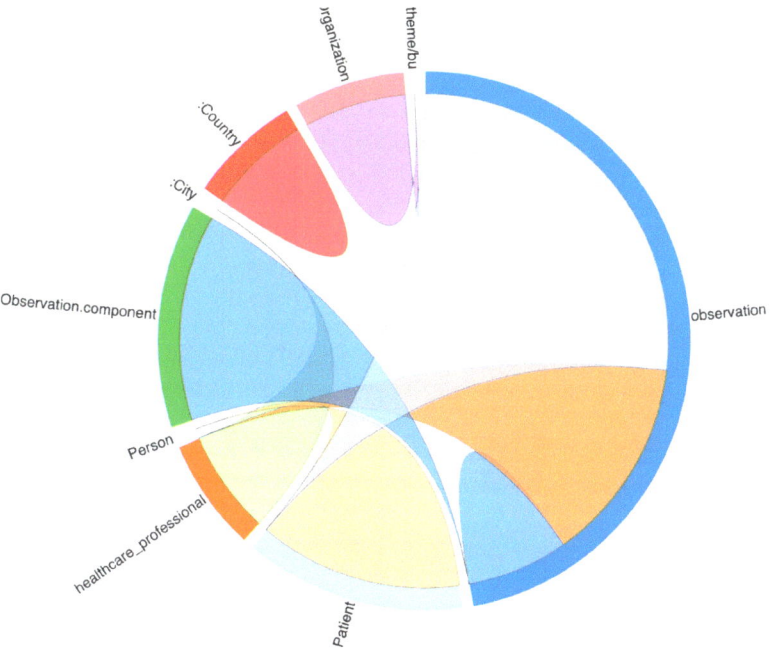

Figure 4. Class relationship with observation.

4.2. Ontology Alignment

Top-level (upper level) ontologies can be used to assist the semantic integration of domain ontologies. Thus, providing domain-independent conceptualization, relations, and axioms (e.g., categories such as Event, Mental Object, Quality, etc.) in order to standardize the upper level of a domain model. This approach enabled us to link the ContSys ontology with other freely available ontology repositories such as Linked Open Vocabulary (LOV) [45] and Biomedical Ontology by the National Center for Biomedical Ontology (NCBO). In ContSOnto, we use the top-level ontology Descriptive Ontology for Linguistic and Cognitive Engineering (DOLCE) [46] as a middle-out solution between the degree of formalization and complexity, contributing to an effective practical solution. DOLCE is one out of three top-level ontologies accredited an ISO standard, i.e., ISO/IEC DIS 21838-3 Information technology—Top-level ontologies (TLO)—Part 3, as recommended by Technical Committee: ISO/IEC JTC 1/SC 32 Data management and interchange.

Despite the benefit of top-level ontologies, we consider and conclude that their alignment and use are not trivial and require some expert effort. The EU project Advancing Clinico-Genomic Trials (ACGT) [47], as well as other healthcare projects, place an emphasis on the need and benefit from top-level alignment. Figure 2 depicts the class hierarchy of ContSOnto ontology and Figure 5 showcases a partial view of ContSOnto class visualization using the web Protégé tool. We highlighted the upper section of Figure 5 green to distinguish the classes (*mentalObject*, *stative*, *event*) as DOLCE classes against the other domain-specific classes taken from ISO 13940:2015 ContSys, which are outlined in blue boxes.

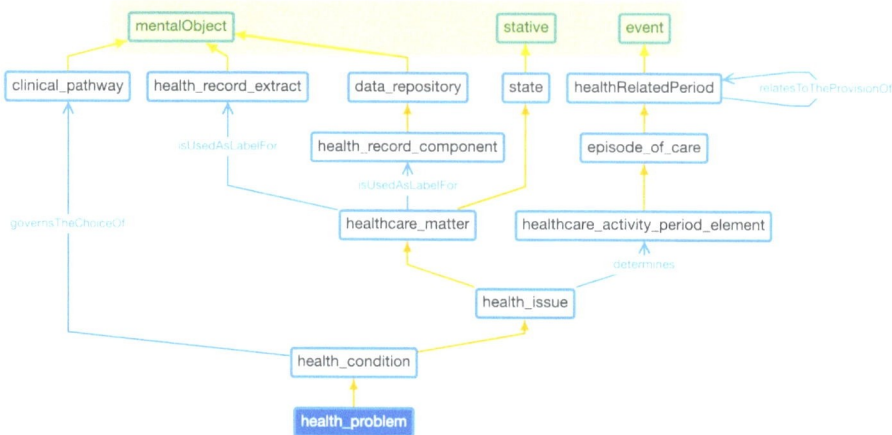

Figure 5. ContSOnto alignment with DOLCE top-level ontology (DOLCE classes are in green).

4.3. Formal Data Model

The expressiveness of our ContSOnto ontology model is ALCHQ(D) as per description logic (DL) scale [48]. We have not exploited the full power of DL-full as supported by OWL-2 language; rather, we used simple rules to make our model compatible with GraphDB rule engine and offer a quick query execution time. This decision was based on the fact that we anticipate that our model will expand exponentially in the future. Finally, in this section, we provide details on the data structure of the class *observation* and property *person.gender* in the resource description framework (RDF) Turtle syntax. The observation class reuses properties as defined by FHIR observation resources. This facilitates our model to be interoperable and semantically aligned to other EHR models using version 4.6 FHIR specification. This is crucial for cross-border studies on intellectual disability (ID) clients in the future. The observation capture measurements and simple assertions are made about a patient, a device or other subject. Subject of observation is *Patient* class. Performer of observation is *healthcare_professional* class. Datatype restriction is encapsulated under property *person.gender*, where data providers have to choose among the gender values "Male", "Female" or "Transsexual" as it a mandatory and important information needed by service providers. It cannot be left blank, and the reasoner will be able to detect if wrong information is inserted into the system. The following excerpt demonstrates an example of this observation of class detail in RDF Turtle syntax.

Observation(class):

> *http://purl.org/net/for-coc#Observatio*
> *CoC:Observation rdf:type owl:Class;*
> *rdfs:subClassOf [rdf:type owl:Restriction;*
> *owl:onProperty observation-definitions:Observation.performer;*
> *owl:someValuesFrom EWS:healthcare_professional],*
> *[rdf:type owl:Restriction;*
> *owl:onProperty observation-definitions:Observation.subject;*
> *owl:someValuesFrom CoC:Patient];*
> *oboInOwl:hasDbXref*
> *"https://www.hl7.org/fhir/observation-definitions.html*
> *#Observation"^^xsd:anyURI;*
> *rdfs:comment "Measurements and simple assertions made about*
> *a patient, device or other subject."@en.*
> *person.gender(property)*
> *https://www.hl7.org/fhir/person-definitions.html#Person.gender*

person-definitions:Person.gender rdf:type owl:DatatypeProperty;
rdfs:range [rdf:type rdfs:Datatype;
owl:unionOf ([rdf:type rdfs:Datatype;
owl:oneOf [rdf:type rdf:List;
rdf:first "Female"^^xsd:string;
rdf:rest rdf:nil]]
[rdf:type rdfs:Datatype;
owl:oneOf [rdf:type rdf:List;
rdf:first "Male"^^xsd:string;
rdf:rest rdf:nil]]
[rdf:type rdfs:Datatype;
owl:oneOf [rdf:type rdf:List;
rdf:first "Transsexual"^^xsd:string;
rdf:rest rdf:nil]])];
rdfs:comment "The gender might not match the biological sex
as determined by genetics, or preferred identification.
Note that there are other possibilities than M and F".

4.4. Inferencing Data Model

ContSOnto OWL contains schema information in addition to links between different classes. This additional information and rules allow users to perform reasoning on the knowledge bases in order to infer new knowledge and expand on the existing knowledge. The core of the inference process is to continuously apply schema-related rules on the input data to infer new facts. This process was considered helpful in this case study for deriving new knowledge and for detecting inconsistencies. An example of an automated inference using HermiT reasoner is depicted in Figure 6.

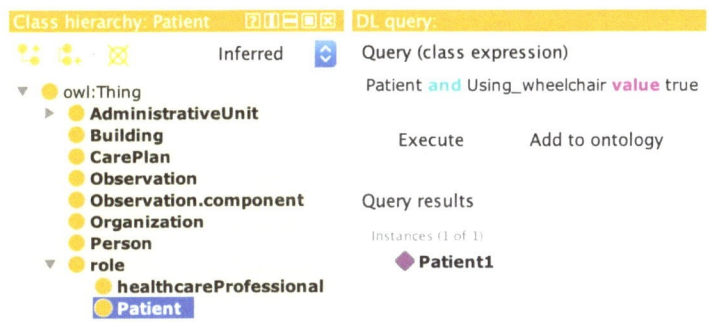

Figure 6. Description Logic (DL) query execution with HermiT reasoner.

4.5. Knowledge Graph

A knowledge graph (KG) can be briefly explained as a graph with interconnected entities. KG became popular around early 2012 when Google started to present their search results as a knowledge graph, which would appear on the right side of the page of a search result [49]. KGs effectively represent relations among entities, so information is connected together, allowing swift search and retrieval.

For those advantages, several studies recently constructed KGs as the data infrastructure to benefit knowledge discovery in the healthcare domain [50]. The KG feature is available in all graph database technologies such as in OntoText GraphDB, Neo4J, and Amazon Neptune [51]. In this particular case study, we obtained our initial ContSOnto KG using Ontotext GraphDB (free version of GraphDB) as shown in Figure 7. In this figure, we can see a personalized knowledge graph of the person named Patrick Kirk from Dublin. The visualization shows that the healthcare professional Dr. J Murphy (i.e., occupational therapist or nurse) is prescribing Patrick a different bed based on his records, which report an incident of a fall from a bed that did not provide appropriate support for Patrick.

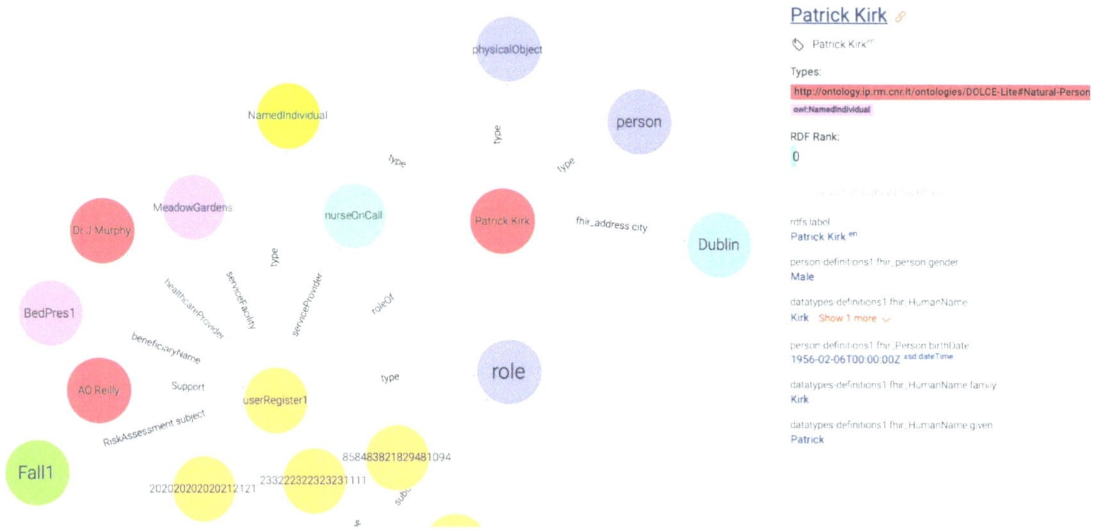

Figure 7. Personalized knowledge graph.

An evaluation of the knowledge graph has been conducted in the following way. At the schema level, accuracy has been checked using the OntoClean methodology as recommended by Guarino, N., and Welty, C. A. (2009) [31]. As part of the formative and summative evaluation process, our clinical partners also reviewed the resource development cycles using PDCA and provided enhancements to the interface language. This work is reported upon in a separate paper by Hussey, P. et al., 2021 [52].

5. Conclusions

We elucidate healthcare data interoperability not as a one-time task to solve, but rather as a continuously evolving process of managing heterogenous data in this rapidly changing information communication technology (ICT) environment. In this paper, we have detailed an approach to achieve a step forward toward addressing the interoperability challenge by adapting existing models and techniques rather than creating additional new models and resources. The approach was crucially grounded in the requirements of the linked data approach in order to generate an interconnected knowledge graph. By implementing such an approach, the usage of graph technologies such as the GraphDB pattern-matching feature to develop a personalized graph was considered crucial, as demonstrated in the following Figure 7. Knowledge graphs help in performing complex queries, which are more efficient than joining operations typical of relational databases' query processes.

In several instances, it is apparent that different organizations, while mapping their data to optimize interoperability and address the heterogeneity challenge, do not distinguish between the various attributes at the schema level. There are three distinctions to be considered at the schema level: (1) the common schema; (2) the core schema; and (3) the context schema [53,54]. The lack of a distinction between the different schemas as listed above creates challenges as the core and common attributes are more often the same; however, the context of use is not. Therefore, when designing information models, it is important to map the ontology-based schema for core and common only. It is very important to omit the context-specific attributes which do not apply to the wider context of use outside of the system under development. The example listed above demonstrates this scenario, where both the Indian and USA FHIR profiles are designed for specific use in the context of the organization. They cannot be applied for reuse in other organizations as their profiles have implicit context-specific schemas and meanings, which are not interpretable by the machine.

As a rule of thumb, we suggest that future semantic schema development should only include that which is common and core, thus leaving the context-specific attributes to be locally modified based on local requirements. In this way, interoperability can be advanced on approximately 80% of the data fields developed using FHIR-based ContSys semantic schema available at GitHub (see https://github.com/subhashishhh/ContSysDoc accessed on 15 March 2023).

During phase 1 development, the CSSDM team has identified opportunities in the current working processes with potential for service improvement. The next step is showcasing the benefit of using CSSDM-integrated interoperable care service architecture to the wider audience. In this way, the benefit of adopting a graph database as part of a data storage and long-term benefit to manage and retrieve service information can be realized. Additional benefits include, but are not limited to, data harmonization and discovering new knowledge to inform targeted interventions. The second phase of development will test CSSDM application from a user satisfaction point of view, using user experience (UX) dimension as proposed by Laugwitz [55] and as was implemented in our previous work on semantic user interface (SemUI) [56]. The questionnaire will be designed to understand different UX dimensions along with the specific traits of user interface. These UX dimensions perform a thorough assessment of the product using six scales with twenty-six terms. These scales were: attractiveness, perspicuity, efficiency, dependability, stimulation, and novelty. The final step will be deploying this system on a cloud server with the help of our industry partner Davra and conduct a performance testing of the CSSDM platform.

Previously, we had implemented CSDM approach in the NHS Scotland HDR UK project (see link for details: https://www.hdruk.ac.uk/projects/graph-based-data-federation-for-healthcare-data-science/ accessed on 15 March 2023 and https://sites.google.com/dcu.ie/csdm/ accessed on 15 March 2023) and also in the EUH2020 project (see link for details: https://www.interopehrate.eu/wp-content/uploads/2019/10/InteropEHRate-D5.9-Design-data-mapper-and-converter-to-FHIR-v1.pdf accessed on 15 March 2023). We are currently in collaboration with FutureNeuro: A Science Foundation Ireland (SFI) Research Centre for Chronic and Rare Neurological Diseases. Our ongoing plan is to implement the CSSDM approach to integrate an evolving epilepsy use case. The SFI center has an established epilepsy EHR (https://www.futureneurocentre.ie/, accessed on 15 March 2023).

Author Contributions: The authors made the following contributions: S.D., methodology, formal modeling and knowledge graph, writing—original draft preparation; P.H., resources and supervision, review, and editing. All authors have read and agreed to the published version of the manuscript.

Funding: This research has received funding from the European Union's Horizon 2020 research and innovation program under the ELITE-S Marie Skłodowska-Curie grant agreement No. 801522, by the Science Foundation Ireland and co-funded by the European Regional Development Fund through the ADAPT Centre for Digital Content Technology, grant number 13/RC/2106_P2 and DAVRA Networks.

Institutional Review Board Statement: Materials used to recruit participants should note that ethical approval for this project has been obtained from the Dublin City University Research Ethics Committee on 9th November 2020 with REC Reference: DCUREC/2020/217.

Informed Consent Statement: Not applicable.

Data Availability Statement: Data models and documentation are available at GitHub repository (see link: https://github.com/subhashishhh/ContSysDoc accessed on 15 March 2023).

Acknowledgments: The authors would like to thank KnowDive group, University of Trento, Italy and Mayukh Bagchi for providing guidance and the idea for this article, and to the two anonymous referees for providing their valuable feedback.

Conflicts of Interest: The authors declare no conflict of interest.

References

1. NHS-England. Department of Health & Social Care, UK. Policy Paper A Plan for Digital Health and Social Care. Available online: https://www.gov.uk/government/publications/a-plan-for-digital-health-and-social-care/a-plan-for-digital-health-and-social-care (accessed on 18 January 2023).
2. Millions of Hours of Doctors' Time Lost Each Year to 'Inadequate' IT Systems. Available online: https://www.bma.org.uk/news-and-opinion/millions-of-hours-of-doctors-time-lost-each-year-to-inadequate-it-systems (accessed on 8 January 2023).
3. ONC. 21st Century Cures Act: Interoperability, Information Blocking, and the ONC Health IT Certification Program Proposed Rule. Available online: https://www.healthit.gov/sites/default/files/facas/2019-03-22_ONC_Cures_Act_NPRM_IB_%20HITAC_IB_Task_Force_508.pdf (accessed on 1 March 2022).
4. *ISO 23903:2021*; Interoperability and Integration Reference Architecture. International Organization for Standardization (ISO): Geneva, Switzerland, 2021.
5. Blobel, B. Challenges and solutions for designing and managing pHealth ecosystems. *Front. Med.* **2019**, *6*, 83. [CrossRef]
6. Blobel, B.; Oemig, F. Solving the modeling dilemma as a foundation for interoperability. *Eur. J. Biomed. Inform.* **2018**. Available online: https://www.ejbi.org/abstract/solving-the-modeling-dilemma-as-a-foundation-for-interoperability-4614.html (accessed on 11 May 2022). [CrossRef]
7. *ISO/IEC 21838-1:2021*; Information Technology—Top-Level Ontologies (TLO)—Part 1: Requirements. International Organization for Standardization (ISO): Geneva, Switzerland, 2021.
8. *ISO 13940:2015*; System of Concepts to Support Continuity of Care. International Organization for Standardization (ISO): Geneva, Switzerland, 2015.
9. HL7 FHIR. Available online: https://build.fhir.org/resourcelist.html (accessed on 8 January 2023).
10. Shang, Y.; Tian, Y.; Zhou, M.; Zhou, T.; Lyu, K.; Wang, Z.; Xin, R.; Liang, T.; Zhu, S.; Li, J. EHR-oriented knowledge graph system: Toward efficient utilization of non-used information buried in routine clinical practice. *IEEE J. Biomed. Health Inform.* **2021**, *25*, 2463–2475. [CrossRef] [PubMed]
11. Das, S.; Hussey, P. FHIR Based ContSys Ontology to Enable Continuity of Care Data Interoperability. In *pHealth*; IOS Press: Amsterdam, The Netherlands, 2022; pp. 139–144. [CrossRef]
12. Bilodeau, A.; Potvin, L. Unpacking complexity in public health interventions with the Actor–Network Theory. *Health Promot. Int.* **2018**, *33*, 173–181. [CrossRef] [PubMed]
13. Leydesdorff, L. The triple helix, quadruple helix, . . . , and an N-tuple of helices: Explanatory models for analyzing the knowledge-based economy? *J. Knowl. Econ.* **2012**, *3*, 25–35. [CrossRef]
14. Gruber, T.R. A translation approach to portable ontology specifications. *Knowl. Acquis.* **1993**, *5*, 199–220. [CrossRef]
15. W3C OWL Working Group. Web Ontology Language (OWL). Available online: https://www.w3.org/OWL/ (accessed on 8 January 2023).
16. Iyamu, T.; Mgudlwa, S. Transformation of healthcare big data through the lens of actor network theory. *Int. J. Healthc. Manag.* **2018**, *11*, 182–192. [CrossRef]
17. The Yosemite Project. Available online: https://yosemiteproject.org/ (accessed on 10 January 2023).
18. InteropEHRate: EHR in People's Hand across Europe. Available online: https://www.interopehrate.eu/ (accessed on 10 January 2023).
19. EU Rolling Plan 2022. Available online: https://joinup.ec.europa.eu/node/705307 (accessed on 10 January 2023).
20. OpenEHR. Archetype Query Language (AQL). Available online: https://specifications.openehr.org/releases/QUERY/latest/AQL.html (accessed on 10 January 2023).
21. Manard, S.; Vergos, N.; Tamayo, S.; Fontane, F. Electronic health record in the era of industry 4.0: The French example. *arXiv* **2019**, arXiv:1907.10322. [CrossRef]
22. Moore, N.; Blin, P.; Lassalle, R.; Thurin, N.; Bosco-Levy, P.; Droz, C. National Health Insurance Claims Database in France (SNIRAM), Système Nationale des Données de Santé (SNDS) and Health Data Hub (HDH). In *Databases for Pharmacoepidemiological Research*; Springer: Cham, Switzerland, 2021; pp. 131–140. [CrossRef]
23. Or, Z.; Gandré, C. Sustainability and Resilience in the French Health System. Institut de recherche et de Documentation en Èconomie de la santé (Irdes). 2021. Available online: https://www3.weforum.org/docs/WEF_PHSSR_France_Report.pdf (accessed on 10 March 2022).
24. New European Interoperability Framework. Available online: https://ec.europa.eu/isa2/sites/default/files/eif_brochure_final.pdf (accessed on 10 January 2023).
25. Michael, M.; Allen, J.; Boyce, T.; Goldblatt, P.; Morrison, J. Health equity in England: The Marmot review 10 years on. *Br. Med. J.* **2020**, *368*, m693.
26. Kankainen, K. Usages of the ContSys standard: A position paper. In *Advances in Model and Data Engineering in the Digitalization Era, Proceedings of the MEDI 2021 International Workshops: DETECT, SIAS, CSMML, BIOC, HEDA, Tallinn, Estonia, 21–23 June 2021, Proceedings 10*; Springer International Publishing: Berlin/Heidelberg, Germany, 2021; pp. 314–324. [CrossRef]
27. Horrocks, I. OWL: A description logic based ontology language. In Proceedings of the International Conference on Principles and Practice of Constraint Programming, Cork, Ireland, 31 August–4 September 2015; Springer: Berlin/Heidelberg, Germany, 2005; pp. 5–8. [CrossRef]

28. Glimm, B.; Horrocks, I.; Motik, B.; Stoilos, G.; Wang, Z. HermiT: An OWL 2 reasoner. *J. Autom. Reason.* **2014**, *53*, 245–269. [CrossRef]
29. ISO/TS 22272:2021; Health Informatics - Methodology for Analysis of Business and Information Needs of Health Enterprises to Support Standards Based Architectures. International Organization for Standardization (ISO): Geneva, Switzerland, 2021.
30. Tao, C.; Jiang, G.; Oniki, T.A.; Freimuth, R.R.; Zhu, Q.; Sharma, D.; Pathak, J.; Huff, S.M.; Chute, C.G. A semantic-web oriented representation of the clinical element model for secondary use of electronic health records data. *J. Am. Med. Inform. Assoc.* **2013**, *20*, 554–562. [CrossRef] [PubMed]
31. Guarino, N.; Welty, C.A. An Overview of OntoClean. In *Handbook on Ontologies. International Handbooks on Information Systems*; Staab, S., Studer, R., Eds.; Springer: Berlin/Heidelberg, Germany, 2009. [CrossRef]
32. Noy, N.F.; Crubézy, M.; Fergerson, R.W.; Knublauch, H.; Tu, S.W.; Vendetti, J.; Musen, M.A. Protégé-2000: An open-source ontology-development and knowledge-acquisition environment. In *AMIA Annual Symposium Proceedings. AMIA Symposium*; Washington, DC, USA, 2003; p. 953. Available online: https://protege.stanford.edu/ (accessed on 10 January 2022).
33. Blobel, B.; Oemig, F.; Ruotsalainen, P.; Lopez, D.M. Transformation of health and social care systems—An interdisciplinary approach toward a foundational architecture. *Front. Med.* **2022**, *9*, 802487. [CrossRef] [PubMed]
34. Blobel, B.; Ruotsalainen, P.; Giacomini, M. Standards and Principles to Enable Interoperability and Integration of 5P Medicine Ecosystems. In *pHealth*; IOS Press: Amsterdam, The Netherlands, 2022; pp. 3–19. [CrossRef]
35. Blobel, B.; Ruotsalainen, P.; Brochhausen, M. Autonomous Systems and Artificial Intelligence-Hype or Prerequisite for P5 Medicine? In *pHealth*; IOS Press: Amsterdam, The Netherlands, 2021; pp. 3–14. [CrossRef]
36. McDonald, K.; Schultz, E.; Albin, L.; Pineda, N.; Lonhart, J.; Sundaram, V.; Spangler, C.S.; Brustrom, J.; Malcolm, E.; Rohn, L.; et al. Care Coordination Measures Atlas. 2014. Available online: https://www.ahrq.gov/ncepcr/care/coordination/atlas.html (accessed on 15 May 2022).
37. Rector, A.L.; Johnson, P.D.; Tu, S.; Wroe, C.; Rogers, J. Interface of infer-ence models with concept and medical record models. In *Artificial Intelligence in Medicine, Proceedings of the 8th Conference on Artificial Intelligence in Medicine in Europe, AIME 2001 Cascais, Portugal, 1–4 July 2001, Proceedings 8*; Springer: Berlin/Heidelberg, Germany, 2001; pp. 314–323. [CrossRef]
38. Das, S.; Hussey, P. ContSOnto: A Formal Ontology for Continuity of Care. *Stud. Health Technol. Inform.* **2021**, *285*, 82–87. [CrossRef] [PubMed]
39. GraphDB. Graphdb Workbench. 2022. Available online: https://graphdb.ontotext.com/ (accessed on 10 January 2022).
40. Josef, H. Cellfie-Plugin User's Guide. 2016. Available online: https://github.com/protegeproject/cellfie-plugin (accessed on 10 January 2022).
41. Gupta, S.; Szekely, P.; Knoblock, C.A.; Goel, A.; Taheriyan, M.; Muslea, M. Karma: A system for mapping structured sources into the semantic web. In *Proceedings of the Semantic Web: ESWC 2012 Satellite Events: ESWC 2012 Satellite Events, Heraklion, Crete, Greece, 27–31 May 2012*; Revised Selected Papers; Springer: Berlin/Heidelberg, Germany, 2015; pp. 430–434. [CrossRef]
42. Chabin, J.; Ciferri, C.D.; Halfeld-Ferrari, M.; Hara, C.S.; Penteado, R.R. Role-Based Access Control on Graph Databases. In *Proceedings of the SOFSEM 2021: Theory and Practice of Computer Science: 47th International Conference on Current Trends in Theory and Practice of Computer Science, SOFSEM 2021, Bolzano-Bozen, Italy, 25–29 January 2021*; Proceedings 47; Springer International Publishing: Berlin/Heidelberg, Germany, 2021; pp. 519–534. [CrossRef]
43. Blobel, B. Authorisation and access control for electronic health record systems. *Int. J. Med. Inform.* **2004**, *73*, 251–257. [CrossRef] [PubMed]
44. Government of Ireland, Department of Health. Health Information Bill 2023. Available online: https://www.gov.ie/en/publication/6f6a6-health-information-bill-2023/ (accessed on 3 May 2023).
45. Vandenbussche, P.Y.; Atemezing, G.A.; Poveda-Villalón, M.; Vatant, B. Linked Open Vocabularies (LOV): A gateway to reusable semantic vocabularies on the Web. *Semant. Web* **2017**, *8*, 437–452. [CrossRef]
46. Gangemi, A.; Guarino, N.; Masolo, C.; Oltramari, A.; Schneider, L. Sweetening ontologies with DOLCE. In *Proceedings of the Knowledge Engineering and Knowledge Management: Ontologies and the Semantic Web: 13th International Conference, EKAW 2002, Sigüenza, Spain, 1–4 October 2002*; Proceedings 13; Springer: Berlin/Heidelberg, Germany, 2002; pp. 166–181. [CrossRef]
47. Stenzhorn, H.; Schulz, S.; Boeker, M.; Smith, B. Adapting clinical ontologies in real-world environments. *J. Univers. Comput. Sci.* **2008**, *14*, 3767. [PubMed]
48. Baader, F.; Horrocks, I.; Lutz, C.; Sattler, U. *An Introduction to Description Logic*; Cambridge University Press: Cambridge, UK, 2017. [CrossRef]
49. Eder, J.S. Knowledge Graph Based Search System. U.S. Patent Application No. 13/404,109, 24 February 2012. Available online: https://patents.google.com/patent/US20120158633A1/en (accessed on 10 March 2022).
50. Zeng, X.; Tu, X.; Liu, Y.; Fu, X.; Su, Y. Toward better drug discovery with knowledge graph. *Curr. Opin. Struct. Biol.* **2022**, *72*, 114–126. [CrossRef]
51. Bebee, B.R.; Choi, D.; Gupta, A.; Gutmans, A.; Khandelwal, A.; Kiran, Y.; Mallidi, S.; McGaughy, B.; Personick, M.; Rajan, K.; et al. *Amazon Neptune: Graph Data Management in the Cloud*; ISWC (P&D/Industry/BlueSky): Monterey, CA, USA, 2018.
52. Hussey, P.; Das, S.; Farrell, S.; Ledger, L.; Spencer, A. A knowledge graph to understand nursing big data: Case example for guidance. *J. Nurs. Scholarsh.* **2021**, *53*, 323–332. [CrossRef]

53. Bella, G.; Elliot, L.; Das, S.; Pavis, S.; Turra, E.; Robertson, D.; Giunchiglia, F. Cross-border medical research using multi-layered and distributed knowledge. In *Proceedings of the 2020 European Conference on Artificial Intelligence, Santiago de Compostela, Spain, 29 August–8 September 2020*; IOS Press: Amsterdam, The Netherlands, 2020; pp. 2956–2963. [CrossRef]
54. Das, S.; Hussey, P. How ontology can be used to achieve semantic interoperability in healthcare. *Eur. J. Public Health* **2022**, *32* (Suppl. S3), ckac129.363. [CrossRef]
55. Laugwitz, B.; Held, T.; Schrepp, M. Construction and evaluation of a user experience questionnaire. In *Symposium of the Austrian HCI and Usability Engineering Group*; Springer: Berlin/Heidelberg, Germany, 2008; pp. 63–76. [CrossRef]
56. Giunchiglia, F.; Ojha, S.R.; Das, S. SemUI: A knowledge driven visualization of diversified data. In Proceedings of the 2017 IEEE 11th International Conference on Semantic Computing (ICSC), San Diego, CA, USA, 30 January–1 February 2017; pp. 234–241. [CrossRef]

Disclaimer/Publisher's Note: The statements, opinions and data contained in all publications are solely those of the individual author(s) and contributor(s) and not of MDPI and/or the editor(s). MDPI and/or the editor(s) disclaim responsibility for any injury to people or property resulting from any ideas, methods, instructions or products referred to in the content.